PHYSIOLOGY
for the
ANESTHESIOLOGIST

PHYSIOLOGY
for the
ANESTHESIOLOGIST

NISHAN G. GOUDSOUZIAN, M.D., M.S.

Assistant Professor of Anesthesia
Harvard Medical School at the
Massachusetts General Hospital
Boston, Massachusetts

AGOP KARAMANIAN, M.D.

Assistant Professor or Anesthesia
Albert Einstein College of Medicine
Montefiore Hospital and Medical Center
New York, New York

APPLETON-CENTURY-CROFTS/NEW YORK

Prentice-Hall International, Inc., London
Prentice-Hall of Australia, Pty. Ltd., Sydney
Prentice-Hall of India Private Limited, New Delhi
Prentice-Hall of Japan, Inc., Tokyo
Prentice-Hall of Southeast Asia (Pte.) Ltd., Singapore
Whitehall Books Ltd., Wellington, New Zealand

Library of Congress
Catalog Card Number: 77-82278

Cover design: Rodelinde Albrecht

PRINTED IN THE UNITED STATES OF AMERICA

0-8385-7858-6

Contents

Preface

The aim of this book is to provide anesthesiologists with an outline of physiology so that they can understand and evaluate in a scientific manner the changes in physiologic parameters that occur during the administration of an anesthetic.

One cannot do justice to a subject as extensive as physiology in such a short volume. Consequently, several aspects have been intentionally omitted for the sake of brevity. We do not ignore the fact that these physiologic parameters also change with anesthesia but we bypassed them because they do not affect in a practical way the administration of an anesthetic. In several situations when explaining the functions of a certain tissue, we have used the simplest and most plausible theory rather than discussing all the pros and cons of that subject. The reader interested in pursuing these controversies should refer to the review articles referenced at the end of each chapter. We have designed this book to be especially helpful to the practicing anesthesiologist whenever he needs to refresh his memory on physiology in a short period of time.

The authors wish to express their sincere gratitude to Daniel Williamson and Raghubar Badola, M.D., for the resplendent drawings in this book and also to the authors and publishers who have allowed us to reproduce their illustrations. We acknowledge the cooperation of Hagop Youssoufian and Margit Salamon for arranging and reviewing the references, and to Hilary Evans, formerly of Appleton-Century-Crofts, who encouraged us to initiate this project and supported us throughout its preparation.

This manuscript would not have been possible without the unstinting assistance and the technical skill of Susan Runci in typing, editing, and correcting the manuscript, which she did so cheerfully. We also express our sincere thanks to Clare Cumiskey, Suzanne Trifone, and Ruth Thomas for typing parts of this work. We are grateful to all the members of the Anesthesia Departments at the Massachusetts General Hospital and the Montefiore Hospital and Medical Center for providing us with the facilities and ancillary services that a book of this caliber requires.

N. G. Goudsouzian
A. Karamanian

PHYSIOLOGY
for the
ANESTHESIOLOGIST

Circulation

Circulation

chapter 1

The Heart

The heart is an intricate pump whose fundamental function is to deliver blood with its nutrients to the tissues at an adequate head pressure. It must function without interruption to maintain the survival of the specific organs. In this respect, the central nervous system is the most sensitive one, because it can suffer permanent damage from transient oxygen deprivation. Therefore, the heart has to beat repetitively for the lifetime of the individual. To accomplish this vital function, it contracts more than 100,000 times per day and circulates more than seven tons of blood daily.

For the heart to be an effective pump, it has to have a sequential pattern of excitation with a subsequent contraction proceeding in an orderly fashion from the atria to the ventricles.

PROPAGATION OF THE CARDIAC IMPULSE (FIG. 1-1)

The normal sinus rhythm starts at the *sinoatrial (SA) node,* which is 2 mm thick and extends vertically downward for 2 cm between the superior vena cava and the right atrium. It consists mainly of spindle-shaped cells smaller than the cardiac muscle fibers and is supplied with both sympathetic and parasympathetic nerve fibers. Autorhythmicity is highly developed at the SA node, whereas its contractile ability is minimal.

The cells of the SA node show spontaneous decay of their resting membrane potential during diastole caused by the influx of sodium into the cells. This steady fall in conductivity continues,[1] until it reaches a threshold potential of -55 mV. Then it discharges rapidly, starting a wave of depolarization that spreads to the other regions of the heart, which eventually leads to cardiac contraction.

From the SA node, the excitatory wave spreads out rapidly over the atrial musculature at a rate of 1 mm per second.

3

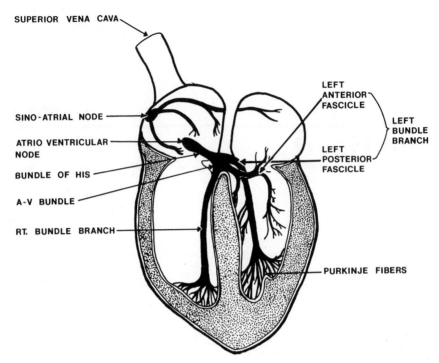

SUPERIOR VENA CAVA

LEFT
ANTERIOR
FASCICLE

SINO-ATRIAL NODE

LEFT
BUNDLE
BRANCH

ATRIO VENTRICULAR
NODE

LEFT
POSTERIOR
FASCICLE

BUNDLE OF HIS

A-V BUNDLE

RT. BUNDLE BRANCH

PURKINJE FIBERS

FIG. 1-1:   Representation of the nodal and conducting tissues of the heart.

Conduction through the atria occurs through three bundles of myocardium containing Purkinje-type fibers: (1) anterior internodal tract; (2) middle internodal tract Wenckebach; and (3) posterior internodal tract. Between all three tracts there are interconnecting fibers that merge just above the atrioventricular (AV) node. Some of the fibers do not enter the AV node, but bypass it. They can reenter the conducting system at a place distal to the AV node.

The impulse traverses the internodal pathway, depolarizes the atria producing the P-wave, and then reaches the AV node. The conductivity at the atrial end of the AV node is very slow. This causes a delay in the propagation of impulses to the ventricles and allows enough time for the excitation of the atria to be completed before the propagated impulse reaches the ventricle.

The ventricular end of the AV node merges with the *AV bundle* (bundle of His). The AV bundle splits into two branches that run down either side of the interventricular septum under the endocardium. The right bundle branch runs to the anterior papillary muscle, where it divides into the Purkinje network. The left bundle branch splits again into an anterior and a posterior branch, each of them going to their respective papillary muscles, where they also divide into the Purkinje network. Some of these Purkinje network fibers cross the cavity of the ventricles. Once the excitatory impulse reaches the AV bundle, it propagates very fast in the bundle, its branches, and the Purkinje fibers (2 to 4 mseconds). Thus, the excitatory wave reaches the endocardial surface of both ventricles almost simultaneously, resulting in a uniform contraction of the ventricles. However, once the excitation reaches the ventricle, the propagation inside the ventricular wall is at a much slower pace (0.3 msecond).

The myocardial fibers are relatively thick. Similar to skeletal muscles, the myofibrils show the A, I, and Z bands. However, at irregular intervals, thick transverse fibers replace the Z bands. These replacement fibers are called intercalated discs. Previously, these intercalated discs were supposed to form a physiologic syncitium through which the excitatory impulses initiated in one part of the heart could rapidly travel through the myocardium. However, studies of the heart with electron microscopy have shown that there is no continuity from cell to cell.[2] The transmission between cells seems to be of an electrical nature in which local current spreads from cell to cell through low-resistance electrical pathways between the interiors of adjacent cells.[3]

Functional Characteristics of the Cardiac Muscle

The heart muscle has three important physiologic properties: (1) rhythmicity, (2) conductivity, and (3) contractility. These properties are developed to different degrees in the various regions of the heart according to their specific function. For example, autorhythmicity is most highly developed in the SA node and to a lesser degree in the AV node. Whereas conductivity is at its fastest in the bundle of His and the Purkinje network, it is slowest at the AV node. In the ventricular muscle, contractility is at its best, while conductivity is very low.

The main reason for this different rhythmicity of the cardiac muscles is the differences in their electrophysiologic properties (Fig. 1-2). The pacemaker cells have an unstable resting potential. Intracellular recordings will show a negative potential of about −60 mV, which gradually drifts upward until it reaches a critical level of about −55 mV. At this threshold, the cell membrane will depolarize. Changing the slope of this diastolic depolarization will result in a change in the heart rate. The conducting cells, similar to the pacemaker cells, have unstable resting potentials. However, the rate of their diastolic depolarization is rather slow. In the normal situation, their rhythmic activity is suppressed because of the faster firing rate of the SA node.

In contrast to the pacemaker cells, the myocardial muscle fibers have a stable resting potential (−90 mV), and they remain the same until the muscle is stimulated from outside.

If the SA node is suppressed, latent pacemaker cells within the heart assume control. The next fibers with the highest rhythmicity start functioning and behave as though they were pacemaker cells. The atria are next in line after the SA node, followed by the AV node and bundle of His, while the

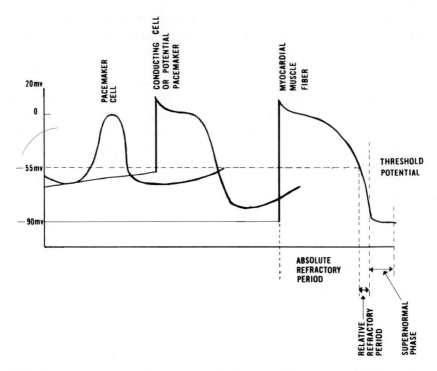

FIG. 1-2: Transmembrane action potential of pacemaker cells, conducting cells, and myocardial muscle fibers. Note the progressive decay of the action potential of the pacemaker cells.

ventricles have the slowest rhythm. Because of their low resting membrane potentials, these reserve pacemaker-type cells drive the heart at a lower frequency than the normal sinus.

The AV node, in addition to its properties of delaying conduction, has the potential to act as a pacemaker. It also transmits atrial impulses up to a certain frequency, thus protecting the ventricles from the rapid impulses that can occur in situations such as atrial flutter. This conduction block capability of the AV node can be increased by increasing the vagal tone and decreased by sympathetic stimulation. In addition, it only can transmit the impulse unidirectionally from the atrium to the ventricle. Retrograde ventricular contraction can occur only in unusual situations.

For the heart to function effectively, every contraction must be followed by relaxation. A tetanic contraction is lethal to the body. To prevent such a possibility, the cardiac muscles have a *prolonged effective refractory period,* which is that period of the cardiac cycle during which a stimulus, no matter how strong, fails to produce a *propagated* electrical response. This occupies about 80 percent of the cardiac systole and extends beyond the peak tension developed in the myocardium. Thus, an abnormal stimulus at this period will start neither a propagated impulse nor a contraction. This effective refractory period is followed by a *relative refractory period* in which a propagated action potential can be elicited but the stimulus required is greater than that required in diastole. Thus, a stimulus at this stage can cause a partial fusion of contractions. Following this relative refractory period, just prior to the diastole, there is a *supernormal period* in which the threshold of excitation is at its lowest, and of short duration. During diastole, excitability is considered to be "normal."

The "all-or-none law" is based on one of the properties discovered early for the cardiac musculature. The law establishes that a threshold stimulus gives rise to a maximal contraction of the heart muscle. Increasing the strength of the stimulus does not lead to any increase in the strength of the contraction. It should be understood that the force of contraction can vary with the initial length of the myocardium, temperature, pH, autonomic tone, and so on. Therefore, the all-or-none law can be rewritten *pertaining to a particular set of conditions,* increasing the strength of the stimulus above the threshold does not lead to an increased contraction.

The cardiac muscle shares the properties of the skeletal muscles in that the tension developed by muscular contraction is directly related to the length of the muscle fibers, and the velocity of its shortening depends on its tension. However, it differs from peripheral muscles in the following ways:

1. Tetanus is not possible in the heart, and, therefore, myocardial contraction is similar to a muscle twitch.
2. The maximum active state develops and declines more slowly in the cardiac muscle.
3. Variations in the strength of myocardial contraction happen as a result of changes in length, tension, and velocity relationships and not by recruitment of more muscle fibers.

Relationship between the Length, Tension, and Velocity of the Myocardium

A simple way to measure the contractile performance of the ventricular muscles in vitro is to use the isolated papillary muscle of the cat because the myocardial fibers are arranged in a parallel formation. One end of the papillary muscle is connected to a force displacement transducer, whereas the other end is connected to a fulcrum. If the fulcrum is prevented from moving, the tension recorded in the transducer is caused by stretching the elastic elements in the muscles without any change in the muscle length.[4] This is known as isometric contraction (Fig. 1-3). In a second set of experiments, the muscle is allowed to contract (isotonic contraction), but the initial length of the muscle is varied by changing the weight on the other end of the fulcrum. The effect of

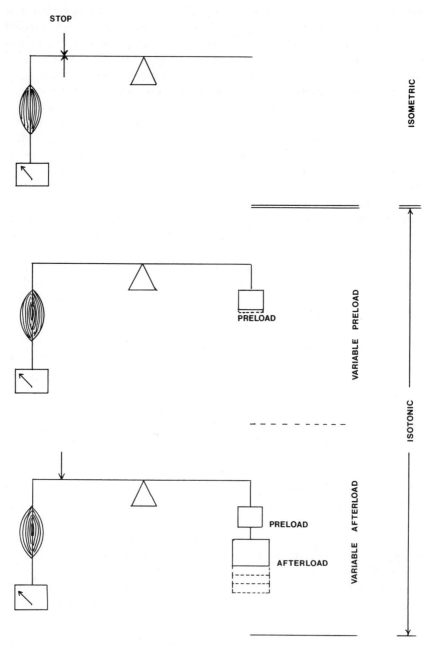

FIG. 1-3: A simple arrangement for studying isometric contraction, preload, and afterload of the isolated papillary muscle.

preload on the velocity of shortening thereby may be studied (dl/dt). To study the effect of afterload, ie, the tension applied to the muscle during contraction, a mechanical stop is incorporated into the fulcrum after the adjustment of the preload, thereby preventing the muscle from stretching further. By this technique, one can study the effect of increasing afterloads on the velocity of shortening and on the tension developed. From these experiments it can be seen that increasing the afterload diminishes the velocity of shortening of the muscle (Fig. 1-4).

By plotting the velocity of shortening against the tension developed, a hyperbolic curve is obtained in the normal heart (Fig. 1-5). If this curve is extrapolated to zero afterload, the velocity of contraction is at a maximum (V_{max}). When the afterload is increased to the point where no demonstrable shortening occurs and only tension results, this point is described as the P_0, ie, the point of maximum isometric tension.

In the human being, these measurements are not easily obtained as in the papillary muscle of the cat. A very good estimate of preload can be obtained by

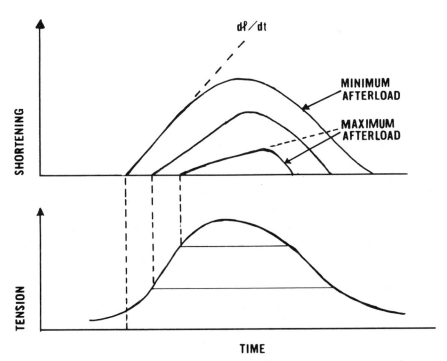

FIG. 1-4: A diagrammatic representation showing the relationships between shortening and time (top) and tension and time (bottom) of the papillary muscle contraction at increasing afterloads. Note the diminution of the velocity of shortening with the increase in the afterload.

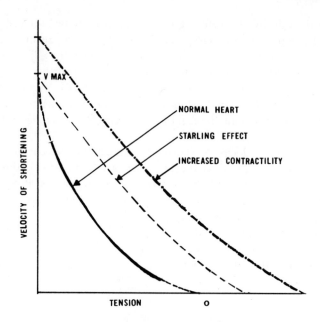

FIG. 1-5: The force–velocity relationship of the normal heart, the moderately stretched myocardium (Starling effect), and sympathetically stimulated heart (increased contractility). Note that with the Starling effect the increase in the maximum tension is developed without any change in the maximum velocity.

determining end-diastolic ventricular volume and pressure (Fig. 1-6), but these are difficult to measure unless a left heart catheterization is performed. Recently with the advent of balloon flotation pulmonary artery catheters, the mean pulmonary capillary wedge pressure can be determined, which is a reliable and useful index of left ventricular filling.[5] The measurement of afterload is much easier in man and is basically the aortic pressure. Less accurately, the arterial diastolic or the mean blood pressure can be used.

With the advent of high-fidelity recording equipment, the instantaneous rate of change of the intraventricular pressure (dp/dt) can be determined. This measurement varies with changes in preload and afterload.[6] The rate of ventricular contraction during the early isovolumetric phase is slow, then increases rapidly to reach its maximum just before the opening of the aortic valves. This point of maximum velocity is known as dp/dt_{max}.

Increasing the initial length of muscle fibers (preload) by raising its diastolic volume will produce an increase in the force of its contraction (Frank–Starling effect). According to the force–velocity diagrams, this mechanism will be expressed as an increase in maximum isometric tension (P_0) developed by the ventricle without any change in the maximum velocity of shortening (V_{max}).

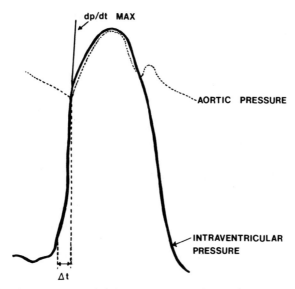

FIG. 1-6: The determination of the maximum rate of rise of intraventricular pressure dp/dt_{max} from intraventricular pressure recording.

Quantitatively the contractile state of the myocardial mechanism can be defined through the force–velocity curves, which express the inverse relationship between the velocity of myocardial shortening and the development of tension within the ventricular wall.[7] Thus, an increase in contractility leads to an upward shift of the integral part as well as an elevation in the extrapolated value of the maximum velocity of shortening (V_{max}) (Fig. 1-5). V_{max} is an extrapolated value. It indicates the velocity of contraction at zero afterload. It cannot be measured directly because every muscle has some intrinsic load. Although it is a reliable and reproducible index of myocardial contractility and is independent of the preload and afterload, being an extrapolated value it is subject to error. Instead, another parameter is used in which the dp/dt is divided by the peak intraventricular pressure. The parameter $dp/dt/IP$ is relatively easy to measure and is accurate and probably as useful as V_{max}.[8]

An increase in contractility can be mediated through the sympathetic nervous system and circulating catecholamines, as well as by cardiac glycosides.

Control of the Heart Beat

The region in the heart with the highest automatic rhythmicity is the SA node, ie, its diastolic depolarization rate is the fastest. This autorhythmicity of the SA node is reduced whenever there is diminution of its blood flow, ie, ischemia from atherosclerosis, or in situations of decreased metabolism, such as hypothermia or hypothyroidism. The SA fires at a faster rate whenever there is an increase in metabolism, such as in fever or hyperthyroidism.

The SA node is under strict autonomic nervous control through its neural connections. Circulatory catecholamines have a less important effect on the SA node than the neural regulation. Beta-adrenergic stimulation increases the slope of the slow depolarization phase so that the threshold is reached more rapidly,[1] resulting in a faster heart rate. In contrast, stimulation of the vagus results in a delay in the firing of the SA node and, hence, results in a slower rate.

The sympathetic and the parasympathetic nervous systems exert a continual tonic effect on cardiac action. It seems that the parasympathetic system is more dominant in the control of normal rate than is the sympathetic system.

The parasympathetic supply of the heart originates in the vagal nuclei in the medulla. The fibers of these nuclei form the main part of the vagus nerve. The vagal cardiac fibers leave the main trunk in the neck to join the cardiac plexus, which is situated at the base of the heart. Here, some of the fibers synapse to form postganglionic fibers, whereas others pass directly as preganglionic to culminate in the intrinsic cardiac ganglia. The postganglionic fibers from the cardiac ganglia are distributed to all the regions of the heart. However, they are more concentrated at the nodal regions. Stimulation of the parasympathetic system leads to an increase in the permeability of the cell membrane to potassium ions, thus delaying the depolarization phase. The final outcome is a slower heart rate, a decrease in atrial contraction, and a decrease in the velocity of conduction at the AV node. With strong stimulation, atrioventricular block and dissociation can occur.

The preganglionic sympathetic fibers originate in the gray column of the first five thoracic segments of the spinal cord. They leave the cord through the white rami to the corresponding spinal sympathetic ganglia. Some synapse at this point, while the remainder reach the three cervical sympathetic ganglia to synapse there. The postganglionic fibers from the superior, middle, and inferior cervical ganglia and from the fourth and fifth thoracic ganglia after passing through the cardiac plexus end up in all segments of the heart.

Stimulation of the sympathetic system increases the rate of depolarization of the pacemaker cells from increased potassium permeability, leading to an increase in the heart rate and an increase in the conduction of the AV node. Epinephrine also enhances the influx of calcium into the cardiac fibers, and this is probably the cause of increased contractility observed with sympathetic stimulation. Epinephrine also enhances the Purkinje fibers to exhibit pacemaker activity, leading to greater susceptibility of the ventricular muscle to fibrillation.

The baroreceptors and the carotid sinus can cause alteration of the heart rate by a reflex mechanism. An acute increase in the arterial pressure will reflexly slow the heart rate in the anesthetized animal. This bradycardia from carotid sinus nerve stimulation is caused primarily by withdrawal of sympathetic stimulation, since it can be blocked by propranolol. However, in an alert man or animal, this bradycardia results from an increase in parasympathetic tone. Thus, this basal parasympathetic tone seems to be higher in the unanesthetized individual.[9]

The Cardiac Cycle

The following text describes the pressure and flow changes of the cardiac cycle in its eight phases (Fig. 1-7).

ATRIAL SYSTOLE (0.15 second)

Atrial systole starts with the spread of excitation in the atria (P-wave of the electrocardiogram); after a very short delay, the atrial muscle contracts, thus emptying the blood from the atria into the ventricle. Obviously, at this stage the AV valves are open. The contraction of the atrium produces the α wave of jugular venous pulse.

ISOMETRIC CONTRACTION (0.06 second)

This phase is characterized by a very rapid rise in the intraventricular pressure from the contraction of the ventricles. It starts from the peak of R-waves of the electrocardiogram (electrical events precede mechanical events), followed by a rise in the intraventricular pressure. As the pressure inside the ventricles exceeds the intraatrial pressure, the mitral and tricuspid valves close, thus producing the first heart sound. The c-wave of the jugular pulse can be seen at this stage from the bulging of the tricuspid valve inside the right atrium. Because the semilunar valves are closed at this stage, there is no flow, nor is there any change in intraventricular volume. As the intraventricular pressure increases, it exceeds the aortic pressure and the semilunar valves open. This is the start of the ejection phase.

MAXIMUM EJECTION PHASE (0.11 second)

Most of the blood ejected during systole flows during this period with a rapid emptying of the ventricles. In this stage, the flow rate into the aorta exceeds the runoff into the peripheral arteries, and the pressure in the aorta continues to rise.

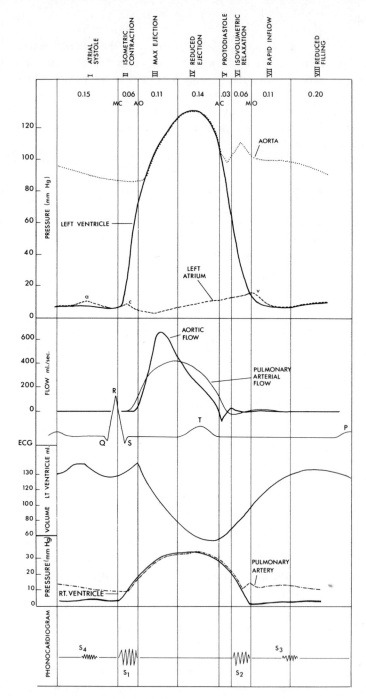

FIG. 1-7: Events in the cardiac cycle. (MC: mitral valve closes. AO: Aortic valve opens. AC: Aortic valve closes. MO: mitral valve opens).

REDUCED EJECTION (0.14 second)

At this stage, the intraventricular pressure is still higher than that of the aortic pressure, and there is still flow from the ventricle to the aorta. However, now the rate of flow is slower. Also at this stage, the runoff from the aorta to the peripheral vessels exceeds the cardiac output. Thus, the intraventricular and intraaortic pressures start to decline.

PROTODIASTOLE (0.03 second)

This phase is a very short period in which the ventricles start to relax with a rapid drop in intraventricular pressure. A brief retrograde flow occurs in the aorta and pulmonary artery, leading to closure of the aortic and pulmonary valves.

ISOVOLUMETRIC RELAXATION (0.06 second)

When this phase is reached, the ventricles relax with the semilunar and AV valves closed, and the pressure inside the ventricles drops rapidly. The v-wave of the jugular venous pulse reaches its highest point at this stage as a result of the inflow of blood from the periphery of the right atrium. At the end of this stage, the atrial pressure exceeds the ventricular pressure leading to the opening of the AV valves. Also, the incisura of the arterial pressure is seen at this stage.

RAPID INFLOW (0.11 second)

At this stage, the blood accumulated in the atria flows rapidly into the relaxed ventricles. Thus, we see the downward slope of the v-wave of the jugular venous pulse. As the ventricles are relaxed, there is a rapid rise in the volume of the ventricle with minimal change in the intraventricular pressure.

REDUCED FILLING (0.2 second)

This is a period of slow filling from the atria to the ventricles and the end of atrial contraction.

Thus, the total duration of the cardiac cycle is 0.86 second, giving us a basal heart rate of 70 beats per minute. In conditions in which there is acceleration of the heart, the diastolic intervals are shortened much more than the systolic ones.

ANESTHETICS AND MYOCARDIAL FUNCTION

As a general rule, all potent anesthetic agents are myocardial depressants. However, with some of these agents, these depressant effects are counteracted by their secondary effects. In the isolated cat papillary muscle at equipotent anesthetic concentrations, enflurane and halothane are the most depressant of the inhalational agents, while diethyl ether is the least depressant as manifested by depressed peak developed tension, maximal dp/dt, and shortened time to peak tension.[10]

In the intact heart, the direct depressant effects of ether and cyclopropane are counteracted by the activation of the sympathetic nervous system, in which contractility is maintained at or near normal. This also seems to be true with fluroxene.[11] However, with halothane, methoxyflurane, enflurane, isoflurane, and chloroform, the depressant effect on myocardial function is dose related.[8]

Nitrous oxide, which has been considered an "innocuous" agent, also has a depressant effect on ventricular function. This has been demonstrated in concentrations as low as 40 percent,[12] and when it is added to morphine anesthesia. With potent inhalational agents, it causes peripheral vasoconstriction, which masks its mild myocardial depressant effects. Of the intravenous agents, barbiturates have a potent myocardial depressant effect. Ketamine has an effect similar to ether and cyclopropane when it depresses myocardial function in isolated systems, but in the intact man it improves myocardial function because of the sympathetic overactivity.[13]

Effect on Heart Rhythm

Most of the anesthetic agents except cyclopropane prolong the atrioventricular conduction time.[14] This in itself will decrease the incidence of arrhythmias. However, the secondary sympathetic or parasympathetic effects may lead to arrhythmias.

The effect of anesthetics on heart rate and rhythm varies according to the agent used as well as its concentration. The dose of beta-adrenergic drug that is required to produce ventricular arrhythmias is lowest with cyclopropane, chloroform, and trichloroethylene, lower with halothane, and is minimally decreased or not changed at all with, ether, enflurane, methoxyflurane, and isoflurane.

REFERENCES

1. Braunwald E: Regulation of the circulation. N Engl J Med 290:1124, 1974
2. Marshall DM: The heart. In Mountcastle V (ed): Medical Physiology. St. Louis, Mosby, 1974, p 850
3. Barr L, Dewey M, Berger W: Propogation of action potentials and the structure of the nexus in cardiac muscles. J Gen Physiol 48:796, 1965
4. Leigh JM, Tyrrell MF: Cardiac performance. In Scurr C, Feldman S (eds): Scientific Foundation of Anaesthesia. Philadelphia, Davis, 1970, p 79
5. Buchbinder N, Ganz W: Hemodynamic monitoring: invasive techniques. Anesthesiology 45:146, 1976
6. Mason DT: Usefulness and limitations of the rate of rise of intraventricular pressure (dp/dt) in the evaluation of myocardial contractility in man. Am J Cardiol 23:516, 1969
7. Sonnenblick EH, Parmley WW, Urschell CW: The contractile state of the heart as expressed by force–velocity relations. J Cardiol 23:488, 1969
8. Merin RG: Effect of anesthetics on the heart. Surg Clin North Am 55:759, 1975
9. Vatner SF, Franklin P, Braunwald E: Effects of anesthesia and sleep on circulatory response to carotid sinus nerve stimulation. Am J Physiol 220:1249, 1971
10. Brown BR, Crout RS: A comparative study of the effects of five general anesthetics on myocardial contractility. Anesthesiology 34:236, 1971
11. Skovsted P, Price HL: Central sympathetic excitation caused by fluroxene. Anesthesiology 32:210, 1970
12. Eisele JH, Smith NT: Cardiovascular effects of 40 percent nitrous oxide in man. Anesth Analg (Cleve) 51:956, 1972
13. Tweed WA, Mymin D: Myocardial force–velocity relations during ketamine anesthesia at constant heart rate. Anesthesiology 41:49, 1974
14. Katz RL, Bigger JT, Jr: Cardiac arrhythmias during anesthesia and operation. Anesthesiology 33:193, 1970

chapter 2

The Electrocardiogram

As the electrical activity spreads over the myocardium, it initiates an electrical field throughout the body that produces the waves of the electrocardiogram. The difference in electrical potential across two points of the body is recorded on a long strip of paper that is run at the rate of 25 mm per second. Thus, the smallest square on the grid strip is 0.04 second and 25 of them (five big squares) are equivalent to 1 second (Fig. 2-1).

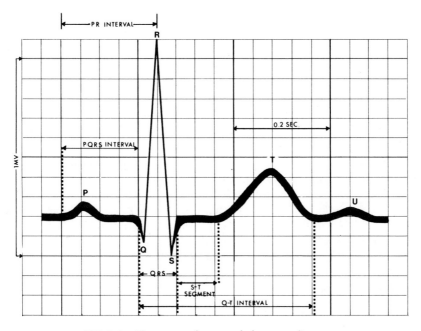

FIG. 2-1: The waves of a normal electrocardiogram.

The spread of the excitation wave (depolarization) in the atria produces the P-wave of the electrocardiogram. It is 0.07 to 0.12 second in duration. The repolarization of the P-wave is not recorded because of its small magnitude, and because of its incorporation in the following ventricular (QRS) complex.

The next wave recorded is caused by depolarization of the ventricle and is manifested by the QRS complex. The Q-wave is the first negative wave. The R-wave is the positive deflection; a second R-wave is noted as R^1. A negative deflection following the R-wave is an S-wave. The duration of the QRS complex is 0.05 to 0.10 second. It represents the time of depolarization from the beginning to the end of ventricular excitation. The P-R interval is the duration from the start of the P-wave to the start of the QRS complex and lasts 0.12 to 0.20 second. This interval indicates the time of excitation between the start of depolarization of the atrium to the start of depolarization of the ventricles. The T-wave is caused by ventricular repolarization and follows the isoelectric RS-T segment. The T-wave is in the same direction as the major deflection of the QRS complex. The repolarization of ventricles is in the opposite direction of depolarization, ie, from epicardium to endocardium. The duration of the Q-T interval is measured from the beginning of the QRS complex to the end of the T-wave and lasts 0.26 to 0.45 second. It represents the time required for complete depolarization and recovery of the ventricles. The U-wave is a small inconstant wave following the T-wave.

THE LEADS OF THE ELECTROCARDIOGRAM

The standard leads of the electrocardiogram record the potential difference between two points of the body. Because of the direction of depolarization, ie, the electrical axis of the heart, the left leg is always positive and the right arm is always negative. Lead I is the potential difference between the left arm and the right arm. It has a horizontal axis. Lead II is the potential difference between the left leg and the right arm. Lead III is the potential difference between the left leg and the left arm. The axes of these three leads form the arms of an equilateral triangle (Einthoven's triangle) (Fig. 2-2).

Unipolar leads can be recorded from the limbs. In these, the positive terminal is attached to the particular limb and the negative (or indifferent) electrode is the sum of potentials of the three limbs together. Unipolar leads are designated as VR for the right arm, VL for the left arm, and VF for the left leg. Since bipolar limbs are the difference between two points, the following formulas result:

$$\text{Lead} \quad I = VL - VR$$
$$\text{Lead} \quad II = VF - VR$$
$$\text{Lead} \quad III = VF - VL$$

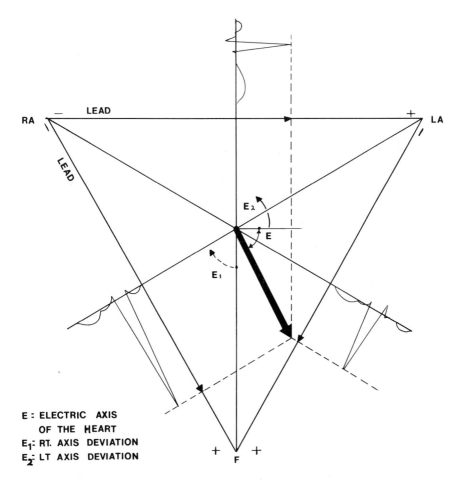

FIG. 2-2:   The determination of the electrical axis of the heart from the standard limb leads of Einthoven's triangle. Any two leads of the standard electrocardiogram can be used.

Also, the three leads of the electrocardiogram form a closed circuit; thus, the algebraic sum of their potential differences at any instant is zero:

$$VR + VL + VF = O$$

The amplitude of the deflection of the unipolar lead is usually very small. To increase their amplitude they are recorded as augmented leads (aVR, aVL, and aVF). Where the neutral electrode is the sum of the two other leads (eg, for aVF the sum of the left and right arms is the neutral electrode), a greater amplitude is achieved by losing slightly from the concept of unchanging potential.

The V-leads of the electrocardiogram are recorded as unipolar leads when the exploring electrode is connected to the positive pole of the electrocardiogram and the neutral electrode is the connection of the wires from the three limbs: right and left arms and left leg (zero potential). Therefore, a positive charge facing the exploring electrode will record as an upward (or positive) deflection and a negative as downward deflection.

The six chest leads are usually recorded at the following areas (Fig. 2-3):

V_1: Fourth right intercostal space at the sternal border
V_2: Fourth left intercostal space at the sternal border
V_3: Midway between V_2 and V_4
V_4: Fifth left intercostal space in the midclavicular line
V_5: Left anterior axillary line same horizontal level as V_4
V_6: Left midaxillary line same horizontal level as V_4
V_3R: Same position as V_3 but to the right of the sternum

The normal lead V_1 has a small R that is due to activation of the septum from left to right. This small R is followed by a deep S-wave in V_1. This is caused by the spread of activation in the wall of the left ventricle from endocardium to epicardium. Similarly, the depolarization of the septum produces the small q-wave in V_6, whereas the depolarization of the left ventricle produces the tall R-wave. Usually at V_3, the R-wave and the S-wave are equal in amplitude (Fig. 2-4). Under normal conditions, the right ventricular depolarization is not recorded because the left ventricle is much thicker than is the right. Thus, the net leftward forces of depolarization dominate over the rightward forces of depolarization. Waves of lower amplitude are denoted by lower case letters and the larger amplitude by capitals. Thus, the QRS in V_1 is described as rS and in V_6 as qR.

To determine a numerical value for the electrical axis of the heart, a triaxial reference system is used. The algebraic sum of the deflection in any two of the standard leads is computed and the points are plotted on the graph. The angle is obtained with reference to the horizontal. On the right-hand side of the horizontal line is the placement for the 0°. The positive values are below this line and the negative values above it. A clockwise displacement of more than 90° is described as right-axis deviation. A counterclockwise displacement above the 0° axis is left-axis deviation (Fig. 2-2). Minor degrees of left-axis deviation can be seen in recumbent position. Abdominal distension or left ventricular hypertrophy can lead to a more severe degree of left-axis deviation. Temporary changes of the axis are also seen during thoracotomy especially with pericardiotomy. In myocardial infarction the electrical axis shifts away from the area of the infarct.

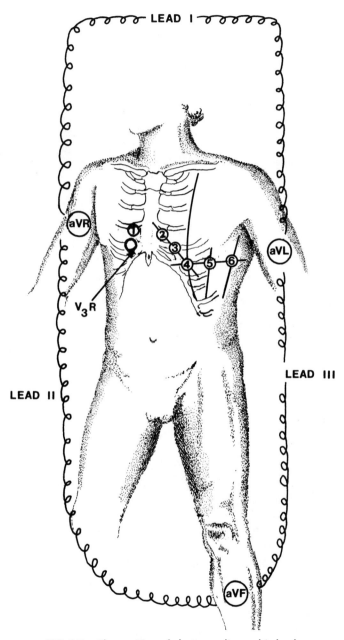

FIG. 2-3: The position of electrocardiographic leads.

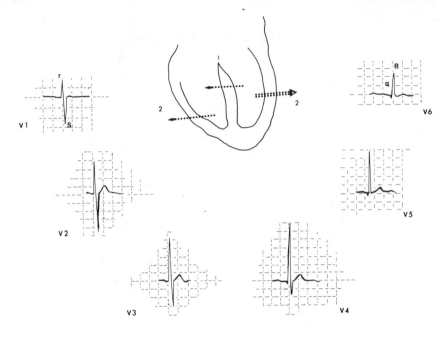

FIG. 2-4: The relationship between the precordial leads and ventricular depolarization in the normal electrocardiogram.

VECTORCARDIOGRAPHY

The cardiac activation can be described by a series of instantaneous vectors. Every 0.02 to 0.03 second, a vector is determined (voltage and direction), and a loop is obtained by connecting the head of the vectors. For the ventricular activation, four resultant vectors are usually satisfactory. It starts by activating the septum represented by a small vector to the right and forward, followed by two vectors from the activation of the ventricles, the first downward and to the left, the second backward and to the left, and finally activation of the posterior basal part of the ventricles ·represented by a small vector backward and upward. Nowadays, with the cathode-ray oscilloscope, a continuous recording of the vectorcardiogram can be obtained for each of the P-, QRS-, and T-complexes at frontal, sagittal, and transverse projections (Fig. 2-5). The value of vectorcardiography at the present stage seems to be limited, and it is used only as a supplement to electrocardiography.

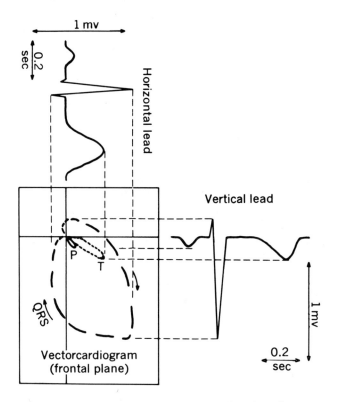

FIG. 2-5: Normal plane vectorcardiogram. (Reproduced with permission from Mosby.[1])

IRREGULARITIES OF THE CARDIAC RHYTHM

Sinus Arrhythmias

A sinus arrhythmia (Fig. 2-6) is a rhythmic variation of the heart rate synchronous with respiration. It is the result of cyclic variation of the vagal tone increasing near the end of expiration, which leads to bradycardia, and of the vagal tone decreasing near the end of inspiration, which leads to tachycardia. It is a physiologic phenomenon most commonly seen in athletes and is abolished with atropine or exercise.

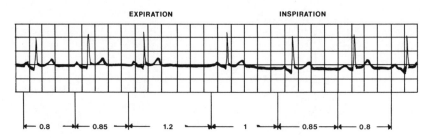

FIG. 2-6:   Sinus arrhythmia.

Sinoatrial Block

This condition (Fig. 2-7) is characterized by a complete absence of any electrical or mechanical activity for one cardiac cycle. Following this long diastole, the next heart beat may originate in the SA node, or in an ectopic focus, such as the AV node or the ventricles.

Supraventricular Arrhythmias

These result from the discharge of a focus of automatic cells from the atria. If this discharge is occasional, then it is known as premature atrial contraction (PAC). More rapid discharges cause atrial tachycardia, atrial flutter, and eventually can lead to atrial fibrillation.

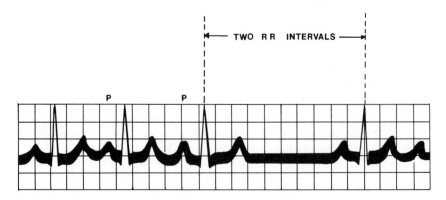

FIG. 2-7:   SA block.

A supraventricular ectopic beat is characterized by an abnormal P-wave, negative or diphasic. The shape of the P-wave depends on the position of the ectopic focus. The P-R interval varies according to the position of the ectopic focus. If it is near the ventricle, then the P-R interval is shortened. However, with premature beats the AV node might be in a relative refractory period whereby the P-R interval is prolonged (Fig. 2-8). Usually, the QRS complex of the ectopic beat has a normal configuration. Also, atrial premature contractions are characterized by the absence of a refractory period. The reason for this absence is that the ectopic impulse depolarizes the sinus, which recovers at its normal rate. Thus, the interval after the ectopic beat is normal.

Sometimes, the AV node will act as a pacemaker and the depolarization of the atria or the ventricles will occur at the same time. In this condition, the P-wave will be absent if it is incorporated in the QRS complex or it might have a negative deflection after the QRS complex from retrograde spread of the P-waves in the atria.

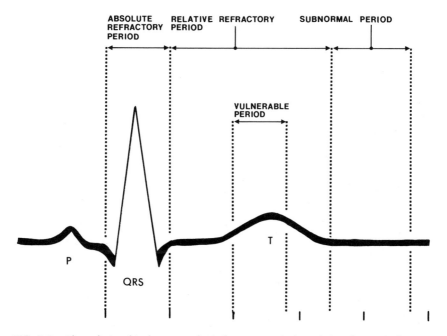

FIG. 2-8: The relationship between the refractory periods and the electrocardiogram. An impulse from an ectopic focus reaching the ventricular muscle during the absolute refractory period will not be able to initiate a contraction. In the relative refractory period, an impulse reaching the AV node will be transmitted with a prolonged conduction time. At the vulnerable period, an ectopic impulse reaching the ventricle can produce a set of ectopic beats. (Modified after Massie Walsh.[2])

Supraventricular Tachycardias

This is usually caused by an ectopic focus in the atria discharging at a rate of 120 to 250 per minute. When the atrial rate exceeds 200 per minute, the ventricular response will be cut in half because of the physiologic delay at the AV node. The exception to this is digitalis-induced atrial tachycardia with block, which has a relatively slow atrial rate with AV delay.

ATRIAL FLUTTER

The discharge from the atrial focus is 250 to 350 per minute. AV block is always present in a 2:1 to 4:1 ratio. The P-wave series produced have a characteristic sawtooth appearance.

ATRIAL FIBRILLATION

The rate of discharge of the atrial ectopic focus is more than 320 per minute. Occasionally, waves of low oscillation can be seen instead of multiple

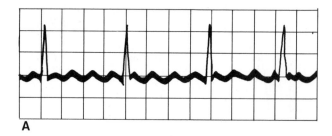

A

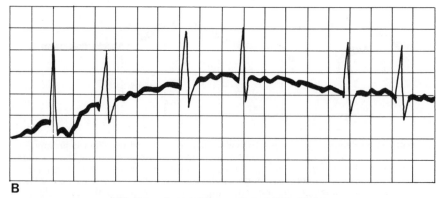

B

FIG. 2-9:   A. Atrial flutter. **B.** Atrial Fibrillation.

P-waves. The P-waves are absent because of the disorganized spread of the excitation waves. The ventricular rate depends on the condition of the AV node and is characterized by complete irregularity (Fig. 2-9).

Atrioventricular Block

Depending on the degree of the blockage, AV blocks are classified into three stages (Fig. 2-10).

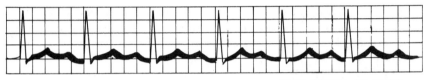

FIRST DEGREE AV BLOCK

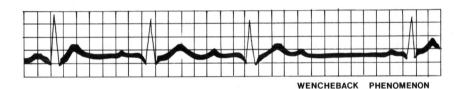

WENCHEBACK PHENOMENON

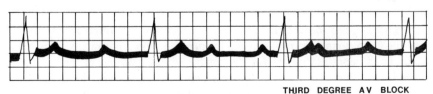

MOBITZ TYPE II

THIRD DEGREE AV BLOCK

FIG. 2-10: The various types of AV blocks.

FIRST-DEGREE AV BLOCK (DELAYED CONDUCTION OR INCOMPLETE AV BLOCK)

With this degree block, all the impulses from the atria are transmitted to the ventricles, but the conduction is delayed at the AV node. The P-R interval is longer than 0.2 second.

SECOND-DEGREE AV BLOCK

This block can be one of two types.

Wenchebach Phenomenon (Type I). In this condition, the P-R interval is prolonged progressively from beat to beat until conduction is completely interrupted and a P-wave is recorded without a QRS complex. The cycle is repeated over and over again. Thus, the ratio between the P-waves and the QRS complex can be 4 : 3 or 5 : 4, and so forth.

Mobitz (Type II). In this condition, there are nonconducted sinus impulses without any prior change in the P-R interval. A greater number of impulses are blocked at the AV junction. Thus, the ratio of P-waves to the QRS complex is 2 : 1 or 3 : 1. The P-R interval can be normal or prolonged in the conducted beats but not variable as in the Wenchebach phenomenon.

THIRD-DEGREE AV BLOCK (COMPLETE HEART BLOCK)

In this condition, there is an absolute blockade between the atria and the ventricles so that there is no relationship between the atrial and ventricular rates. The atria beat at a rate of 70 per minute and the ventricles at their inherent rate of 30 to 40 per minute, except in congenital heart block in which the rate is 60 per minute. The shape of the QRS complex depends on the origin of the ventricular beat. If it is at the main AV bundle, then the QRS complexes are normal. If, however, the origin of the excitatory impulse is at one of the bundle branches, then it resembles a bundle branch block or premature ventricular contractions.

Wolff–Parkinson–White Syndrome (Preexcitation Syndrome)

This is a rare congenital condition in which the P-R interval is shortened and the QRS complex is prolonged. This preexcitation syndrome is supposed to result from impulses that are rapidly conducted down on one of the bundles of Kent in addition to the AV node. This preexcitation also produces the delta-wave, which is a peculiar slurring of the upstroke of the first portion of the

QRS complex (Fig. 2-11). It is a benign condition but can be associated with bouts of supraventricular tachycardia from reciprocal stimulation of the atria through the accessory bundles.

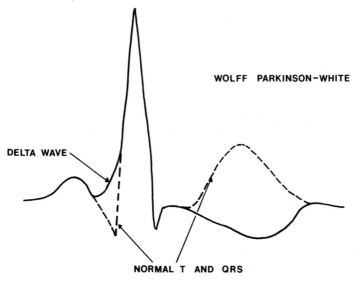

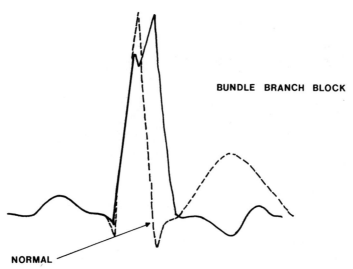

FIG. 2-11: Differences between the Wolff–Parkinson–White syndrome and the bundle-branch-block pattern.

Ventricular Extrasystoles

These are due to a discharge from an ectopic focus situated in the branches of the bundle or in the Purkinje system. Because of this abnormal origin, the recorded impulse is similar to bundle branch block. They are broad and bizarre with a T-wave in the opposite direction of the QRS complex (Fig. 2-12). Fifty percent of the time a compensatory pause can be detected after a ventricular premature contraction. This occurs because when the normal impulse from the SA node reaches the ventricle, the latter is in the refractory period and that impulse is blocked. However, the second impulse from the atria reaches the ventricle in the excitable period and the AV conduction is normal. Therefore, the sum of the intervals after the normal beat and the one following the ventricular extrasystole is equal to two normal cardiac cycles. This does not occur all the time because the ventricular extrasystoles might be conducted retrogradely, activating the atria and disturbing the sequence of P-to-P activation.

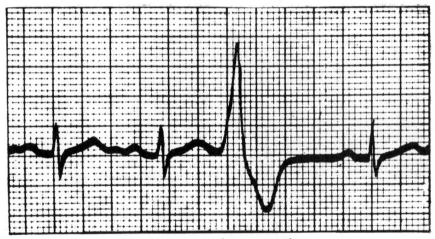

FIG. 2-12:   A ventricular premature beat.

Ventricular Tachycardia

This condition occurs when an ectopic focus fires rapidly, at the rate of 70 to 180 per minute, and the QRS complex resembles ventricular ectopic beats.

Ventricular Fibrillation

In this dangerous condition, the ventricular muscles show rapid tremulous ineffectual contractions, which, if not treated immediately, prove fatal.

ABNORMALITIES OF THE ELECTRICAL ACTIVITY OF THE HEART

Atrial Hypertrophy

Inasmuch as the SA node is situated in the right atrium, it is depolarized before the left atrium. The direction of depolarization of the atria is caudal and to the left, parallel to lead II. For this reason, the P-waves are very apparent in this lead.

In right atrial hypertrophy, the amplitude and duration of the right atrial component of the P-wave overshadow those of the left component, and a tall, peaked P-wave results. This contrasts with left atrial hypertrophy, where the peak of the P-wave arising from the left atrium can be seen. Thus, we have a notched P-wave (mitral P-wave).

Left Ventricular Hypertrophy (Fig. 2-13)

In this condition, the R-waves are more marked in the leads facing the left ventricle (ie, V_5 or V_6 and the S-waves in V_1). It is assumed that left ventricular hypertrophy is present when the total of the amplitude of the R-waves in V_5 or V_6 and of the S-waves in V_1 is greater than 3.5 mV. Also, in this condition, because of the prominence of the left ventricle, there is a left axis rotation. Occasionally, a strain pattern manifested by an upward convexity and inverted T-wave in the leads that have tall R-waves is seen.

Right Ventricular Hypertrophy

In this condition, the forces of depolarization of the septum are added to the hypertrophied right ventricle in the leads facing the right atrium. Thus, in V_1 and V_2 the peaks of the R-waves are taller than the depths of the S-waves. Also, the electrical axis of the heart is shifted to the right (right-axis deviation). An axis more than 105° is considered pathognomonic for right ventricular hypertrophy. This is in contrast to the left-axis deviation in left ventricular hypertrophy, in which it is a less reliable sign.

Bundle Branch Block

If one of the main branches of the bundle of His is blocked, the only way in which the impulse can reach the affected ventricle is through the slowly conducting ventricular wall. Thus, the duration of the QRS complex is more than 0.1 second in bundle branch block.

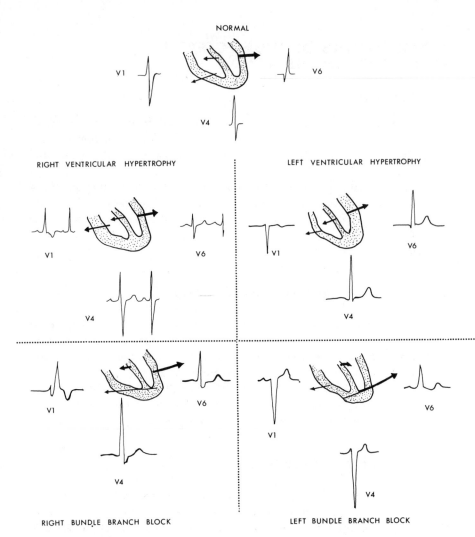

FIG. 2-13: Depolarization of the ventricles in the normal, right ventricular hypertrophy, left ventricular hypertrophy, right bundle branch block, and left bundle branch block. Note the septal depolarization from left to right in all situations except with left bundle branch block. The magnitude of the force is demonstrated by the thickness of the arrows.

RIGHT BUNDLE BRANCH BLOCK

The depolarization of the septum is in a normal direction. Therefore, the R-wave has a normal configuration in V_1 and the Q-wave is normal in V_6. Also, the depolarization of the left ventricle is normal. Thus, the S-wave in V_1 and the R-wave in V_6 are normal. However, the late right ventricular depolarization, which is now unopposed by left ventricular forces produces a large voltage that appears as a slurred R-wave in V_1 and aVR and as a late slurred S-wave in V_5, and/or V_6 and in aVL.

LEFT BUNDLE BRANCH BLOCK

The septum normally depolarizes from left to right. However, this does not happen in left bundle branch block. The first portion of the heart to be activated is the right side of the septum, and the depolarization of the septum spreads from left to right. Thus, we have a small Q-wave in V_1 and a small R-wave in V_6. Depolarization of the right ventricular wall is as usual. Thus, we have a small R-wave in V_1 and a small S-wave in V_1. Finally, the left ventricle is activated through the septum and intramyocardial spread, and we get a broad notched secondary R-wave (R^1 in V_5 or V_6 and slurred S-waves in V_1).

Myocardial Infarction and Ischemia (Fig. 2-14)

If the coronary artery is progressively compressed, the first change noted in the electrocardiogram is a deep and symmetric inversion of the T-wave. The reason for this ischemic type of T-wave inversion is supposed to result from delayed recovery of the epicardial region. Therefore, there is a reversal of the order of repolarization. These T-wave changes can be reversed by resuming the circulation.

More compression of the coronary arteries leads to the elevation of the ST segment, caused by a strong current of injury leading to a marked depression of the resting isopotential line. To be clinically significant, these ST-segment changes should be more than 1 mm above the base line. These ST-segment changes are temporary in nature, and they return to normal when the blood flow is reestablished to the myocardium. In cases of a myocardial infarct, the ST segment becomes isoelectric within 2 to 7 days.

If the flow in the coronary artery is completely interrupted, the area of the myocardium supplied by that vessel becomes infarcted. This infarcted area will have no electrical activity of its own but will simply conduct to the surface the potentials found inside the cavity of the heart. Therefore, a deep Q-wave will be seen in the leads looking at an infarcted area. Clinically, a Q-wave whose amplitude is more than one-third greater than that of its corresponding R-wave and whose duration is more than 0.04 second is diagnostic of a myocardial infarction.

EFFECTS OF DRUGS AND ELECTROLYTES ON THE ELECTROCARDIOGRAM

Digitalis causes a shortening of the Q-T interval and a sagging of the ST segment. This sagging is characterized by a downward slope from the

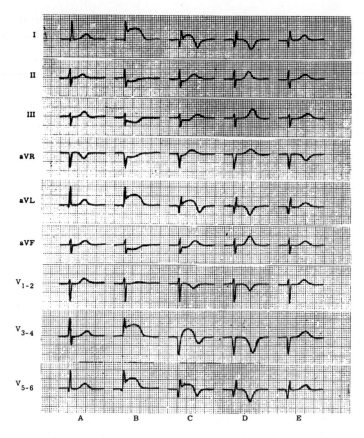

FIG. 2-14: Serial electrocardiographic changes following infarction of the anterior portion of the ventricular wall. **A.** Normal tracing. **B.** Very early pattern (hours after infarction). There is a ST-segment elevation in leads I, aVL, and V_3 to V_6, and there is reciprocal ST depression in leads II, III, and aVF. **C.** Later pattern (many hours to a few days following infarction). The Q-waves have appeared in leads I, aVL, V_5, and V_6. QS complexes are present in V_3 and V_4. This indicates that the major transmural infarction is underlying the area recorded by V_3 and V_4. ST-segment changes persist but are of lesser degree, and the T-waves are beginning to invert in those leads in which the ST segments are elevated. **D.** Late established pattern (many days to weeks after infarction). The Q-waves and the QS complexes persist; the ST segments are isoelectric. The T-waves are symmetric and deeply inverted in leads that had ST elevation and tall in leads that had ST depression. This pattern may persist for the remainder of the patient's life. **E.** Very late pattern. This may occur many months to years after the infarction. The abnormal Q-waves and QS complexes persist. The T-waves have gradually returned to normal. (Reproduced with permission from Lange[3])

isoelectric junction starting at the end of the QRS complex. This is a normal result of digitalis use and is known as the digitalis effect. However, an overdose of digitalis leads to atrial or ventricular ectopic beats, and thus ectopic supraventricular or ventricular tachycardia can occur. Various forms of heart block

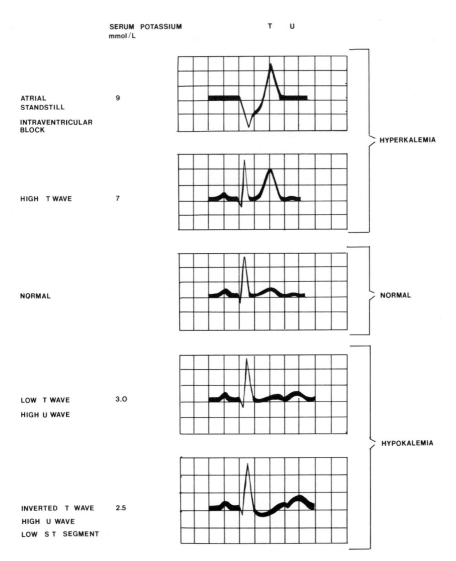

FIG. 2-15: Electrocardiographic changes with hypokalemia and hyperkalemia.

are also seen. Most of the effects of digitalis toxicity can be reversed with potassium supplementation.

Hypokalemia is initially manifested by a prominence of the U-wave (Fig. 2-15). Later, the amplitude of the T-wave is reduced and the ST segments begin to sag. With severe hypokalemia (serum potassium 2.5 mEq per liter) the T-wave may be isoelectric and the prominent U-wave will give the false impression of a prolonged ST segment.

In *hyperkalemia,* the T-waves become tall and peaked with a tent-like appearance. With increasing level of serum potassium (8 mEq per liter), the P–R interval becomes prolonged with widening of the QRS complex. At very high levels, the P-waves disappear and the QRS complex merges with the tall T-wave, producing a distorted appearance. This condition is usually followed by ventricular fibrillation and standstill.

Hypocalcemia leads to prolongation of the ST segment without any change in the T-waves, and *hypercalcemia* causes a shortening of the ST segment.

REFERENCES

1. Milnor WR: The electrocardiogram. In Mountcastle VB (ed): Medical Physiology, 13th ed. St. Louis, Mosby, 1974 p. 890
2. Massie E, Walsh TJ: Clinical Vectoricardiography and Electrocardiography. Chicago, Year Book, 1960
3. Goldman MJ: Principles of Clinical Electrocardiography, 9th ed. Los Altos, Calif, Lange, 1976

BIBLIOGRAPHY

Chung EK: Principles of Cardiac Arrhythmias. Baltimore, Williams & Wilkins, 1973
Grant RP: Clinical Electrocardiography. New York, McGraw-Hill, 1970
Hamer J: An Introduction to Electrocardiography. London, Pitman, 1975
Littman D: Textbook of Electrocardiography. Hagerstown, Md, Harper & Row, 1972
Schamroth L: An Introduction to Electrocardiography. Oxford, Blackwell, 1973

chapter 3

Regulation
of Cardiac Output

The 300 trillion cells of the body require a constant internal environment (milieu interieur) to carry on their own specific functions. Thus, the heart as a pump must supply them with their nutrients and at the same time remove their waste products. To achieve this, the heart circulates the total blood volume around the body once every minute.[1] At the same time, fluid, which is equivalent to 45 times the blood volume, diffuses from the capillaries into the interstitial spaces and back.[2] It has been observed that if the cardiac output falls below one-third of its normal value, then the functioning of the tissues becomes seriously impaired from hypoxia.

NORMAL VALUES

The normal cardiac output of a young healthy adult is 6 liters per minute. However, it is usually expressed as the cardiac index, which is the cardiac output per square meter of body surface area.

$$\text{Cardiac index} = \frac{\text{Cardiac output (liters per minute)}}{\text{Body surface area (sq meters)}}$$

Thus, the cardiac index of the standard, healthy 70-kg man with a surface area of 1.73 sq meters is 3.5 liters per minute. It is about 7 to 10 percent less in females. It decreases with age, and it reaches 2.5 liters per minute in people over 60 years of age.

MEASUREMENT OF CARDIAC OUTPUT

There are three methods that are most commonly used for measuring cardiac output.

Fick Principle

$$\text{Cardiac output} = \frac{\text{Oxygen consumption}}{\text{Arteriovenous oxygen difference}}$$

The oxygen consumption is measured by allowing the individual to breathe from a respirometer containing a known oxygen mixture. The expired gases are collected in a Douglas bag (nondiffusible bag). The volume and the concentration of the expired gases are measured. From these two the oxygen consumption per unit time (milliliters per minute) is derived. An arterial blood sample and a mixed venous sample from a pulmonary artery catheter are withdrawn. The oxygen content is determined in the two samples, and the difference between the two becomes the denominator of the equation.

Indicator Dilution Method

This method depends on the principle that if a nondiffusible dye is injected in a central vein, the rapidity with which it is distributed in the arterial system is directly proportional to the cardiac output.

The dye most commonly used is indocyanine green (Cardio-green). It is injected rapidly into a central vein. The concentration of the dye is measured continuously through a peripheral arterial catheter by a spectrophotometer. From the area under the curve before the recirculation, the cardiac output is derived (Fig. 3-1).

$$\text{Cardiac output} = \frac{\text{Amount of dye injected} \times \text{calibration factor}}{\text{Area under the curve}}$$

Recently, a computer program has been developed to calculate the area under the curve and derive the cardiac output almost instantaneously.

Thermodilution Method

This is performed by using a four-lumen Swan–Ganz catheter.[3, 4] The catheter is positioned in such a manner that the distal tip lies in the pulmonary artery. Then the proximal port will lie in the right atrium. Blood is withdrawn to fill the dead space of the catheter. A bolus of saline with a known temperature is injected into the right atrium through the proximal port. The thermistor present in the pulmonary artery (just proximal to the deflated balloon of the

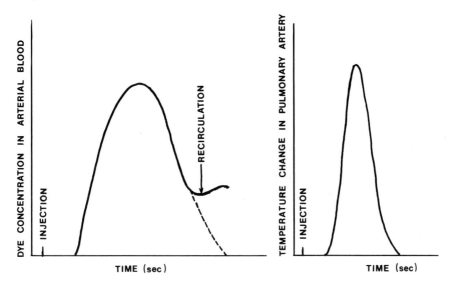

FIG. 3-1: Diagrammatic representation of dye dilution curves and thermodilution curves obtained during cardiac output measurement. Note the steeper rise and decline of the thermodilution curve, indicating negligible recirculation.

Swan–Ganz catheter) will measure the temperature change. The cardiac output is computed from the temperature–time curve. Because recirculation is negligible with this technique, repeated cardiac output measurements can easily be performed in intensive care units or cardiac catheterization laboratories.

FACTORS CONTROLLING CARDIAC OUTPUT

The cardiac output is the product of the heart rate and the stroke volume. The heart rate is under strict control from the autonomic nervous system. Stimulation of the sympathetic nervous system increases the heart rate (chronotrophic effect), while the parasympathetic nervous system decreases it. The sympathetic nervous system also affects the other components of the cardiac output, ie, stroke volume, where it improves the strength of contraction of muscle fibers (inotropic effect). However, the factors that mostly affect the cardiac output are peripheral in origin, such as the venous return, total blood volume, and arterial blood pressure. Obviously, the contractile state of the myocardium is of utmost importance. A weak heart will be unable to cope with circulatory demands, thus leading to congestive heart failure.

Heart Rate

It seems that the heart has a relatively unimportant effect on the regulation of cardiac output.[5] In normal, resting individuals, increasing the heart rate
does not lead to an increase in cardiac output.[6] However, this mechanism is
important for the increase in cardiac output during exercise. Also, in patients
with low cardiac output and bradycardia, raising the heart rate to the upper
levels of normal augments the cardiac output, since an increase in heart rate is
associated with an inherent increased inotropic state even when this rise is not
induced by adrenergic stimulation.[7]

Stroke Volume

In a young adult with a heart rate of 70 beats per minute, each of his
ventricles will contain about 120 ml of blood at the end of diastole; 70 ml of
these will be expelled with each systole, constituting his stroke volume. Three
main factors determine the stroke volume.

PRELOAD

This forms the basis for the Frank–Starling mechanism, which states that
the work performed by the ventricle is a function of end-diastolic ventricular
volume. As the fiber length of the heart muscle increases, the energy of contraction also increases up to a certain length. With further lengthening beyond this
optimal length, the energy of contraction diminishes (or the cardiac work).
This has been clarified by electron microscopy, which shows that, with
increased lengthening of the myocardium, the sarcomeres become slightly
elongated. Thus, the number of sites for chemical interaction between adjacent
actin and myosin filaments is increased.[8] Several factors can affect the stretching of the ventricular muscle at the end of diastole. Among these are venous
return to the heart, intrapericardial pressure, atrial contraction, and venous
tone.

MYOCARDIAL CONTRACTILITY

During diastole, extracellular calcium is concentrated near the cell
membrane, whereas intracellular calcium is sequestrated in the sarcoplasmic
reticulum. Excitation of the cell membrane and depolarization are accompanied
by a rapid entry of extracellular calcium into the cell, and, more importantly, a
release of intracellular calcium occurs. During relaxation, the intracellular calcium is recaptured by the sarcoplasmic reticulum, and an outflowing of calcium

across the cell membrane occurs. One theory suggests that during diastole there is a troponin–tropomyosin complex inhibiting interaction between the two major proteins actin and myosin. Thus, the released calcium during depolarization deactivates this troponin–tropomyosin complex and a contraction occurs.[9]

Myocardial contractility depends on many factors. Ionized calcium availability to the heart muscle will affect the strength of contraction. Potassium has an opposite effect. It depresses the contractile mechanism of the muscle cell in addition to the conduction block that it produces, and these effects are counteracted by calcium. Norepinephrine, the adrenergic neurotransmitter of the heart, can be a strong stimulus for contractility by acting on the myocardial beta receptor.[9] The baroreceptor reflexes seem to have minimal or absolutely no effect on the control of myocardial contractility in the conscious intact organism. However, they seem to be functional in anesthetized animals.

AFTERLOAD

The term "afterload" refers to the load or tension that the heart is called on to develop during contraction. In the isolated cardiac muscle, when the afterload is increased, the velocity of shortening decreases and vice versa (Figs. 1–4). Therefore, at a constant preload and contractility, a reciprocal relationship exists between afterload and shortening. In the intact ventricle where the afterload is the systolic pressure, raising the left ventricular systolic pressure leads to diminution of stroke volume and vice versa.[10] The intracardiac pressure, besides being dependent on intracavitary pressure, depends on the ventricular diameter. This relationship between pressure and wall tension was studied by LaPlace. His theory states that circumferential tension is the product of the pressure per square centimeter and the radius of cylinder ($T = Pr$). Because the cardiac radius is increased in heart failure, the tension on the myocardial wall rises with a consequent increase in afterload. This mechanism acts diametrically opposite to Starling's law, in which the increased stretch within its limits improves the contractile ability.

Afterload has an important role in maintaining the circulatory equilibrium. For example, a rise in the arterial pressure will augment afterload, which in turn will depress the myocardial shortening, and hence the cardiac output. Thus, through this negative feedback mechanism arterial pressure is restored to its previous level.

CARDIAC OUTPUT IN VARIOUS CONDITIONS

The cardiac output varies[1] according to the physiologic and pathologic needs of the body.

Physiologic

POSTURE

When a person is moved quietly and passively from a sitting or recumbent to a standing position, his cardiac output decreases by 20 to 30 percent. This results from the pooling of blood in the lower parts of the body while standing. However, if the individual rises actively, the tensing of his muscles from active contraction will increase the output. It is interesting to note that the heart is in a more dilated position when the individual is recumbent compared to what it is in the standing position. When he stands up, the stroke volume decreases while the heart accelerates.[11]

EXERCISE

Any movement of the body will increase the cardiac output. The extent of the rise in the cardiac output will parallel the increase in oxygen consumption from the exercising muscles. In the average human being, a maximum amount of exercise will increase the cardiac output fourfold. This is accomplished by doubling the heart rate and doubling the stroke volume.[11] However, a trained athlete can increase his/her cardiac output sixfold.

MEALS

A heavy meal will increase the cardiac output by about 25 percent.

SLEEP

The sleeper's cardiac output is reduced by 20 percent.

CYCLIC CHANGES

In females the cardiac output is lower during the menstrual periods and ovulation and rises higher on premenstrual and postmenstrual days.

ENVIRONMENTAL CHANGES

Exposure to a hot atmosphere leads to an increase in cardiac output as a result of cutaneous vasodilatation in an effort to increase heat loss. There is also stimulation of the sweat glands, which in turn will increase the cardiac output. Exposure to a cold environment will also lead to a rise in cardiac output as a result of the body shivering.

PREGNANCY

The cardiac output increases during pregnancy from 30 to 50 percent above the nonpregnant levels. Several factors contribute to this augmented cardiac output, ie, increase of uteroplacental circulation, rise in maternal oxygen consumption, arteriovenous shunts in the placenta, and hyperthyroidism.

Pathologic

ANXIETY AND EXCITEMENT

Severe anxiety can increase the cardiac output more than 50 percent due to sympathetic overactivity.

ANOXIA

Two phases are recognized. First, an increase from vasodilatation in the hypoxic tissues in an effort to compensate for the anoxia. This stage is followed by a drop in the output because of the failing of the myocardium due to a lack in its oxygen supply.

FEVER

Similar to body metabolic requirements, with every degree Celsius rise in body temperature the cardiac output rises by 12 percent (7 percent for each degree Fahrenheit).

HYPERTHYROIDISM

The increase in the cardiac output in this condition is due to hypermetabolism and also from the hyperdynamic circulatory state caused by increased sympathetic nervous activity. The opposite situation exists with hypothyroidism (Chap. 25).

ANEMIA

Reduction of hemoglobin to less than 5 gm per 100 ml increases the output twofold.

ARTERIOVENOUS SHUNTS

The cardiac output increases in the presence of arteriovenous shunts in order to provide adequate tissue perfusion to the affected area.

OTHERS

Several diseases cause an increase in cardiac output such as beri-beri, Paget's disease, and septic shock. It is decreased in severe myocardial infarction, chronic valvular disease, hypothyroidism, and severe shock. However, in essential hypertension the cardiac output is within normal limits.

EFFECT OF ANESTHETIC AGENTS ON CARDIAC OUTPUT

Several factors influence the cardiovascular effect of an anesthetic agent including:

1. The concentration of the anesthetic agent. Usually the minimum alveolar concentration (MAC)* is used as a basis for comparison.
2. The effect of time, with concomitant circulatory adaptation.
3. The ventilatory pattern, spontaneous or controlled, and the arterial carbon dioxide content.
4. The effect of associated surgery.
5. The presence of any associated disease.

In healthy individuals during the first hour of anesthesia, ether, fluroxene, and cyclopropane allow the cardiac output to remain near or above control (awake) values, whereas halothane depresses cardiac output by decreasing the stroke volume.

The effect of increasing the inspired anesthetic concentration varies according to the agent used. With halothane the depression of cardiac output is marked and linear with the rise of its concentration. With cyclopropane this linear drop in output is less marked.[15] In contrast to halothane raising, the inspired ether or fluroxene concentration will increase the cardiac output. With these two latter agents the diminution in stroke volume is more than compensated by an increase in the heart rate.

---

* *Minimum Alevolar Concentration (MAC) is the concentration of inhalational anesthetic agent at which 50 percent of the subjects do not react to skin incision.*

With prolonged anesthesia (5 hours), circulatory adaptation with stimulation occurs. The output values increase 20 to 40 percent with halothane, fluroxene, and ether and 10 percent with cyclopropane. The lesser rise in cardiac output with cyclopropane is caused by the failure of the heart rate to accelerate significantly with this agent.[12]

The diminution of cardiac output with halothane is less if the patient breathes spontaneously rather than with controlled respiration. This probably results from beta-sympathetic stimulation, which accompanies the rise of arterial carbon dioxide levels, and also from the lack of positive intrathoracic pressure,[13] which impedes the venous return.

With enflurane (Ethrane), the cardiac output is well maintained at or near normal levels. If hypercapnia occurs with enflurane anesthesia, a marked rise in cardiac output is noted.[14]

With ketamine the cardiac output is also increased by about 30 percent. This increase in output is not solely caused by rate changes. There occurs a corresponding increase in stroke volume.[15] This probably is a result of central autonomic response. However, there is a probability that the baroreceptors are also involved, especially in the chronotropic effect.

REFERENCES

1. Guyton AC, Jones CE, Coleman TG: Circulatory Physiology Cardiac Output and Its Regulation, 2nd ed. Philadelphia, Saunders, 1973
2. Pappenheimer JR: Passage of molecules through capillary walls. Physiol Rev 33:387, 1953
3. Buchbinder N, Ganz W: Hemodynamic monitoring: invasive techniques. Anesthesiology 43:146 1976
4. Forrester JS, Ganz W, Diamond G, et al: Thermodilution cardiac output determination with a single flow directed catheter. Am Heart J 83:306, 1972
5. Braunwald E, Ross D, Sonnenblick EH: Mechanisms of contraction of the normal and failing heart. N Engl J Med 277:962, 1967
6. Ross J, Linhart JW, Braunwald E: Effect of changing heart rate in man by electrical stimulation of the right atrium. Circulation 32:549, 1965
7. Mason DT, Spann JF, Zelis R, et al: Alterations of hemodynamic and myocardial mechanisms in patients with congestive heart failure. In Friedberg CK (ed): Congestive Heart Failure. New York, Grune, 1970
8. Braunwald E: Structure and function of the normal myocardium. Br Heart J 33:Suppl 3–8, 1971.
9. Braunwald E: Regulation of the circulation. N Engl J Med 290:1124, 1974
10. Sonnenblick EH, Downing SE: Afterload as a primary determinant of ventricular performance. Am J Physiol 204:604, 1963
11. Mitchell JH, Blomqvist G: Maximal oxygen uptake. N Engl J Med 284:1018, 1971
12. Eger EI, Smith NT, Cullen DJ, et al: A comparison of the cardiovascular effects of halothane, fluroxene, ether, cyclopropane in man. Anesthesiology 34:25, 1971

13. Bahlman SH, Eger EI, Halsey MJ, et al: The cardiovascular effects of halothane in man during spontaneous ventilation. Anesthesiology 36:494, 1972
14. Marshall BE, Cohen PJ, Klingemaier CH, et al: Some pulmonary and cardiovascular effects of enflurane (ethrane) anaesthesia with varying $PaCO_2$ in man, Br J Anaesth 43:996, 1971
15. Tweed WA, Minuck M, Mymin D: Circulatory responses to ketamine anesthesia. Anesthesiology 37:613, 1972

chapter 4

Arterial Blood Pressure

In the normal, healthy young adult, the ideal systemic arterial pressure is considered to be 120 mm Hg systolic and 80 mm Hg diastolic. However, in the great majority of healthy adults the systolic varies between 100 and 150 mm Hg and the diastolic between 60 and 90 mm Hg. These values are lower in infants and they increase with age. The blood pressures of women are 5 to 10 mm Hg lower than males until the age of 50, after which there is no appreciable difference. In normal humans, both the systolic and diastolic pressures increase with age. However, the systolic rise is greater than the diastolic.[1] This is partly due to the diminished elasticity of the arteries occuring with age.

The mean arterial pressure is the average pressure throughout the cardiac cycle. Because of the shape of the arterial pressure wave, the mean pressure is nearer to diastolic than systolic. The mean pressure can be integrated or derived electronically. For a rough approximation, the following formula can be used:

$$\text{Mean arterial pressure} = \frac{\text{Systolic pressure} + 2 \times \text{diastolic pressure}}{3}$$

This mean pressure represents the effective pressure that drives blood throughout the circulatory system.

MEASUREMENT OF BLOOD PRESSURE

Direct Measurement

This is done by inserting a cannula into an artery and connecting it to a mercury manometer or a strain gauge transducer. The signal from the transducer can be arranged to record on a strip of paper or can be displayed on an oscillograph. If the cannula is obstructing the flow of the artery or if the artery beyond is ligated, an *end pressure* is recorded in which all the kinetic energy is transformed into pressure energy. However, if a T tube is used instead of a straight cannula, the recorded side pressure is less than that of the end pressure, the reason being that not all of the kinetic energy is transformed into pressure energy; part of it remains as kinetic energy of flow (Bernouelli's principle).[2]

Indirect Measurement

AUSCULTATORY METHOD

Any technique that is to be used in a general clinical situation should be noninvasive. In 1905, Korotkoff described the sounds that can be heard over the brachial artery during deflation of the cuff. Since that time his findings have been used as the criteria for systolic and diastolic blood pressure measurement. This method is based on the principle that the blood flow in the main arteries is laminar in character and is inaudible. However, if the flow is arrested by a cuff and then the pressure of the cuff is released slowly, audible sounds can be heard when the pressure of the cuff falls below the systolic pressure and blood starts flowing in the brachial artery. These sounds occur because in the narrowed artery the velocity of the flow through the constriction exceeds the critical velocity and results in turbulence. These sounds undergo changes and are described in four phases.

Phase I: Sudden appearance of a clear *tapping* sound synchronous with the heart beat. This sharp phase of the Korotkoff sound is probably due to short bursts of relaxation oscillation of the arterial wall.[3] Usually this sound starts faintly and becomes louder as the pressure drops in the cuff to 10 to 15 mm Hg. At this point, the arterial flow occurs only at the peak of systole.

Phase II: With the next 15- to 20-mm Hg fall in pressure, a *murmurlike* sound is heard. Now the flow is interrupted for a shorter time, and this intermittent flow gives a murmurlike (swishing) quality to the sound.

Phase III: The murmurlike sounds become *clearer* and louder.

Phase IV: The sounds become *muffled* for the next 5-mm Hg fall in cuff pressure. At this point the vessel is still constricted and the turbulence is rather continuous, which imparts the muffled (or blowing) quality to the sounds.

Phase V: Silence. The diastolic pressure usually correlates better at the point where the sounds become muffled (Phase IV) rather than when they become silent. The muffling occurs at pressures 7 to 10 mm Hg higher than direct intraarterial diastolic pressures.[4] The separation of the last two phases is more apparent in exercise or in children in whom the chances of intraarterial turbulence is high.[1] If the difference between these two points is marked, it is better to record both of them. Also, the auscultatory murmurlike sound at Phase II may be so low that it becomes inaudible, and this in turn might lead to an underestimation of systolic blood pressure. This possibility can be avoided by checking first with the palpatory method.

For these readings to be reasonably accurate, the size of the cuff must be comparable to the size of the arm. As a general rule, the inflatable bag should cover at least half of the arm; ideally it should be 20 percent wider than the diameter of the limb on which it is to be used. Thus, in an adult a bag 12 to 14 cm is satisfactory, while a child of 8 years will require a cuff of 8 cm, a child less than 4 years a cuff of 5 cm, and an infant a cuff of 2 cm. If the individual is very obese or if the pressure is taken in the thigh, a bigger cuff will be needed (18 cm), because in these situations a higher amount of pressure will be required to compress the extra tissues.

PALPATORY METHOD

This is the pressure at which the radial pulse is first felt. By this technique the pressure measured is 3 to 5 mm Hg lower than the ausculatory method.

OSCILLOMETRIC METHOD

The iscillometer consists of two concentric cuffs, the upper one of which is small (Fig. 4-1). An aneroid manometer measures either the pressure in the cuffs or the pressure difference through a two-way stopcock. First, the pressure in the cuffs is pumped up while the cuffs are interconnected. Then the pressure is deflated slowly and the manometer switched to differential. At pressures above systolic, there is no differential pressure between the cuffs, and no oscillations are detected. When the pressure drops below the systolic, the intermittent flow of blood in the distal artery expands it. This expansion is detected through the differential manometer. At pressures below diastolic, no swings in the manometer can be detected because the artery is expanded all the time.

ULTRASOUND METHOD (DOPPLER EFFECT)

The crystals that detect the ultrasound are deposited distal to the cuff over the artery. By transmitting and receiving the ultrasounds the flow through the arteries can be identified. They have the advantage that they are accurate when the flow in the arteries is diminished as in hypotensive states or in infants in whom the auscultatory sounds are very weak.

In all indirect pressure measurements the lateral pressure of the brachial artery is obtained. This is in contrast to the direct methods used in which the end pressure is measured. The direct method gives a higher value because it combines the following pressures:[5]

1. The lateral pressure in the elastic arterial wall
2. The energy derived from conversion of kinetic energy of the blood to pressure as it meets the obstruction
3. Pressure reflected from the obstruction

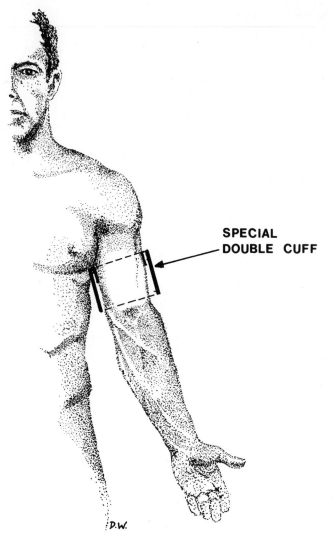

SPECIAL
DOUBLE CUFF

D.W.

FIG. 4-1:   Arrangement of the oscillometer cuffs.

REGULATION OF THE ARTERIAL BLOOD PRESSURE

The arterial blood pressure is the product of cardiac output and peripheral resistance. Increasing either one of them without changing the other will increase the arterial blood pressure.

Diminution in the elasticity of the main arteries per se does not lead to an increase in the mean arterial blood pressure. However, it does increase the pulse pressure from the diminished ability of the rigid walls to damp out the oscillations produced by the heart.

The cardiac output is the product of the heart rate and the stroke volume. Thus, changing either one of them will consequently alter the blood pressure, eg, the stroke volume can be increased by raising the filling pressure of the heart through increased blood volume or by venoconstriction. Similarly, tachycardia, with constant stroke volume, leads to a rise in blood pressure.

The biggest resistance to the arterial flow is at the arteriolar level. The pressure is these small arteries drops from 95 mm Hg to 35 mm Hg (Fig. 4-2). Relative to the arterioles, the resistance of the arteries, capillaries, and veins is small. Thus, the biggest determinant of the arterial blood pressure is the tone of the smooth muscles in the walls of the arterioles. This tone can be markedly altered by the sympathetic nerve endings that release noradrenaline at their terminals. Also, these vessels are sensitive to humoral agents.

Control of Blood Pressure

There are two main control mechanisms for adjusting the blood pressure. The first is through the autonomic nervous system, which responds to acute changes in blood pressure. The second is poorly understood, operates through

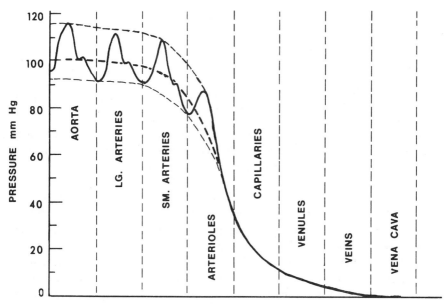

FIG. 4-2: Pressures at different sites in the systemic circulation.

the kidney, and is involved in situations of prolonged changes in arterial blood pressure.

AUTONOMIC SYSTEM

The baroreceptors form the afferent part of this reflex system. Being located at strategic points in the aortic arch and carotid arteries, they respond to changes in arterial blood pressure.[6] These receptors respond to stretch rather than to pressure changes, and their sensitivity to pressure changes is greatest near the normal arterial pressure. The efferent part of the baroreceptor reflex is through the parasympathetic fibers of the vagus leading to slowing of heart rate. Also, inhibition of the sympathetic vasoconstriction center leads to a decrease in peripheral arterial and arteriolar resistance. This is a typical example of a *negative feedback* mechanism, in which a change in one direction results in changes in the opposite direction leading to stability of the system.

The cerebral and the coronary vessels have a relatively poor sympathetic innervation. Thus, they are affected very little by the baroreceptor reflexes. The net result of a drop in blood pressure is shifting of the circulatory blood volume from the less vital tissues, such as muscle, splanchnic area, and skin, to the vital organs, such as the heart and liver.

If a person rises from a supine position, there will be a tendency for the venous return to the heart to be diminished. This will lead to hypotension and fainting if these rapid reflexes did not compensate by increasing the heart rate, the peripheral resistance, and venous tone.

THE HUMORAL SYSTEM

Goldblatt found that if one of the renal arteries has been partially occluded, the systemic arterial blood pressure rises in the next few weeks to hypertensive levels. This occurs because the kidney is trying to keep its blood supply constant.

Also, in prolonged hypertension, the baroreceptors seem to be reset at a higher level. They work quite normally, acting as a buffer and preventing any deviation from the new hypertensive level.

Although there are several theories explaining this mechanism, the most acceptable seems to be the renin–angiotensin theory. The juxtaglomerular cells of the kidney contain granules that have similar characteristics to renin. When the renal blood flow is diminished, the number of these granules decreases and renin is released into the circulation. Renin is a proteolytic enzyme and acts on α_2-globulin in the plasma to form the decapeptide angiotensin I. Angiotensin I is hydrolyzed in the plasma to the octopeptide angiotensin II. Angiotensin II by itself is a powerful vasoconstrictor. The pressor responsiveness of the arterioles to angiotensin II is greatly enhanced by sodium loading and blunted by sodium depletion.[7] It also leads to the release of aldosterone from the adrenal cortex, which leads to salt and water retention by the kidney.

THE PERIPHERAL RESISTANCE

This is the frictional resistance offered by the circulatory system to the flow of blood in it. It is not due to the scraping of the blood over the rough vascular wall.[8]

Laminar and Turbulent Flow

The blood flow in most of the large blood vessels is laminar. Within the blood vessel, an infinitely thin layer of plasma comes in contact with the vessel wall and that layer of plasma does not move at all. It is held there by cohesive forces. Thus, no friction exists between this layer and the vessel wall. However, the next concentric layer inside this stagnant layer moves at a slow velocity. The next layer moves at a higher velocity so that the velocity is highest at the center of the vessel. Thus, the layers of fluids are sliding over each other (Fig. 4-3). This lack of slipperiness of the adjacent layers is the cause of the frictional resistance to flow. Thus, the most important function of the heart is to overcome these cohesive forces.

In 1846, Poiseuille, a French physician and physiologist, described the laminar constant flow of newtonian liquids through rigid cylindrical tubes,[9]

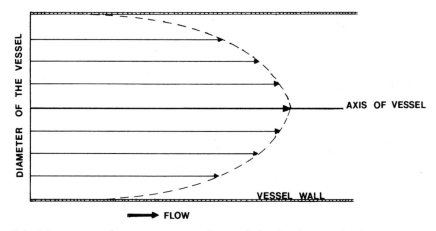

FIG. 4-3: Laminar flow pattern. Note the parabolic distribution of velocities, ie, the outermost layer is stagnant while the layer at the axis of the vessel has the highest velocity.

and this is expressed mathematically in the Poiseuille–Hagen formula:

$$\text{Flow} = \frac{\text{Pressure difference at the ends of the tube} \times \pi \times \text{radius of the tube}^4}{8 \times \text{coefficient of viscosity} \times \text{length of tube}}$$

Thus, the resistance of the flow is directly proportional to the length of the tube and the viscosity and is indirectly proportional to the fourth power of the diameter of the tube. Increasing the radius of the tube twice will lead to a 16-fold increase in the flow of the liquid.

Laminar flow occurs up to a certain velocity. At higher velocities, the pattern of laminar flow breaks down and the particles move in irregular and variable paths forming eddies. The critical point in which the transition occurs from laminar to turbulent flow is defined by Reynold's number.[10]

$$\text{Reynold's number} = \frac{\text{Flow velocity (cm/second)} \times \text{tube diameter (cm)} \times \text{liquid density (g/cm}^3)}{\text{Viscosity of liquid (poise)}}$$

Thus, increased velocity or wider tube diameter encourages turbulence, while increased viscosity discourages turbulence.

If the result of Reynold's formula is a number above 2000, turbulence usually occurs. However, a mixture of laminar and turbulent, flow occurs at Reynold's numbers above 1000. Laminar flow is silent, whereas turbulence creates sound. In man, laminar flow is the rule, except in the ascending aorta at the peak of systolic ejection. Also, this critical velocity is exceeded when the arteries are compressed and forms the basis of the auscultatory measurement of the blood pressure. In anemia, in which the viscosity is diminished, turbulence occurs, leading to the well-known systolic murmurs that are heard over the precordium.

These rules about the types of flow are for rigid tubes. Although they are applicable to blood vessels, one must realize that the blood flow in the vessels is pulsatile rather than constant. Also, blood is not an absolute newtonian fluid, ie, its viscosity can vary according to the velocity gradient. However, the magnitude of this effect is minimal in blood vessels more than 0.5 mm in diameter.

Vascular Resistance

The relationship between vascular resistance, flow, and pressure can be expressed by an equation similar to Ohm's law of electric current.

$$\text{Resistance} = \frac{\text{Pressure difference}}{\text{Flow}}$$

There are several units for expressing peripheral resistance. However, for simplicity, it is expressed as R units, which is obtained by dividing the pressure in mm Hg by the flow measured in ml per second.

If we assume that the mean pressure generated by the left ventricle into the aorta is 105 mm Hg while the pressure in the right atrium is 5 mm Hg and the cardiac output is 6 liters per minute (100 ml per second), then the peripheral resistance in the systemic circuit becomes:

$$R = \frac{105 - 5}{100} = 1 \text{ R unit or mm Hg per ml per second.}$$

This means that the heart should produce a difference of pressure of 1 mm Hg to push 1 ml of blood per second through the resistance offered by the systemic circulation.

In the pulmonary side of circulation, the pressure difference generated by the right ventricle is 20 mm Hg. Then the peripheral resistance of pulmonary circuit is R = 20 ÷ 100 = 0.2 R. Thus, it requires 80 percent less effort by the right ventricle than the left to pump the same amount of blood through the pulmonary circulation.

The greatest drop in the peripheral arterial pressure occurs along the arterioles. The pressure along the arterial side of the arterioles is about 90 mm Hg, while at the capillary end it is about 35 mm Hg. Thus, the resistance offered by the arterioles is 90 − 35 ÷ 100 = 0.55, ie, more than half of the resistance of the systemic circulation is at the arteriolar level. The main reason for the high arteriolar resistance is due to the arterioles' narrow caliber and not to their thick muscular walls.

Although the arterioles have a larger diameter than the capillaries, they offer about three times more resistance than the capillaries. The resistance offered by a single capillary is higher than that of a single arteriole, but the total capillary resistance is small because of the huge number of capillaries that lie in a parallel fashion.

Vessel Length

Usually the vessels of the body do not change their length; therefore, this factor contributes very little to the total peripheral resistance.

HYPOTENSION AND SHOCK

It is very difficult to define the difference between hypotension and shock. In the clinical sense, the term "in shock" is used to describe a patient displaying symptoms of acute hypotension accompanied by pallor, weakness, sweating, and a rapid thready pulse,[11] and most of these symptoms are due to sympathetic overactivity. However, from the physiologic standpoint, shock is defined as an abnormal state of the circulation in which the tissue perfusion is inadequate to meet the metabolic needs of the body.

CARDIOVASCULAR REFLEXES DURING HYPOTENSION

If hypotension is induced by a sudden hemorrhage in which 10 to 20 percent of the blood volume is lost within minutes, a set of cardiovascular reflexes occur to compensate for this hypotensive episode. A generalized activation of the sympathetic efferent fibers occurs, leading to tachycardia, contraction of the resistance and capacitance vessels, and to diminution of cardiac vagal efferent activity.[6] These reflex adjustments of the cardiovascular system are principally mediated through the carotid sinus mechanism. The aortic baroreceptors are involved at the higher than normal blood pressures and may play only a secondary role.[12] Also, a small component of these reflexes arise from cardiopulmonary receptors (eg, atrial beta receptors).

The first response is generalized vasoconstriction mediated by the above-cited mechanism. This vasoconstriction is marked in the kidneys, viscera, and skin, giving to the latter a cold pale look. Only the cerebral and coronary vessels are spared from this generalized vasoconstriction because their sympathetic innervation is rather poor. As a matter of fact, the coronary vessels are dilated in response to increased myocardial metabolism caused by the augmented cardiac activity. This widespread vasoconstriction involves the venous system also, thus mobilizing most of the blood present in the veins and helping them maintain the filling pressures of the heart.

In the kidneys, both the afferent and the efferent vessels are constricted, but this constriction is more marked in the efferent vessels. Glomerular filtration and renal plasma flow is diminished. Urine output is diminished, and sodium retention occurs. The resultant effect of all these regionally selective vasoconstrictions is to divert the blood from the kidneys, skin, muscles, and splanchnic beds to areas of the body that cannot tolerate much anoxia, such as the heart and the brain. With advanced hypotension, shunting of blood occurs at the medullary portion of the kidney bypassing the cortical glomeruli. If this hypotension is prolonged, severe renal tubular damage occurs. In man, the renal circulation is far more likely to suffer in shock from stagnation than the other viscera.

Hemorrhage stimulates adrenal medullary secretion. This may lead to stimulation of the reticular system of the brain, making the patient restless and very apprehensive. However, with severe hypotension, patients become apathetic from cerebral ischemia.

Delayed Compensatory Reactions

With arteriolar constriction, the capillary pressure drops. This leads to an increase in the movement of fluid from the interstitial spaces to intravascular space at the venular end of the capillaries. This decrease in the extracellular volume gives one the sensation of thirst.

If the amount of blood lost in the healthy individual is moderate (in the vicinity of 1 liter), the plasma volume is restored in 20 to 40 hours.[13] The initial rate replacement is rather fast, about 2.0 ml per minute, but the rate of this refill is one of constantly decreasing magnitude. Albumin is also mobilized from its extravascular stores at a rapid rate and might reach 4.0 g per hour in the first 4 hours. Subsequently, the ingress of albumin is at a much slower rate, suggesting the synthesis of new albumin in the liver.

Hemorrhage also leads to an increase in aldosterone secretion from increased renin activity and from increased ACTH secretion. Also, vasopressin (antidiuretic hormone) secretion is stimulated because of the decreased discharge from the atrial baroreceptors. The increased aldosterone and vasopressin levels in turn lead to sodium and water retention in the body's effort to maintain interstitial volume (Chap. 27).

Shock

When the flow of blood in the tissues becomes too low to meet the oxygen requirements of the body, the tissues turn to anaerobic glycolosis whereby large amounts of lactic acid are produced. In advanced cases of shock, the blood lactic acid levels may reach a level as high as 10 mmol per liter from a norm of 1 mmol per liter. This metabolic acidosis is also associated with severely hypercapnic mixed venous blood[14] from the sluggish circulation. The acidosis, combined with the hypoxia from diminished blood flow at the carotid and aortic bodies, stimulates the chemoreceptors, leading to hyperventilation.

It appears that if treatment is started prior to a certain point, the patient in shock recovers. If, for any reason treatment is delayed beyond this point, no matter how aggressive it is, the cardiac output remains depressed and the patient enters into a stage of *irreversible shock*[11] in which the peripheral resistance drops, bradycardia occurs, and the patient eventually dies.

The exact cause of this irreversibility is unknown. However, there are several perpetuating causes for it.

1. Myocardial ischemia[15] is one of these. The inadequate perfusion of the myocardium during shock, in spite of the coronary vasodilatation, leads to an irreversible myocardial depression, and the cardiac output cannot be restored to a normal level despite reexpansion of blood volume.
2. Cerebral depression. The decreased cerebral blood flow leads to ischemia of the vasomotor and cardiac centers leading to vasodilatation and bradycardia. This leads to a further drop in the blood pressure and in cerebral blood flow, thus perpetuating the vicious circle. The foregoing are two typical examples of positive feedback mechanisms.

3. Acidosis, combined with the metabolites and hypoxia, relaxes the precapillary more than the postcapillary sphincters. Thus, the direction of the flow of fluids in the interstitial spaces is reversed, and interstitial edema occurs. It has been demonstrated that if the serum lactate level rises above 4 mmol per liter, survival becomes exceedingly rare.[16]

4. Bacterial toxins. Endotoxin released from gram-negative organisms from the bowel have been incriminated in the perpetutation of irreversible shock. It seems that in shock there is a breakdown of the barriers that prevent the entry of bacteria and their toxins into the bloodstream from the intestinal tract and liver.

CIRCULATORY REGULATION AND GENERAL ANESTHESIA

The value of compensatory reactions of the body in response to hemorrhage can be easily demonstrated by denervation of the baroreceptors in dogs. These animals tolerate hemorrhage very poorly. With the same amount of blood loss, the denervated dogs will drop their blood pressure more than three times that of intact conscious dogs. If other intact animals are anesthetized and exposed to the same amount of blood loss, their hypotension will be similar to the denervated, conscious, bleeding dogs. This indicates that the impairment of circulation induced by general anesthesia is equivalent to complete baroreceptor denervation.[17]

It is well known that hemorrhage causes intense peripheral vasoconstriction in which the muscular, mesenteric, and the renal beds actively participate. The severe constriction of the latter might lead to renotubular necrosis. However, this renal vasoconstriction seems to occur in anesthetized dogs only. In contrast, in conscious animals renal vasodilatation does occur despite the intense vasoconstriction in the mesenteric and the peripheral vessels. This latter effect seems to be mediated by prostaglandins.[18]

DELIBERATE HYPOTENSION

This refers to the situations in which the systemic arterial pressure is reduced during anesthesia and surgery with the aim of reducing bleeding and facilitating surgery. It is achieved by decreasing the systemic vascular resistance through a sympathetic blockade either by high subarachnoid block or ganglionic blocking agents. A similar effect can be obtained by the use of agents that act directly on the smooth muscles of blood vessels, such as sodium nitroprusside. The hypotension is often helped by a myocardial depressing agent such as halothane or propranolol.

The main difference between shock and deliberate hypotension is that in shock the peripheral resistance is increased in most of the organs, whereas in deliberate hypotension the peripheral resistance is diminished, and thus the regional blood flow is improved in the majority of the organs. The cardiac output is increased if hypotension is induced in the anesthetized patient by pentolinium[19] or sodium nitroprusside[20] from diminution in peripheral vascular resistance and increased return to the heart. Whereas if hypotension is induced by high spinal or deep halothane, the cardiac output declines mainly from myocardial depression and loss of sympathetic tone of the heart.

Organ Perfusion During Deliberate Hypotension

MYOCARDIUM

The coronary circulation depends on myocardial oxygen demands, and this is determined by the heart rate, the systemic arterial pressure, and the velocity of contraction of the ventricle.[21] By reducing the blood pressure and the cardiac work, ganglionic blockers lead to a decrease in cardiac work and its oxygen consumption. This fall in cardiac work is in parallel with the fall in arterial pressure. Thus, the coronary circulation remains adequate during induced hypotension.

BRAIN

If mild hypotension is deliberately induced, cerebral vasodilatation occurs through autoregulation restoring blood flow to normal. The lowest limit at which it seems that this cerebral blood flow autoregulation becomes ineffective is when the arterial blood pressure has decreased by about one-third. This corresponds to a systolic pressure of about 60 mm Hg[22] measured at the level of the auditory canal. Also, most of the volatile anesthetics used cause cerebral vasodilatation (Chap. 24).

KIDNEY

With a drop in arterial pressure, the renal filtration decreases, and below 70 mm Hg systolic arterial pressure urine output ceases. However, at this level the renal perfusion remains adequate to meet its internal demands (Chap. 29).

LIVER

During any type of hypotension almost complete desaturation of the splanchnic circulation occurs. Thus, blood of the portal vessels reach the liver completely desaturated. Therefore, during hypotension, the liver depends entirely on the hepatic arterial flow for its oxygenation.

LUNGS

Similar to shock patients, dead space values of 60 to 70 percent of the tidal volume have been recorded under induced hypotension.[23]

REFERENCES

1. Hamilton M, Pickering GW Roberts F: The aetiology of essential hypertension. I. The arterial pressure in the general population. Clin Sci 13:11, 1954
2. Ganong WF: Review of Medical Physiology, 7th ed. Los Altos, Calif, Lange, 1975, p 429
3. Ur A, Gordon M: Origin of Korotkoff sounds. Am J Physical 218:524, 1970
4. Kirkendall WM, Burton AC, Epstein F, et al: Recommendations for human blood pressure determinations by sphygmomanometers. Circulation 36:980, 1967
5. Best CH, Taylor NB: In Brobeck JC (ed): Physiological Basis of Medical Practice. Baltimore, Williams & Wilkins, 1973
6. Folkow B, Neil E: Circulation. New York, Oxford, 1971 p. 320
7. Brunner H, Gavras H: Clinical implications of renin in the hypertensive patient. JAMA 233:1091, 1975
8. Roddie IC: Physiology for Practitioners. Edinburgh, Churchill Livingston, 1975, pp 155–164
9. Poiseuille JLM: Recherche expérimentales sur le mouvement des liquides dans les rubes de très-petit diamètres. Mémoires Présentes par divers savants, à l'Acad Sci de l'Institut de France 9:433, 1846
10. Reynolds O: An experimental investigation of the circumstances which determine whether the motion of water shall be direct or sinuous, and of the law of resistance in parallel channels. Philos Trans 174:935, 1883
11. Tyrrell MF: Hypotension. In Scurr C, Feldman S (eds): Scientific Foundations of Anesthesia. Philadelphia, Davis, 1970, p 117
12. Oberg B, White S: Role of vagal cardiac nerves and arterial baroreceptors in the circulatory adjustments to hemorrhage in the cat. Acta Physiol Scand 80:395, 1970
13. Moore FD: The effects of hemorrhage on body composition. N Engl J Med 273:567, 1965
14. Halmagyi DF, Kennedy M, Varga D: Hidden hypercapnia in hemorrhagic hypotension. Anesthesiology 33:594, 1970
15. Crowell JW, Guyton AC: Evidence favouring a cardiac mechanism in irreversible haemorrhagic shock. Am J Physiol 201:893, 1961
16. Broder G, Weil MH: Excess lactate: an index of reversibility of shock in human patients. Science 143:1457, 1964
17. Vatner SF, Braunwald E: Cardiovascular control mechanisms in the conscious state. N Engl J Med 293:970, 1975
18. Vatner SF: Effects of hemorrhage in regional blood flow distribution in dogs and primates. J Clin Invest 54:225, 1974
19. Fahmy NR, Laver MB: Hemodynamic response to ganglionic blockade with pentolinium during N_2O halothane anesthesia in man. Anesthesiology 44:6, 1976

20. Wildsmith JA, Marshall RL, Jenkinson JL: Haemodynamic effects of sodium nitroprusside during nitrous oxide/halothane anaesthesia. Br J Anaesth 45:71, 1973
21. Rowe GD: Responses of the coronary circulation to physiologic change and pharmacologic agents. Anesthesiology 41:182, 1974
22. Strunin L: Organ perfusion during controlled hypotension. Br J Anaesth 47:793, 1975
23. Eckenhoff JE, Hale Enderby GE, Larson A, et al: Pulmonary gas exchange during deliberate hypotension. Br J Anaesth 35:750, 1963

chapter 5

The Peripheral Circulation

The systemic vascular system is made up of the aorta, central arteries, the peripheral arterioles, the capillaries, and the veins.

AORTA AND CENTRAL ARTERIES

With each stroke, the left ventricle ejects about 70 ml of blood during systole. At the protodiastolic phase, the aortic valve closes after a momentary retrograde flow (see Fig. 1-7). During diastole, the flow of blood continues forward to the peripheral arteries because of its initial momentum and also because of the elastic recoil of the arteries releasing their potential energy created by distension during systole. Since the lumen of these arteries is wide, the resistance that they offer to blood flow is minimal. This is proved by the fact that the mean pressure drop from the aorta to the radial artery is less than 5 mm Hg.

ARTERIOLES

Usually, the arterioles are defined as precapillary vessels with a prominent muscular coat and a diameter less than 200 microns. They contribute most of the systemic vascular resistance, the blood flow to the peripheral tissues is altered by varying the number of arterioles open at any one time.

CAPILLARIES

It has been demonstrated that true capillaries do not arise directly from the arterioles, but they are branches of the *metarterioles*. The metarterioles are

65

preferential channels for blood flow. They arise at right angles from arterioles, but they differ from true arterioles by the fact that they have only a partial covering of smooth muscles. A network of capillaries carries blood from one or more metarterioles. A few muscle cells surround the origin of the capillaries and are called precapillary sphincters (Fig. 5-1). Contraction of these muscle cells can stop the blood flow to these capillaries and direct the blood to other preferential channels (vasomotion).

All the controls of the cardiovascular system are geared for ensuring adequate supply to oxygen and nutrients to the capillaries. This is the only place in which the exchange between blood and tissue fluids takes place.

The volume of the capillary system at rest is relatively small (about 300 ml), but the number of open capillaries can increase severalfold. For example, the number of active capillaries in the skeletal muscle can increase 100-fold during exercise. Also, when the number of active capillaries is increased, the distance that oxygen and nutrients have to travel is lessened. In this way the delivery of oxygen to the tissues is accelerated.

Early in 1896, Starling described the exchange of materials between blood and interstitial fluid across the capillary[2] and stated that it depended on three factors: (1) the hydrostatic pressure on each side of the capillary wall; (2) the oncotic pressure of plasma protein; and (3) the properties of the capillary wall. Water and liquid-soluble materials can diffuse freely through the capillary membrane, while they are relatively impermeable to large molecular weight substances such as plasma proteins.

The pressure at the arteriolar end of the capillaries is about 30 mm Hg and is 15 mm Hg at the venous end. The oncotic pressure or the colloid osmotic

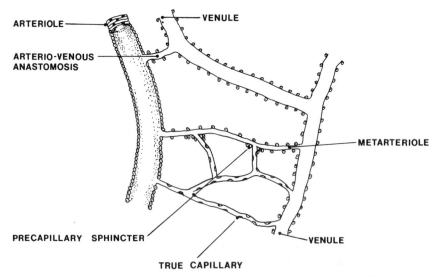

FIG. 5-1: Microcirculatory channels. (Modified after Zweifach.[1])

pressure of plasma is about 26 mm Hg, and this depends exclusively on plasma protein concentration. The plasma protein concentration is 7 g per 100 ml, and most of the colloid osmotic pressure is due to albumin because of its higher molar concentration. The colloid osmotic pressure is very low in the interstitial tissue (about 1 mm Hg). Thus, the effective oncotic pressure is 25 mm Hg.

Another force that opposes the transfer of fluid across the capillaries is the interstitial fluid pressure, which is very difficult to determine and seems to be from 0 to 2 mm Hg.

If we take a hypothetical example (Fig. 5-2) in which the pressure at the **arteriolar end** of the capillary is 35 mm Hg, then the net filtration is:

Hydraulic pressure	35
Colloid oncotic pressure	−25
Interstitial fluid pressure	−2
Net filtration pressure =	8 mm Hg

Therefore, fluid moves from inside the capillary to the interstitial fluid spaces.

At the **venular end** of the capillary the net pressure filtration is:

Hydraulic pressure	15
Colloid pressure	−25
Interstitial pressure	−2
Net filtration pressure =	−12 mm Hg

Now the pressure is from the opposite direction, so fluid will move to the inside of the capillary.

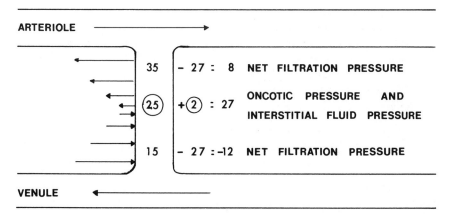

FIG. 5-2: Starling's hypothesis on fluid exchanges across the capillaries. The numbers represent pressures in mm Hg. Note the diffusion toward the interstitium at the arteriolar end of the capillary and the opposite direction in the venular end.

The amount of fluid exchanged through this system is 45 times the blood volume each minute. However, transport within the tissue spaces is more complex than this simple system because the interstitial space is not a homogeneous fluid compartment but an organized material resembling a gel in which molecules of medium or large size do not diffuse freely.

VEINS

The return of blood from the capillaries to the heart is a passive process in a supine subject and depends mainly on the difference between capillary pressure and right atrial pressure (0 mm Hg during diastole). However, when standing, blood has to flow against gravity, and other factors come into play, such as (1) the pumping effect of the muscles as they compress the veins; (2) the valves inside the veins preventing retrograde flow of blood; and (3) the increased sympathetic tone, which increases the venous pressure. Occasionally the large veins are termed capacitance vessels because of the large amount of blood they contain, which consists of 60 to 70 percent of the total blood volume.

LYMPHATIC SYSTEM

The lymphatic system starts by closed "blind" capillaries in between the interstitial tissue space. They are lined by a single layer of endothelial cells. These capillaries join together to form lymph trunks that connect to the lymph glands. Through a system of complex plexus, these join to form collecting ducts, which eventually combine to form the thoracic ducts that empty into the venous system. The main function of the lymphatic system is to clear the interstitial spaces of protein, lipids, and foreign materials.

Pressure is low in the lymphatic system (1 to 3 mm Hg). It moves mainly by external compression, and the valves present therein prevent retrograde flow. The amount of lymph flow is 2 to 4 liters per day. During capillary exchange, a small amount of plasma protein diffuses into the interstitial spaces (leakage), and virtually all of it is returned to the venous system through the lymphatic channels.

THE SEQUELAE OF CHANGES IN VASCULAR TONE

Changes in vascular tone can affect peripheral perfusion and cardiac function in different ways depending on the sites of vasoconstriction[3] or vasodilatation, eg:

1. Generalized arteriolar constriction will raise the systemic vascular

resistance, leading to a rise in arterial blood pressure and a reflex diminution in cardiac output.

2. Constriction of the precapillary vessels will diminish capillary hydrostatic pressure, and therefore fluid will shift from tissues to capillaries with an eventual increase in cardiac output.

3. Constriction of the postcapillary vessels will raise the capillary hydrostatic pressure, and fluid will be shifted from capillaries to tissues with an eventual decline in blood volume and cardiac output.

4. Acute venoconstriction will shift a few hundred milliliters of blood from the peripheral veins to the central veins, resulting in an increased venous return (preload) to the heart, which in turn will raise the cardiac output.

Also the ratio between the pre- and postcapillary resistance changes with time and by several other factors. For example, in acidosis the arteriolar sphincters lose their tone before their venular counterparts. The venoconstriction continues apparently due to lower pH at which the venous system normally functions; therefore, blood pools in the peripheral circulation[4] and the decreased return to the heart will further diminish the cardiac output.

CONTROL OF THE PERIPHERAL CIRCULATORY SYSTEM

The circulatory system has a complex and intricate system of regulatory mechanisms. The main purpose of these regulatory mechanisms is to provide an adequate blood supply to the effector organ without jeopardizing the vital organs, such as the brain and the heart. These intricate mechanisms start at the tissue level from the simple direct effect of the metabolites on tissue perfusion to a complicated autonomic response involving all parts of the circulatory system mediated through the central nervous system.

Local Control Mechanisms

The arteriolar blood vessels have an intrinsic myogenic activity. This inherent myogenic activity is more pronounced at the precapillary resistance level and is responsible for the basal vascular tone. The cells of these smooth muscles can act as pacemakers and generate a response that spreads from cell to cell.[5] This myogenic activity is increased by stimulation of the local vasomotor nerves and by catecholamines.

However, a more important factor for regulating local blood flow is vasodilatation from a relative lack of oxygen in the tissues. It is possible that the high oxygen consumption of the muscle fibers will produce a relative anoxia of the smooth muscles, leading to their relaxation, hence vasodilatation. Also, there is the possibility that the tissue metabolites, such as adenosine triphosphate, acetylcholine, or hydrogen ion, produce vasodilatation by reducing myogenic activity.

A rise in the arterial blood pressure will have a tendency to dilate the arterioles. This stretching of the cell membranes augments the tone of the vascular smooth muscles. This vasoconstriction provides a positive feedback mechanism with a further rise of the blood pressure. However, in the actual situation the active tissue metabolite will overcome this vasoconstriction and the perfusion of the active tissue will increase. Thus, the net result will be shifting of blood from nonactive tissues to the more active areas.

Autonomic Controls

Under normal conditions, the sympathetic discharge to the vascular smooth muscle is very slow, on the order of 1 to 3 impulses per second and provides only 15 to 20 percent of the total vascular resistance at rest.[5] This sympathetic vasoconstrictor tone is directly correlated with the frequency of efferent stimuli.

The number of sympathetic vasoconstrictor fibers varies according to the regions of the body, eg, cerebral vessels have a very sparse innervation, while the skin, skeletal muscle, and the mesenteric vessels have a very rich supply. As a general rule, arteries and arterioles are provided with more sympathetic fiber terminals than the veins and venules. If the sympathetic supply to a limb is interrupted by denervation, vascular tone starts to reestablish within a few minutes and blood flow is back to normal in a few weeks. This is due to the fact that the smooth muscles establish the tone by themselves through a spontaneous activity of their fibers, and also these vessels become very sensitive to circulating catecholamines after denervation.

In addition to the sympathetic vasoconstrictor fibers, there are sympathetic vasodilator fibers, which are cholinergic in nature and are mostly present in skeletal muscles where they supply the arterioles only. They are involved in vasodilatation during muscular activity. This vasodilatation can even be seen with the anticipation of exercise. However, direct local action of metabolic products is a much more potent stimulus than the sympathetic vasodilatation.

Also there are few parasympathetic vasodilator fibers that supply mainly the external genitalia and are involved in erection.

Humoral Control

Epinephrine and norepinephrine are the principal catecholamines involved in vascular responses. Epinephrine is the principal secretion of the adrenal medulla, while norepinephrine is the transmitter of sympathetic vasoconstricting fibers. Adrenergic effects are usually classified into two main types: alpha (α) and beta (β). Alpha receptors, which lead to vasoconstriction, are stimulated by norepinephrine and are blocked by phentolamine and phenoxybenzamine. Beta responses are further subdivided to β_1 effects, which lead to cardiac inotropy and β_2 responses that produce bronchodilatation and vasodilatation.[6] The number of each type of receptor differs from one vascular bed to another, and the result will depend on which type of receptor is more prevalent in that area. For example, epinephrine, which stimulates the alpha and beta receptors, causes vasoconstriction in the spleen, kidney, and mesentery but will dilate the myocardial, hepatic, and skeletal vessels as well. This is attributed to the higher number of alpha receptors in the first group and the predominance of beta receptors in the second group. In man, the net effect of epinephrine is a decrease in total peripheral resistance, vasodilatation of the heart and skeletal muscle with an increased myocardial autorhythmicity, and contractility and conductivity (beta effect), whereas norepinephrine, which has strong alpha effect, will produce hypertension by increasing the peripheral resistance through vasoconstriction. In the normal human being, the effect of the circulating catecholamines on the vascular smooth muscles seems to be minimal compared to neurogenic influences.

Other vasoactive agents like bradykinin, angiotensin II, vasopressins, and prostaglandins are present in the blood. However, their value in the control of normal circulation has never been clearly defined.

Reflex Control

Several reflexes arising from different areas of a cardiovascular system are involved in maintaining the adequacy of circulation. The most important afferent components of these reflexes include baroreceptors, pulmonary arterial receptors, cardiac receptors, and chemoreceptors.

BARORECEPTORS

The arterial stretch receptors are present in the two carotid sinuses as well as the arch of the aorta. The carotid sinus is a dilatation of the internal carotid at its origin. At the sinus, the arterial wall is modified so that most of the muscular layer is replaced by elastic tissue. It is supplied by the corresponding sinus nerve, which is a branch of the glossopharyngeal nerve. Aortic baroreceptors are supplied by the left aortic nerve. A rise of intraarterial pressure stretches the relatively thin walls of the sinus and stimulates the afferent endings.

The number of afferent impulses from the baroreceptors is proportional to the distending pressure. Within limits, the higher the pressure is, the higher the number of firing impulses will be. In the normal situation, in which the flow is pulsatile, the firing rate is higher during the rising and peak phases of the pulse pressure (Fig. 5-3). Baroreceptors respond to absolute changes in pressure and also to the rate of change in pressure. In clinical hypertension, the sensitivity of the carotid sinus receptor is reduced, ie, it is reset to function at a higher level.

Thus, elevation of the blood pressure will increase the rate of discharge in the carotid and aortic nerves, which will relay the information to the cardioinhibitory and vasomotor centers. The efferent pathway to the arterioles is through the sympathetic system, leading to a decrease in arteriolar and venous tone by a reduction in the frequency of efferent sympathetic constrictor impulses. The cardiac component of the reflex seems to be mediated through the parasympathetic system[7] (not the sympathetic), leading to a slower heart rate and decreased myocardial activity. Thus, the net effect is a drop of the arterial blood pressure and a concomitant diminution in heart rate.

PULMONARY ARTERIAL RECEPTORS

These are present at the bifurcation of the pulmonary artery, and they have a function similar to arterial baroreceptors in sensing the pulmonary artery pressure.[8] Besides raising the arterial pressure, a fall in pulmonary artery pressure will also lead to an increase in the rate and depth of respiration.

CARDIAC RECEPTORS

They are present in the right and left atria and their afferent nerve is the vagus.[9] There seem to be two types of receptors: one stimulating the sympathetic system, the other inhibiting it. The Bainbridge reflex, which can be elicited in anesthetized dogs, is an increase in the heart rate after large doses of intravenous saline solution and seems to be due to activation of these receptors.

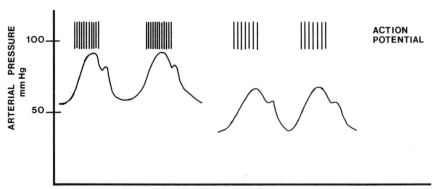

FIG. 5-3: Action potential in carotid sinus nerve at various levels of blood pressure (diagrammatic).

The atrial receptors are located in the atria near the opening of the veins. They can sense changes in central venous pressure, and their afferent signals reach the hypothalamic center that controls antidiuretic hormone secretion with its consequent effect on blood volume.[10]

There are also ventricular stretch receptors, but their function under normal conditions is undetermined.

CHEMORECEPTORS

Chemoreceptors are highly vascular bodies present at the bifurcation of common carotid arteries and at the aortic area. They have epitheloid cells and nerve endings that are sensitive to the chemical composition of the arterial blood. The afferent fibers of the carotid bodies are branches of glossopharyngeal nerves, whereas the afferent fibers of the aortic bodies are branches of the vagus.

Chemoreceptors are stimulated by changes in the tension of blood gases. Their respiratory response is much more marked than their cardiovascular response. Chemoreceptors are sensitive to a fall in arterial oxygen tension or to a rise in arterial carbon dioxide tension (probably a pH effect). They also respond to hypotension. The cardiovascular effects of the stimulation of chemoreceptors are peripheral arterial vasoconstriction, bradycardia, and catecholamine secretion from the adrenals. However, their primary effect is respiratory, leading to a marked increase in rate and depth of breathing.

Central Nervous System Control

SPINAL CORD

In man or animals with transected spinal cord, increased sympathetic responses are seen arising from the hollow viscera. Thus, distension of bladder will cause an intense vasoconstriction mediated by the spinal cord and sympathetic outflow leading to severe hypertension. These reflexes can be blocked by spinal anesthesia.

MEDULLA

The medullary vasomotor centers are present in the floor of the fourth ventricle. There is a lateral pressor area that produces vasoconstriction, cardioacceleration, and myocardial stimulation, and a medial depressor area that transmits inhibitory impulses to the lateral portion. The medullary centers are responsible for the continuous vasoconstrictor tone. Thus, transection of the cord at a lower cervical region causes a fall of blood pressure from vasodilatation. After a time, the spinal reflexes take over and the blood pressure returns to its original level.

HYPOTHALAMUS

This is the center of coordination and integration for all the complex responses that occur in thermoregulation, defense reactions, and exercise. Localized hypothalamic stimulation (fields of Forel) produces changes in the cardiovascular system similar to those seen during exercise.[11] Also, generalized sympathetic adrenergic stimulation, accompanied by skeletal vasodilatation (cholinergic sympathetic), can be elicited from localized stimulation of the hypothalamus. These responses are rather similar to those seen in defense reactions.[12]

The hypothalamus is also the center for the coordination of chemoreceptor responses. The bradycardia and the vasoconstriction seen from the stimulation of chemoreceptors is absent if the hypothalamus is ablated. For the baroreceptor reflexes, the presence of hypothalamus is not essential.

CEREBRAL CORTEX

There is no doubt that the cerebral cortex has an integral influence on almost all of the autonomic responses. Typical examples are the sympathetic effects of emotional stress, blushing, or the cardiovascular response of the athlete before the start of a race. This has been typically demonstrated by Rushmer et al,[11] the startled cardiovascular response to exercise begins when the animal hears the loud noise of the switch of the treadmill.

The cortical centers that can affect the autonomic functions seem to be mostly localized in the sensory-motor cortex, the ungulate-gyrus. The ways by which the cerebral cortex controls the response of the hypothalamic and medullary centers are rather obscure, but there is no doubt that they interact continually and in conjunction through mutually interdependent loop circuits that stitch together the various parts of the brain into a functional whole.[13]

Axon Reflex

A typical example of an axon reflex is the triple response of the skin (Fig. 5-4). If the skin is stroked by a blunt point, a response with three components is seen:

1. Red line of vasodilation along the line of stroke. This vasodilation results from injury to the capillaries.
2. Flare response extending for a few centimeters around the first. This is due to an axon reflex. The impulse travels in the normal direction in a pain nerve fiber toward the spinal cord. However, some of the impulses, change

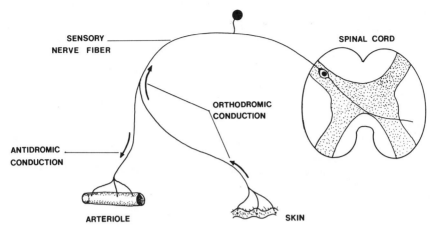

FIG. 5-4: The pathways involved in the axon reflex.

their direction when they reach the axon and travel peripherally ("antidromic") to the cutaneous blood vessels, leading to their dilatation. The flare response can be seen if the spinal connection of the pain fiber is severed. However, it is absent if sufficient time is given for the nerve to degenerate.

3. The last component of the triple response is a wheal along the initial line resulting from the accumulation of fluid in the tissues. Histamine injected intradermally does cause a similar type of response.

REFERENCES

1. Zweifach BW: Functional Behavior of the Microcirculation. Springfield, Ill, Thomas, 1961
2. Starling EH: The Fluids of the Body. Chicago, Ill, Keener, 1909
3. Smith NT, Corbascio AN: The use and misuse of pressor agents. Anesthesiology 33:58, 1970
4. Lillehei RC, Dietzman RH, Mosas S, et al: Treatment of septic shock. Mod Treatment 4:321, 1967
5. Braunwald E: Regulation of the circulation. N Engl J Med 290:1420, 1974
6. Lefkowitz RJ: B-adrenergic receptors: recognition and regulation. N Engl J Med 295:323, 1976
7. Heymans C, Neil E: Reflexogenic Areas of the Cardiovascular System. Boston, Little, Brown, 1958
8. Eckberg DL, Fletcher GF, Braunwald E: Mechanisms of prolongation of the R-R interval with electrical stimulation of the carotid sinus nerve in man. Circ Res 30:131, 1972
9. Milnor WR: The cardiovascular control system. In Mountcastle VB (ed): Medical Physiology. St. Louis, Mosby, 1974

10. Hays RM: Antidiuretic hormone. N Engl J Med 295:659, 1976
11. Rushmer RF, Smith OA, Lasher EP: Neural mechanisms of cardiac control during exertion. Physiol Rev 40:27, 1960
12. Folkow B, Lisander B, Tuttle RS, Wang SC: Changes in cardiac output upon stimulation of the hypothalamic defense area and the medullary depressor area in the cat. Acta Physiol Scand 72:220, 1968
13. Peiss CN: Concepts of cardiovascular regulation past, present and future. In Randall WC (ed): Nervous Control of the Heart. Baltimore, Williams & Wilkins, 1965

chapter 6

The Coronary Circulation

When we compare the coronary circulation to other regional circulations of the body, we find that the myocardium is at a severe disadvantage[1] for the following reasons. First, there is an absence of functional anastomoses between the two major coronary arteries. Second, the oxygen extraction from the coronary circulation is very high, and the coronary venous blood is less than 25 percent saturated with oxygen. Thus, the only way to increase oxygen delivery to the myocardium is by coronary vasodilatation. Third, the blood supply to the myocardium is interrupted during systole from the mechanical compression of the coronary vessels in contrast to other organs having a continuous blood perfusion. Finally, the coronary arteries are extremely vulnerable to degenerative atherosclerotic changes and these changes are usually widespread;[2] and the coronary arteries are among the worst affected.

ANATOMY OF CORONARY VESSELS (FIG. 6-1)

The two coronary arteries arise from the sinuses behind the cusps of the aortic valve at the root of the aorta. The right coronary artery runs downward into the right portion of the AV groove and supplies branches to the posterior surface of both ventricles. The left coronary artery, which is larger than the right at 2 mm from the atrium, gives off a large interventricular branch that decends into the anterior interventricular groove. This artery supplies both ventricles. The left coronary artery runs into the left AV groove accompanying the coronary sinus and supplies branches to the left atrium and to the base of the left ventricle. The main coronary arteries are distributed along the surface of the heart, whereas the small branches penetrate the muscle. These deeper vessels are the ones that are compressed during cardiac contraction. The right coronary artery usually supplies the right ventricle and the posterior part of the interventricular septum, while the left coronary artery supplies the left ventricle and the anterior portion of the interventricular septum.

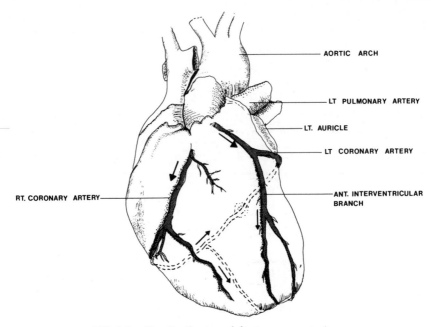

FIG. 6-1:   The distribution of the coronary arteries.

Despite the presence of small anastomoses between the coronary arteries, functionally they are end arteries. Therefore, obstruction of the flow in one of the large coronaries leads to the death of the tissues supplied by that artery.

Similar to skeletal muscles, the ratio of capillaries to myocardial fibers is 1:1. Even in the presence of cardiac hypertrophy, this ratio remains constant. In cardiac hypertrophy, the number of individual cardiac fibers remains the same while their diameters increase. Thus, each capillary must supply a greater bulk of muscles, and the distance that the nutrients have to travel to reach the center of the muscle is increased. These two factors limit the amount of cardiac hypertrophy that can occur without developing any ischemia.

The **venous drainage** of the heart is through superficial and deep systems. The larger part of the superficial system joins to form the coronary sinus; a smaller part of the superficial system drains into the right auricle of the heart through the anterior cardiac veins. The deep venous drainage is largely made up of the sinusoidal vessels that empty directly into the heart chambers. Also, there are the thebesian veins, which are small communicating channels between the coronary vessels and the cardiac cavities. The greater part of the venous drainage of the heart (70 percent) is through the coronary sinus. The little amount of blood that is drained by the deep system that empties into the left side of the heart constitutes a small part of the anatomic arteriovenous shunt.

CORONARY FLOW

The coronary flow is measured in the human being by a modification of Fick's principle developed by Kety and Schmidt:[3]

$$\text{Coronary blood flow} = \frac{\text{Nitrous oxide uptake of myocardium}}{\text{Arteriovenous coronary nitrous oxide difference}}$$

While the individual is breathing a mixture of nitrous oxide and oxygen, blood samples are continually taken from a peripheral artery and from the coronary sinus by a cannula inserted through a peripheral vein. The quantity of nitrous oxide taken up by the myocardium is calculated from its tension in the coronary venous blood and from its solubility coefficient in the heart muscle.

By this technique it has been found that the resting left coronary flow in man is approximately 80 ml per 100 g of left ventricle per minute with total flow of about 250 ml per minute, which represents about 5 percent of the total cardiac output. In strenuous exercise, the coronary flow can increase up to 500 percent.[4] The resting oxygen consumption of the heart is about 40 ml per minute or 15 percent of the total body oxygen consumption. Normally, about two-thirds of the oxygen content of the coronary arterial blood is extracted through its passage to the myocardium. Thus, normal oxygen content in coronary sinus blood is 4 to 5 ml per 100 ml, and this value remains constant with increased myocardial work.

The coronary artery flow can also be measured by electromagnetic flowmeters and radioisotope techniques.

Phasic Variations in Coronary Flow

During systole, the myocardial tissue pressure rises, leading to compression and the shutting off of the arteries penetrating the muscle. Thus, the flow in the left coronary is sharply reduced and even flows backward for a very short interval (Fig. 6-2). At the end of systole with the closure of aortic valve, the coronary flow rises to a maximum to decline slowly during diastole. About 75 percent of the total coronary flow occurs during diastole.[5] As the branches of the coronary vessels traverse the heart from the epicardium to the endocardium, the vessels supplying the subendocardial portion of the left ventricle are the ones most likely to be compressed by the myocardium during systole. Consequently, the subendocardial region of the left ventricle is more prone to ischemic damage and is the most common site for myocardial infarction. Tachycardia with the associated decrease in diastolic interval might aggravate further this endocardial ischemic pattern, especially if the coronary arteries are already narrowed from arteriosclerosis and are unable to dilate during diastole.

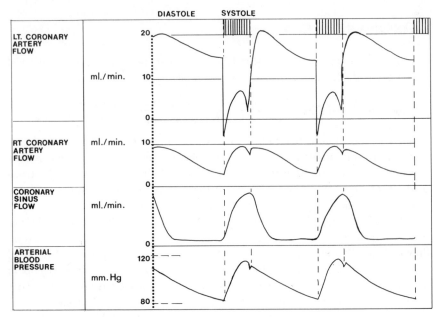

FIG. 6-2: The phasic changes in the flow of both the coronary arteries and coronary sinus during the cardiac cycle. Note the marked diminution in left coronary artery flow during systole.

In contrast to the left ventricle, the flow in the right coronary artery is not disturbed during systole. The main cause is that pressure in the aorta and the coronary vessels is higher than the pressure developed in the right ventricle.

Regulation of Coronary Circulation

Similar to other areas of the body, the major resistance to coronary flow is at the level of small arterioles,[6] not in the superficial large arteries.[7] These arterioles are the ones that respond to the metabolic needs of the myocardium, which is the most important factor that influences coronary flow.

The metabolism of the myocardium is predominantly aerobic.[8] Thus, the coronary flow is directly proportional to the amount of work that the myocardium is performing. Inasmuch as the heart extracts a large amount of oxygen from the blood at rest (10 to 12 ml per 100 ml), oxygen consumption can be increased only by raising its flow by vasodilatation. The mechanism by which this coronary flow is adjusted to the metabolic requirements of the myocardium is unknown. It is probably through the local action of a metabolic product, possibly adenosine,[9] which is a very active coronary vasodilator, is locally available, and is destroyed rapidly in the blood and lungs.

The prime determinants of myocardial blood flow are heart rate and blood pressure.[10] There is a very close and direct relationship between heart rate and coronary blood flow.

The arterial blood pressure is the driving force that influences the coronary circulation. In the normal blood pressure range, an increase in blood pressure will increase the coronary flow. However, this lasts for a short time and the coronary flow returns to its basal value because of the increased tone of the coronary vessels (autoregulation). Also, a fall in arterial pressure leads to a decrease in oxygen tension in the myocardium, and the ensuing accumulation of metabolites will produce coronary vasodilatation. However, with severe hypotension this vasodilatation will be insufficient to restore coronary flow. Thus, myocardial contraction will be impaired, leading to a vicious circle, which, if not treated adequately, can end in death.

The effect of the autonomic nervous system on the coronary vessels seems to be weak and insignificant under normal circumstances. Stimulation of the sympathetic nerves of the heart leads to an increase in coronary blood flow with an associated increase in heart rate and in the contractile force of the heart. However, this coronary vasodilatation is due to an increase in the metabolic requirement of the heart. If ventricular fibrillation is induced, thus diminishing the external work of the heart to a minimum, then the stimulation of the sympathetic nerve fibers leads to a mild vasoconstriction. Alpha and beta receptors have been demonstrated, with alpha receptors mediating vasoconstriction and beta receptors mediating vasodilatation. In contrast to anesthetized preparations and earlier beliefs, a substantial coronary vasoconstrictor tone has been demonstrated in conscious dogs. This vasoconstrictor tone is mediated through the alpha-adrenergic system and can be abolished by activation of the arterial baroreceptor or chemoreceptor reflexes.[11]

In contrast to epinephrine, acetylcholine causes coronary vasodilatation in the fibrillating heart, whereas it decreases coronary flow in the functioning myocardium by causing bradycardia.

The coronary blood flow is also raised in anemia and hypoxemia. The coronary blood flow seems to correlate better with coronary venous than with arterial oxygen content; at a critical level of coronary venous oxygen content 5 to 6 ml per 100 ml of blood coronary vasodilatation can be seen.

MYOCARDIAL METABOLISM

The metabolism of the normal heart is predominantly aerobic. However, it is also capable of anaerobic metabolism and can consume carbohydrates, proteins, and fats.[6]

The oxygen consumption of the arrested heart is minimal. With fibrillation, the oxygen consumption increases but still is much lower than that of the contracting myocardium. Increasing either the heart rate or the blood pressure leads to further increases in myocardial metabolism. As a matter of fact, the products of heart rate and systolic blood pressure or the "time–tension index" is commonly used as an index of myocardial work, since it is very closely related to myocardial oxygen consumption. It has been established that the heart expends more energy in overcoming "pressure work" than it does "volume work."[10]

The myocardium consumes oxygen to perform several types of work. Some of these are obvious; others are less apparent. The following are the principal determinants of myocardial oxygen consumption.[12]

1. Intrinsic work. This is the work performed during the isometric contraction phase and is mostly dependent on intraventricular volume and pressure.
2. Rate of myocardial shortening (contractility). The rate of the contraction of myocardium (dl/dt) or the rate of the rise of intraventricular pressure (dp/dt) parallels the oxygen consumption of the myocardium.

    The previous two factors are the main determinants for the "pressure work" of the heart.
3. Heart rate. An increase in the heart rate will raise the myocardial oxygen consumption by either direct effect, in which an increase in the frequency of contraction also means an increase in the number of times that tension is executed, thus increasing oxygen consumption; or by indirect effect, in which an increase in the heart rate per se will augment the myocardial contractility, which in turn increases oxygen requirements.
4. External work. This is basically the "volume work" of the ventricle. It consumes far less energy than any of the first three factors.
5. Activation energy. This represents less than 1 percent of the total oxygen utilization. It is the energy used for initiating the electrical events of the heart and the active diffusion of ions.
6. Basal myocardial metabolism. This is the energy utilized by the arrested heart that is necessary for its viability as well as for maintaining the ionic environment of the cell. This resting energy requirement is in direct relation to the circulating levels of the thyroid hormones.

LIGATION OF A CORONARY ARTERY

If the flow in a large coronary artery of an animal is interrupted by ligation, the pressure drops to about 20 mm Hg distal to ligation, indicating the inefficient anastomoses between the coronary arteries. If the animal survives the acute episode, the pressure distal to the occlusion starts rising by the 12th hour. After a day, it reaches about 40 mm Hg and in 3 weeks returns to the preligation level, thus indicating the presence of anastomoses that are very late in responding to an acute occlusion. This is in contrast to other vascular beds in which after a sudden occlusion the anastomotic channels open up within minutes. This difference between the response of the anastomotic channels of peripheral vessels and the coronary vessels to sudden occlusion is not understood except that it is a design feature.[1]

CORONARY ARTERY DISEASE

The basic problem with patients who have coronary artery disease is that, when the demand on circulation is increased, they are unable to increase their coronary flow as normal subjects can do. Also, people with angina have an unequal flow of blood in different regions of the heart, and, if blood flow is inadequate for normal resting metabolism, myocardial ischemia will occur. This ischemic episode may be associated with elevated end-ventricular diastolic pressure, which is reflected as a rise in pulmonary wedge pressure.

Nitrites usually produce relief in anginal attack. This relief of anginal attack is probably due to a decrease in the cardiac work from a drop in arterial blood pressure and a decreased venous tone with a consequent diminution of venous return. Although intracoronary artery injection of nitrites during coronary arteriography has been shown to relieve catheter-induced large coronary artery spasm, systemic nitrite administration is not associated with increased coronary flow but rather produces a slight decrease.[13]

ANESTHESIA AND CORONARY ARTERY FLOW

Animal studies and a few human studies have demonstrated that coronary blood flow and oxygen consumption parallel changes in cardiovascular function.[14] Halothane, by depressing myocardial contractility, decreases cardiac work and myocardial oxygen consumption, leading to coronary vasoconstriction. This vasoconstriction does not produce myocardial hypoxia. This is probably an autoregulatory mechanism preventing "unnecessary" hyperperfusion.[15] Similar effects are observed with other anesthetic agents that depress cardiac function (eg, methoxyflurane and fluroxene). With anesthetic agents that increase cardiac performance (ether, cyclopropane), there is a pari passu increase in oxygen consumption.

With all anesthetic agents, the normal lactate concentration and oxygen extraction of the coronary venous blood suggest adequate myocardial oxygenation. Therefore, this coronary vasoconstriction secondary to myocardial depression without any evidence of lactate accumulation indicates that this vasoconstriction is not harmful but rather beneficial to the heart with ischemic coronary artery disease, similar to the effect of propranolol. However, myocardial depression might adversely affect these patients. The associated diminution of arterial pressure might decrease the perfusion pressure in the coronary arteries, further diminishing the flow in these narrowed arteries, especially during diastole.

REFERENCES

1. Roddie IC: Physiology for Practitioners. Edinburgh, Churchill, Livingstone, 1975
2. Enos WF, Holmes RH, Beyer JI: Coronary disease among United States soldiers killed in action in Korea. JAMA 152:1090, 1953
3. Kety SS, Schmidt CF: The nitrous oxide method for the quantitative determination of cerebral blood flow in man; theory, procedure and normal values. J Clin Invest 27:476, 1948
4. Khouri EM, Gregg DE, Rayford CR: Effect of exercise on cardiac output, left coronary flow and myocardial metabolism in the unanesthetized dog. Circ Res 17:427, 1965
5. Gregg DE, Khouri EM, Rayford CR: Systemic and coronary energetics in the resting unanesthetized dog. Circ Res 16:102, 1965
6. McGregor M, Fam WM: Regulation of coronary blood flow. Bull NY Acad Med 42:940, 1966
7. Wynands JE, Sheridan CA, Batra MS, et al: Coronary artery disease. Anesthesiology 33:260, 1970
8. Bing RJ: Cardiac metabolism. Physiol Rev 45:171, 1965
9. Rowe GG, Afonso S, Gurtner HP, et al: The systemic and coronary hemodynamic effects of adenosine triphosphate and adenosine. Am Heart J 64:228, 1962
10. Rowe GG: Responses of the coronary circulation to physiologic changes and pharmacologic agents. Anesthesiology 41:182, 1974
11. Vatner SF, Braunwald E: Cardiovascular control mechanisms in the conscious state. N Engl J Med 293:970, 1975
12. Sonnenblick EH, Lynn S, Kelton C: Myocardial energetics: basic principles and clinical applications. N Engl J Med 285–668, 1972
13. Rowe GG: The nitrates as an antianginal drug. In Gensini GG (ed): The Study of the Systemic Coronary and Myocardial Effects of Nitrates. Springfield, Ill, Thomas, 1972
14. Merin RG: Effect of anesthetics on the heart. Surg Clin North Am 55:759, 1975
15. Wolff G, Claudi B, Rist M, et al: Regulation of coronary blood flow during ether and halothane anaesthesia. Br J Anaesth 44:1139, 1972

chapter 7

Cutaneous and Splanchnic Circulation

CUTANEOUS CIRCULATION

Besides covering the body, the skin, has a very important function in thermoregulation. Through the skin, most of the heat generated by the body is dissipated. The blood flow to the skin predominantly reflects the requirements of thermoregulation and is seldom influenced by local metabolic events, eg, changing from a cold environment to a warm environment, and the amount of skin flow can increase from 1 ml to 120 ml per 100 ml of skin per minute. Also, the blood flow of the skin is variable from one area to another, eg, the blood flow to the fingers and ear lobes is the highest in the body, the palm and face have less blood flow, and the least is in the forearm and the legs.[1] The areas of the highest blood flow are more responsive to thermoregulatory responses than the ones with less blood supply.

The blood reaching the skin may have a different temperature than that of core temperature. This is due to two peculiar anatomic arrangements of cutaneous arteries. First, these arteries pierce the underlying muscles before reaching the skin. Thus, they transmit directly the excess heat produced in the muscles to the skin. Second, these cutaneous vessels are the same branches of the arteries that run next to the venae comitantes from the skin and the muscles. Therefore, the blood reaching the skin is warmed or cooled according to the temperature of the drained tissues.[2]

In exposed areas of the body, such as the fingers, toes, palms, and ear lobes there are a great number of arteriovenous anastomotic connections. They are very well innervated, and they have similar nervous connections as the arterioles. They open at very hot environmental temperatures, increasing the blood flow to the skin. Also, they open on exposure to extreme cold. Thus, the excess flow warms the skin at the expense of the rest of the body, protecting the limb from frostbite.

The cutaneous blood vessels constrict in response to adrenergic nerve stimulation or to circulatory epinephrine and norepinephrine. The only type of nerve supply to the skin is through the sympathetic nervous system. This includes also the innervation to the sweat glands, which is also sympathetic in origin, but is cholinergic in nature. The vessels of the distal parts of the limbs are innervated by sympathetic vasoconstrictor fibers, whereas the proximal areas of the skin are innervated through the sympathetic fibers to the sweat glands. No vasodilator fibers have been identified in the cutaneous blood vessels. Vasodilatation is achieved either by decreasing the vasoconstrictor tone or by activating the cholinergic pathways to sweat glands, which apparently release bradykinin formed by the enzymes of the sweat glands.[3] Skin color reflects the amount of blood present in the capillary loops of the skin papillae and in the subpapillary venous plexus. When the blood supply of the superficial skin vessels is diminished, the skin takes on a pale and transparent look, while the deeper venous plexus gives it a leaden tint. Conversely, with rapid cutaneous blood flow the red oxyhemoglobin will give a reddish hue or the characteristic blush to the skin.

Pain leads to diffuse cutaneous vasoconstriction from generalized adrenergic discharge. However, the most effective vasoconstrictor stimulus to the skin is exposure to cold. Local or central cooling initiates profound vasoconstriction, which is mediated through the hypothalamus.[4] Conversely, heating leads to reflex vasodilatation, which is also mediated through the hypothalamus, and is effected by withdrawal of sympathetic constrictor tone to arterioles and arteriovenous anastomoses and possibly by the release of bradykinin.[5]

All of the known general anesthetic agents increase the blood flow to the skin at light levels of anesthesia[3] presumably from inhibition of the temperature-regulating center. At deeper levels of anesthesia, the cutaneous blood flow returns to control levels with fluroxene and halothane but remains increased with ether and cyclopropane.[6]

SPLANCHNIC CIRCULATION

The splanchnic circulation is divided into three main components: hepatic, mesenteric, and splenic. The special feature of the circulation in this region is that the combined venous outflow of the latter two (mesenteric and splenic) forms the major inflow of the first (hepatic) through the portal vein.

Hepatic Circulation

The liver has a double source of blood supply: (1) the portal vein, which is formed by the junction of superior mesenteric and splenic veins and drains most of the viscera; and (2) the hepatic artery, which is a branch of the celiac axis. The portal vein contributes about 70 percent of the total hepatic flow, while the remainder of the blood supply is derived from the hepatic artery.[7] This highly saturated arterial blood supplies about two-thirds of the oxygen uptake of the liver, while the remainder is provided by the portal veins.

In man the hepatic blood flow is measured by a method based on the Fick principle. Bromosulphalein or indocyanine green are taken up from the blood as they pass through the liver. The extrahepatic removal of these dyes is minimal. The dyes are infused continuously to maintain a constant peripheral concentration. The arteriovenous difference is measured by obtaining a sample from the arterial blood and, simultaneously, another sample is withdrawn from the hepatic vein through a transvenous catheter. With these techniques, the estimated total hepatic flow is about 100 ml per minute per 100 g liver,[7] and the total flow through the liver 1.5 liters per minute, which is equivalent to one-fourth of the total cardiac output. The sinusoids of the liver are its exchange vessels.

The hepatic arterioles and the portal venules enter the peripheral part of the sinusoids while the blood is drained through the central lobular vein (Fig. 7-1). These join to form sublobular veins, which join to form the hepatic veins proper, which eventually empty into the inferior vena cava.

The mean portal venous pressure in man is about 10 mm Hg while the hepatic venous pressure is 5 mm Hg. In contrast, the hepatic artery branches that reach the sinusoids have a pressure of 90 mm Hg, and thus a marked drop in arterial pressure occurs along the hepatic arterioles. This occurs through

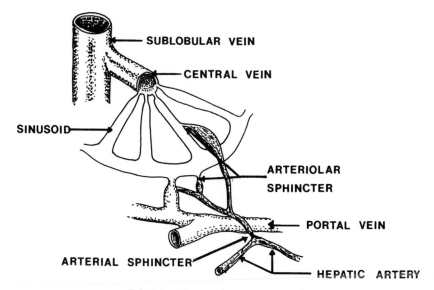

FIG. 7-1: The intrahepatic vascular bed.

functional sphincters located at the entrance of the hepatic arterioles at the sinusoids. Similarly functioning sphincters are present at the entrance of the portal venules and at the junction of sinusoids with the central veins of the liver lobules.[8] Through the rhythmic and asynchronous contraction and relaxation of these functional spincters, a particular sinusoid can receive arterial or portal blood or any mixture of the two.

The hepatic artery is innervated through the hepatic plexus. The smooth muscle of the intrahepatic portal veins are innervated by adrenergic vaso-constrictor nerve fibers derived from the 3rd to 11th thoracic ventral roots through the splanchnic nerve. Splanchnic nerve stimulation leads to an increase in hepatic arterial and portal venous pressure with a concomitant reduction in the flow of each. In addition to this predominant alpha-adrenergic vasoconstric-tor response, beta receptors can be identified after the administration of alpha blockers. Normally, the hepatic blood volume constitutes about 10 percent of the total blood volume, and about 50 percent of this blood can be expelled by stimulation of the sympathetic supply of the liver.

Several factors affect the hepatic blood flow. Autoregulation probably occurs via the hepatic artery only. A marked drop in systemic arterial pressure will decrease hepatic blood flow. Hypercapnia[9] or hypoxia will have the same effect on hepatic flow from splanchnic vasoconstriction as a result of cate-cholamine release. Also, hyperventilation produced by mechanical ventilation can reduce liver blood flow.[10] In hemorrhagic hypotension from the diffuse adrenergic discharges, constriction of the mesenteric and the hepatic arterioles will reduce the hepatic blood flow. In addition, the intrahepatic portal vessels will constrict, leading to a rise of portal pressure and further diminishing the liver blood flow. In severe shock, the diminution of hepatic blood flow can be so severe that patchy necrosis of the liver can occur. A rise of systemic venous pressure will lead to dilatation of the portal vein radicles and the blood content of the liver increases. This becomes marked in situations of congestive heart failure in which the enlarged liver can be palpated through the abdomen.

Mesenteric Circulation

The mesenteric vascular bed seems to behave in a passive manner. Above a critical pressure of 15 mm Hg, an increase in intravascular pressure leads to a decrease in vascular resistance with a concomitant increase in the flow. This is caused by dilatation of blood vessels and the opening up of new capillaries from the increased intraluminal pressure. In contrast, below a critical closing pressure (15 mm Hg), the flow in the mesenteric vascular bed ceases.[11]

Also, the mesenteric flow is related to intestinal activity, the mean flow increasing with increased intestinal activity. However, because of the mechanical effect, the arteriolar inflow diminishes and venous outflow increases during the individual phases of segmental contractions. These changes are reversed during relaxation.

With severe passive changes in intraluminal pressure that occur during intestinal obstruction, segmental contraction ceases at intraluminal pressures of 15 to 20 mm Hg. With higher pressures circulation slows first on the venous side then on the arterial side. This progressive venous obstruction is the cause of massive leakage of plasma and blood into the gut wall and lumen seen in this pathologic condition.

Splenic Circulation

In several animal species, the splenic capsule and the trabeculae are provided with smooth muscles that contract on sympathetic stimulation, expelling its blood into the general circulation. Thus, the spleen acts as a reservoir of blood rich in red blood cells. However, this contraction of the spleen has never been demonstrated in man.

Although the spleen does not function as a blood reservoir in man, it is a part of the reticuloendothelial system and is engaged in production of mononuclear leukocytes and antibody formation and also helps in removing aging red cells.

After splenectomy, the functions of the spleen are taken over by other lymphoid and reticuloendothelial organs. However, for a transient time, red cells with nuclear remnants and inclusion bodies can be seen in circulation with an increase in leukocyte and platelet counts.[12] The spleen ordinarily destroys rather than forms cells. Asplenic patients are prone to be inflicted with overwhelming and often fatal sepsis, which is sometimes associated with disseminated intravascular coagulopathies.[13]

Effect of Anesthetics on Splanchnic Circulation

All anesthetic agents and techniques diminish splanchnic blood flow (SBF). However, the mechanism of this decrease in flow differs from one agent to another.

Cyclopropane reduces SBF by about one-third by increasing the splanchnic vascular resistance, whereas the perfusion pressure (systemic arterial pressure) is not changed.[14] With cyclopropane the excess lactate in portal blood is increased. Both this increased vascular resistance and the excess lactate production is blocked by ganglionic blocking agents, indicating that these are sympathetic effects.

Halothane reduces SBF by decreasing the perfusion pressure[15] secondary to the diminution of cardiac output and systemic vasodilatation. The splanchnic vascular resistance is little affected by this agent.

Spinal anesthesia (sensory level T_5) reduces SBF without changing vascular resistance. The diminution of SBF parallels the diminution in perfusion pressure.

Methoxyflurane reduces hepatic blood flow by two different mechanisms:[16] (1) by decreasing the perfusion pressure and (2) by raising the hepatic vascular resistance through a selective and specific contraction of hepatic artery.

Nitrous oxide by itself does not seem to have any specific effect on SBF. With techniques using thiopental, N_2O, and muscle relaxants, SBF seems to depend mostly on the ventilatory status. Hypercapnia is associated with a diminution in SBF from sympathetic vasoconstriction. Normocapnia does not change SBF, whereas the SBF diminishes with hypocapnia, probably due to mechanical factors, such as a rise in intraabdominal pressure and peripheral pooling of blood.

During any of these anesthetic techniques, the hepatic blood flow decreases more than its oxygen consumption. Conceivably, this might result in anaerobic metabolism, which can be manifested by an increase in lactate production. However, this does not occur except with cyclopropane, indicating that with the other agents no adverse effects have occurred from this disproportionate decrease in blood flow. The two techniques that reduce blood flow proportionally more than the comparative diminution in O_2 consumption are N_2O: curare, associated with hypocapnia, and methoxyflurane. Therefore, in the patient with marginal splanchnic circulatory adequacy, these latter two techniques must be suspect. Cyclopropane should be avoided because of the increased lactate production. Techniques that provide a high ratio of splanchnic flow to O_2 consumption may be preferable, ie, halothane, spinal, or N_2O:curare with normocapnia.[17]

REFERENCES

1. Hertzman AB: Vasomotor regulation of cutaneous circulation. Physiol Rev 39:280, 1959
2. Milnor WR: Regional circulation. In Mountcastle VB (ed): Medical Physiology. St. Louis, Mosby, 1974
3. Heistad DD, Abboud FM: Factors that influence blood flow in skeletal muscle and skin. Anesthesiology 41:139 1974
4. Benzinger TH: Heat regulation: homeostasis of central temperature in man. Physiol Rev 49:671, 1969
5. Rowell LB: Human cardiovascular adjustments to exercise and thermal stress. Physiol Rev 54:75, 1974
6. Eger EI, Smith NT, Cullen DJ: A comparison of the cardiovascular effects of halothane, fluroxene, ether, and cyclopropane in man. Anesthesiology 34:25, 1971

7. Greenway CV, Stark RD: Hepatic vascular bed. Physiol Rev 51:23, 1971
8. Elias H, Sherrick JC: Morphology of the Liver. New York, Academic, 1969
9. Epstein RM, Wheeler HO, Frumin M, et al: The effect of hypercapnia on estimated hepatic blood flow, circulating splanchnic blood volume, and hepatic sulfobromophthalein clearance during general anesthesia in man. J Clin Invest 40:592, 1961
10. Strunin L: Organ perfusion during controlled hypotension. Br J Anaesth 47:793, 1975
11. Selkurt EE, Johnson PC: Effect of acute elevation of portal venous pressure on mesenteric blood volume, interstitial fluid volume and hemodynamics. Circ Res 6:592–599, 1958
12. Crosby WH: Hyposplenism: an inquiry into normal functions of the spleen. Ann Rev Med 14:349, 1963
13. Likhite VL: Immunological impairment and susceptibility to infection after splenectomy. JAMA 236:1376, 1976
14. Price HL, Deutsch S, Cooperman LH, et al: Splanchnic circulation during cyclopropane anesthesia in normal man. Anesthesiology 26:312, 1965
15. Epstein RM, Deutsch S, Cooperman LH, et al: Splanchnic circulation during halothane anesthesia and hypercapnia in normal man. Anesthesiology 27:654, 1960
16. Libonati M, Malsch E, Price HL, et al: Splanchnic circulation in man during methoxyflurane anesthesia. Anesthesiology 38:466, 1973
17. Batchelder BM, Cooperman LH: Effects of anesthetics on splanchnic circulation and metabolism. Surg Clin North Am 55:787, 1975

chapter 8

Placental and Fetal Circulation

THE UTEROPLACENTAL CIRCULATION

In the nonpregnant uterus, the uterine blood flow is relatively small (50 ml per minute) and is closely related to the metabolic activity of the myometrium and endometrium, fluctuating with the menstrual cycle. The uterine blood flow during pregnancy (600 ml per minute) is divided between the placenta and uterine wall. With current techniques it is impossible to differentiate between the two. The maternal increase in cardiac output is much higher than what is required for the needs of the fetus. The cardiac output rises 30 to 50 percent above the nonpregnant control levels. The causes of this increased output include hypervolemia, arteriovenous shunts in the placenta, and an increase in maternal oxygen consumption due to the mild hyperthyroid state. The peak increase in cardiac output occurs during the 25th through 32nd weeks and declines near term. The cause of this decline is due to the senescence of the placenta, which occurs in the last trimester of pregnancy, and also to compression of the inferior vena cava by the pregnant uterus, especially if these measurements are done in the supine position.[1]

The placental circulation is maternal in origin, made up of the intervillous spaces and the vessels supplying these spaces (Fig. 8-1). Both the radial and spiral arteries of the uterus open directly into the intervillous spaces and they spurt their blood like a fountain into the intervillous spaces at a pressure of 60 to 70 mm Hg.[2] However, the end pressure in the intervillous spaces is 6 to 10 mm Hg. The placental veins have thin walls, are devoid of valves, and are liable to external compression. The contraction of the uterine muscles compresses the intrauterine blood vessels, decreasing the flow in the arteries and stopping it completely in the veins. Thus, the intervillous pressure rises with every uterine contraction.

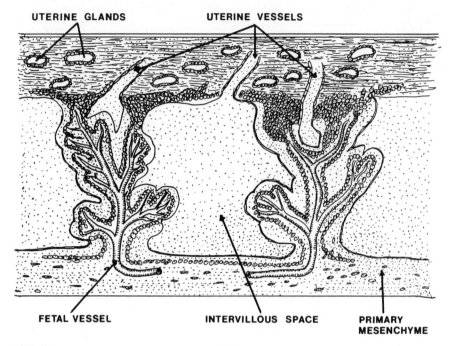

UTERINE GLANDS   UTERINE VESSELS

FETAL VESSEL   INTERVILLOUS SPACE   PRIMARY
                                                      MESENCHYME

FIG. 8-1: Diagrammatic representation of the arrangement of umbilical and uterine vessels and the intervillous spaces.

During early pregnancy, the arteriovenous oxygen difference is relatively small, because of disproportionate increase in uterine blood flow in excess of tissue oxygen needs. This effect is probably hormonal in nature, resulting from the increased estrogen and progesterone levels in the circulation.[3] However, at the late stages of pregnancy, despite more than a tenfold increase in uterine blood flow, more oxygen is extracted from the uterine vessels. The reason for this need is that at this stage the increase in the size of the fetus is much faster than the increase in blood flow. Thus, the oxygen saturation of uterine venous blood falls.

Near the end of normal gestation, arteriosclerotic changes can be seen in the walls of the placental arteries with a diminution in the arterial openings in the base of the placenta. These changes are more marked in pregnancies complicated by hypertension or eclampsia.

In the presence of hypotension, the uterine blood flow is diminished and signs of fetal asphyxia can be observed. These disappear with the restoration of blood volume. Ephedrine is also effective in increasing uterine blood flow in correcting fetal hypoxia and acidosis following spinal hypotension. Methoxamine, despite its ability to correct the blood pressure, accentuates the fetal hypoxia and acidosis. Metaraminol ranks between ephedrine and methoxamine in its effectiveness in correcting fetal deterioration due to spinal hypotension. It

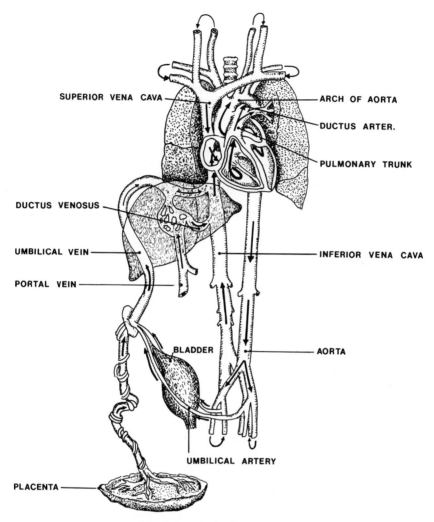

SUPERIOR VENA CAVA

ARCH OF AORTA

DUCTUS ARTER.

PULMONARY TRUNK

DUCTUS VENOSUS

UMBILICAL VEIN

INFERIOR VENA CAVA

PORTAL VEIN

BLADDER

AORTA

UMBILICAL ARTERY

PLACENTA

FIG. 8-2: The fetal circulation.

improves the fetal P_{O_2} and P_{CO_2}, indicating a better placental perfusion, but does not affect the progressive metabolic acidosis of the fetus.[4]

FETAL CIRCULATION (Fig. 8-2)

The placenta is the fetal lung. About 55 percent of the combined outputs of two ventricles of the fetus reaches the placenta through the umbilical arteries, where the exchange of nutrients occurs. The blood returns to the fetus by way of a single umbilical vein with an oxygen saturation of about 80 percent. Part of this blood mixes in the liver with the portal vessels, whereas most of it is directed by the ductus venosus to the inferior vena cava. The inferior vena caval blood, when it reaches the right atrium, is preferentially directed by the valve of the inferior vena cava to the left atrium through the *foramen ovale*. The left atrium pumps this blood to the left ventricle, which forces it into the aorta to be distributed mostly in the branches of the ascending aorta. A smaller amount of blood from the superior vena cava passes to the right ventricle, where it is pumped out to the pulmonary arteries. The pressure in the pulmonary artery is higher than the aortic pressure because of the collapsed lungs. Thus, most of the blood pumped by the right ventricle is diverted through the *ductus arteriosus* to the lower part of the aorta. As the ductus joins the aorta distal to the vessels supplying the head and neck, the blood with the lowest saturation is diverted mostly to the umbilical arteries to be oxygenated in the placenta. A smaller part of this poorly saturated blood perfuses the lower part of the fetus. In contrast, the relatively highly saturated blood of the left ventricle supplies the head of the fetus.

However, this separation of the two streams is not absolute and mixing does occur, and this difference of oxygen saturation in the carotid and descending aorta blood cannot always be found.

Exchange Across the Placenta

Although a countercurrent flow pattern at the placenta of ewes and rabbits has been seen, this seems to be absent in the primate placenta. Thus, the fetal blood is exposed at the intervillous space to maternal blood of intermediate composition between arterial and venous blood (Fig. 8-3).

The arterial oxygen tension of the uteroplacental arteries similar to peripheral arteries is 95 mm Hg (100 percent saturation), while in the veins it is 33 mm Hg. The oxygen tension in fetal blood is nearer to the maternal venous level, where the oxygen tension is 28 mm Hg in the umbilical vein. Thus, the fetus is at a disadvantage because of the low oxygen tension in its arterial system. However, other factors seem to offset this balance:

1. The fetal red blood cells contain fetal hemoglobin (hemoglobin F), which has a low affinity for 2,3-diphosphoglycerate (2,3-DPG) and a high affinity for oxygen. Thus, at a normal umbilical Po_2 of 28 mm Hg, the fetal hemoglobin is 80 percent saturated, while the adult hemoglobin (hemoglobin A) at the same Po_2 is only 50 percent saturated (Fig. 8-4).
2. The hemoglobin concentration is higher in the fetus 17 g per 100 ml (maternal, 12 g per 100 ml). Thus, the oxygen-carrying capacity of fetal blood is much higher in the fetus 23 ml per 100 ml (maternal, 16 ml per 100 ml) blood.

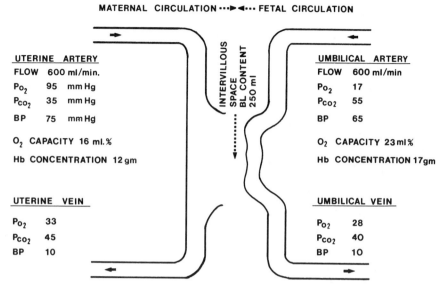

FIG. 8-3: The approximate comparative values of respiratory and circulatory parameters in the placenta.

3. The cardiac output relative to body weight is high in the fetus. Thus, the amount of blood to which tissues are exposed per unit tissue is relatively high.
4. The head and neck receive blood with higher oxygen saturation.
5. Last but not least, the fetus or the newborn seems to have a remarkable resistance to hypoxia, the mechanism of which is poorly understood.

The normal transplacental Pco_2 gradient is about 5 mm Hg. Near term, the maternal Pco_2 drops to about 33 mm Hg due to hyperventilation. Consequently, the fetal Pco_2 also drops, reaching a value similar to an adult but higher than the mother.

The fetus has normal acid–base values in intrauterine life. However, during labor the contraction of the uterus impedes the flow in the placenta and a mild acidosis occurs. A pH of 7.20 is considered the lowest limit of normal, whereas a range of 7.20 to 7.24 is termed "preacidotic."[5]

Labor and Delivery

During labor, the intrauterine pressure rises from about 10 mm Hg during relaxation to 20 to 60 mm Hg during contraction.[6] At the beginning of

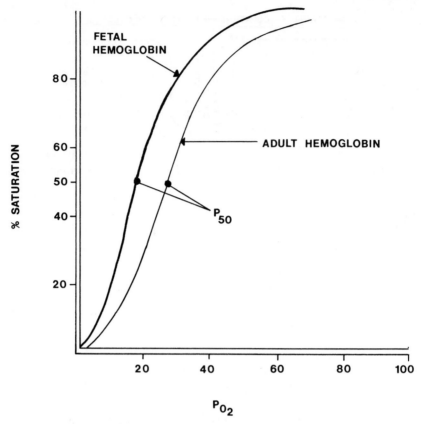

FIG. 8-4: The oxygen dissociation curves of adult and fetal hemoglobin. Notice the lower P_{50} value of fetal hemoglobin (20 mm Hg) compared to adult hemoglobin (28 mm Hg) indicating the greater affinity of fetal hemoglobin to oxygen.

contraction, the uterine veins are compressed. With the increase in pressure, the spiral arteries are shut off. Therefore, a period of relaxation is required between contractions for equilibration to occur between maternal and fetal circulations. During the uterine contractions, there is a tendency for the fetal heart rate to accelerate, probably resulting from sympathetic activation secondary to the stress of contraction. However, if the placental function is impaired or the uterine contractions are too frequent, then the fetus is liable to become asphyxiated. Similarly, if the umbilical cord is entangled with the fetus inside the uterus, it is more liable to be occluded during contractions. Also, maternal hypoxia or hypotension reflects itself on fetal oxygenation. In the early stages of hypoxia, the fetal heart rate will decrease (decelerate) during contractions and will increase (accelerate) during relaxations. These signs will precede acidosis. In the later stages, the deceleration of the fetal heart rate will become more

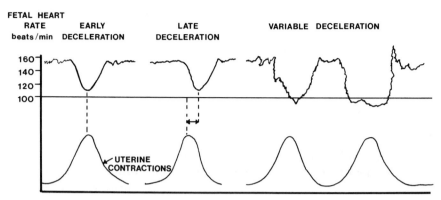

FIG. 8-5: The deceleration patterns in fetal heart rate recordings.

prolonged, extending into the phase of uterine relaxation, and this stage is usually accompanied by fetal acidosis.[5] Clinically, the auscultation for fetal heart sounds is performed between the uterine contractions. Thus, detection of fetal asphyxia is more liable to be delayed if one depends on auscultation rather than recording and continuously monitoring the fetal heart rate.

Several abnormal fetal heart rate patterns are recognized[7] (Fig. 8-5).

VARIABLE DECELERATION WITH AN ABNORMAL BASE-LINE HEART RATE

The deceleration may start before, with, or after the beginning of contraction. The deceleration is usually a severe one, falling below 100 beats per minute. It is supposed to be caused by compression of the umbilical cord. Atropine diminishes this deceleration but does not abolish it. If the heart rate falls below 60 beats per minute, a temporary or even a permanent cardiac arrest may ensue.

LOSS OF BEAT-TO-BEAT VARIATION

Normally the fetal heart rate shows a mild variation, indicating an adequately functioning nervous system and an integrated sympathetic and parasympathetic system. Damage to the central nervous system will abolish this beat-to-beat variability. This might be seen with depressant drugs, such as diazepam, with local anesthetics, narcotics, and barbiturates.

LATE DECELERATION

In this condition, the deceleration occurs uniformly after the onset of contraction. The heart rate returns to normal at the end of contraction. This is said to result from myocardial hypoxia due to uteroplacental insufficiency. With any of these conditions, the prognosis is worse if they are accompanied by fetal acidosis.

The mature fetus has a well-developed autonomic nervous system capable of mediating chemoreceptor and baroreceptor reflexes.[8] Thus, mild episodes of hypoxia are well tolerated with tachycardia as a response. However, after several hypoxic episodes, these reflexes become blunted and prolonged bradycardias occur as the fetus loses the ability to respond by tachycardia.[5]

The accurate interpretation of the abnormalities in the fetal heart rate is sometimes difficult, and the only way for a definite diagnosis of fetal asphyxia is by determinating fetal pH. This can be readily performed by obtaining capillary blood from the scalp of the fetus. A conical endoscope is introduced into the partially dilated cervix. A puncture incision is made with a guarded blade, and the drop of blood that appears is collected into heparinized glass capillary tubes. Determinations of pH, P_{CO_2}, and P_{O_2} are performed by the micro-Astrup techniques.

Transfer of Drugs Across the Placenta

Blood gases, water, and small diffusible molecules pass freely across the placenta under normal circumstances. For the transfer of larger molecules, such as drugs, the following special features are of importance.[4]

1. Molecular weight. For substances with molecular weights more than 600, the transfer is determined mainly by the lipid solubility of the drugs.
2. Dissociation constant. Highly ionized substances such as succinylcholine cross the placenta with difficulty.
3. Drug concentration. The higher the concentration of the drug in maternal circulation is, the higher the gradient and the faster the transfer of the drug will be.
4. Placental enzymes. Some enzymes are present in the placenta, such as amine oxidase that dissociates the catecholamines, impeding their transfer across the placenta.
5. Lipid solubility. Substances with high lipid solubility cross the placenta more readily.

All anesthetic gases and vapors cross the placenta relatively easily; however, their concentrations in cord blood are lower than the maternal blood. Also, thiopental and meperidine cross the placenta. The brain of the fetus is rather immature and is deficient in myelin. It has been shown that drugs with poor lipid solubility such as morphine depress the brain of the newborn rat more easily than the adult rat brain. Muscle relaxants do not readily cross the placental barrier except gallamine, which has been demonstrated in cord blood in significant amounts. Of the local anesthetics, lidocaine and mepivacaine are lipid soluble and can cross the placental barrier. Of lidocaine administered for lumbar epidural anesthesia, the fetal concentration is 52 percent of the maternal level, whereas with bupivacaine it is 64 percent. Addition of epinephrine to the local anesthetic solution diminishes the maternal as well as the fetal blood level of these drugs.[10]

The maternal and fetal circulatory status will affect the transferance of drugs across the placenta, eg, with maternal hypotension, the rate of transfer will be diminished from decreased flow in the uterine circulation. Also, strong and continuous uterine contractions can isolate the maternal from the fetal circulation.

Circulatory Changes at Birth

With the delivery of the fetus, the episodic breathing present antenatally becomes continuous. The exact cause of this change in the pattern of breathing is unknown.[11] Although cold exposure and tactile and gravitational stimuli enhance ventilation, the continued breathing movement probably depends on the large rise in cerebral arterial oxygen tension.

The respiratory movements create a markedly negative intrapleural pressure (-30 to -50 mm Hg), which leads to expansion of the lung and consequent drop in the pulmonary resistance to less than one-fifth of its in utero value, leading to a marked increase in pulmonary blood flow. Also, the placental circulation is cut off, leading to a rise in peripheral arterial resistance. Therefore, the rise in arterial pressure and the fall in pulmonary pressure leads to the reversal of the shunt at the ductus.

However, these changes are not abrupt. The lumen of the pulmonary arterioles increase only gradually. Thus, in the first hour of extrauterine life, the flow in the ductus is bidirectional. At 15 hours of age, the shunt becomes entirely left to right.

With the drop of pulmonary resistance and the increase in the flow of the pulmonary arteries, the blood returned to the left atrium increases, leading to a rise in the left atrial pressure above right atrial levels and to the closure of the foramen ovale.

The closure of the ductus arteriosus depends mainly on the arterial oxygen tension. The increase in the arterial oxygen tension will lead to closure of the ductus, while hypoxemia leads to the opening of the ductus and resumption of the shunt. Also, the ductus constricts in response to epinephrine and norepinephrine, and this response is blocked by adrenergic-blocking agents, whereas the response to oxygen tension is not blocked by adrenergic blockers.

The response of the ductus to hypoxia is opposite to that of the pulmonary arterioles. In the fetus, this is advantageous in that it diverts a greater fraction of the cardiac output to the placenta. However, in the newborn infant this has the opposite effect. In the latter, a hypoxic episode leads to a rise in pulmonary vascular resistance and opening of the ductus arteriosus, with a reverse shunt at the ductus (ie, right to left) that aggravates the hypoxia.[12]

In the normal infant, the functional closure of the ductus is complete within 2 days, while the anatomic closure of the ductus arteriosus and the foramen ovale takes a few weeks. Also the peculiar response of the pulmonary arteries to hypoxia is seen for about 10 days in the postnatal period. This seems to be more related to chronologic postnatal age than to the maturity of the fetus.

Anesthetic Agents and the Uterus

All of the commonly used anesthetic agents, with the exception of nitrous oxide, depress the uterine muscles. This depressant effect is dose related and at light levels of anesthesia can be reversed by oxytocin. At high inspired halothane concentrations, fetal acidosis associated with hypoxia occurs in addition to the profound uterine relaxation. The hypoxia-associated acidosis is secondary to the reduction of uterine blood flow secondary to maternal hypotension and diminution in her cardiac output, despite the presence of accompanying uterine vasodilatation.[13]

Of the anesthetic techniques used for therapeutic abortion, general anesthesia with nitrous oxide plus intravenous thiopental and meperidine or paracervical block cause the least amount of blood loss when compared to halothane and fluroxene.[14]

REFERENCES

1. Ueland K, Novy MJ, Peterson EN, et al: Maternal cardiovascular dynamics. IV. The influence of gestational age on the maternal cardiovascular response to posture and exercise. Am J Obstet Gynecol 104:856, 1969
2. Harris JWS, Ramsey EM: The morphology of human uteroplacental vasculature. Carnegie Institute of Washington Publication 625. Contrib Embryol 38:61, 1966
3. Killam AP, Rosenfeld CR, Battaglia FC, et al: Effect of estrogens on the uterine blood flow of oophorectomized ewes. Am J Obstet Gynecol 115:1045, 1973
4. Shnider SM, de Lorimier AA, Steffenson JL: Vasopressors in obstetrics. Fetal effects of metaraminol infusion during obstetric spinal hypotension. Am J Obstet Gynecol 108:1017, 1970
5. Beard RW: The detection of fetal asphyxia in labor. Pediatrics 53:157, 1974
6. Lind J: Physiology of neonatal circulation. Acta Anaesth Scand Suppl 37:5, 1970
7. Finster M, Petrie RH: Monitoring of the fetus. Anesthesiology 45:198, 1976
8. Yeh SY, Forsythe A, Hon EH: Quantification of fetal heart beat-to-beat interval differences. Obstet Gynecol 41:355, 1973

9. Mirkin BL: Perinatal pharmacology: placental transfer, fetal localization, and neonatal disposition of drugs. Anesthesiology 43:156, 1975
10. Brown WU, Jr, Bell GC, Lurie AO, et al: Newborn blood levels of lidocaine and mepivacaine in the first postnatal day following maternal epidural anesthesia. Anesthesiology 42:698, 1975
11. Boddy K, Dawes GS: Fetal breathing. Br Med Bull 31:3, 1975
12. Pang LM, Mellins RB: Neonatal cardiorespiratory physiology. Anesthesiology 43:171, 1975
13. Palahniuk RJ, Shnider SM: Maternal and fetal cardiovascular and acid–base changes during halothane and isoflurane anesthesia in the pregnant ewe. Anesthesiology 41:462, 1974
14. Cullen BF, Margolis AJ, Egen EI: The effects of anesthesia and pulmonary ventilation on blood loss during elective therapeutic abortion. Anesthesiology 32:108, 1970

chapter 9

Physiologic
Adjustment to Exercise

When an individual exercises, an intricate and complex set of circulatory, respiratory, and metabolic changes takes place in his body. While the muscles are moving, the cardiovascular system must adjust itself to provide these active muscles with the necessary nutrients to remove their metabolites and at the same time maintain homeostasis.

LOCAL CHANGES IN THE MUSCLES

During active contraction of the muscles, the blood flow in the muscle stops. However, during its intermittent relaxation, the blood flow can increase up to 30-fold. This is accomplished by increasing (up to 100-fold) the number of open capillaries. The opening of these capillaries, besides increasing the surface for exchange, has the added advantage of shortening the distance in which the diffusion of oxygen and nutrients takes place between the capillaries and the muscle fibers from about 50 microns at rest to about 5 microns in exercise.

This vascular diltation is mediated through the central nervous system and can be proven by the fact that this increased flow occurs before the start of exercise.[1] However, several other local factors help to maintain this high flow. Tissue hypoxia, excess carbon dioxide, and excess metabolites, such as lactic acid and adenylic acid, are involved. Also, the rise in muscle temperature dilates the blood vessels further. The acidosis and the elevated temperature have the added advantage that they shift the oxygen dissociation curve for hemoglobin to the right. Thus, more oxygen is given up by the hemoglobin molecule. All these changes increase the arteriovenous oxygen difference across the active muscles up to three times.

The capillary vascular dilatation raises the capillary pressure. This plus the accumulation of osmotically active metabolites in the interstitial spaces increases the fluid accumulation in the interstitial spaces. This leads to a tremendous increase in the lymph flow.

CARDIOVASCULAR ADJUSTMENTS

To compensate for this active vasodilatation and the excess demand of the exercising muscle, the cardiovascular system adjusts by increasing the cardiac output and by vasoconstricting the inactive areas such as the skin and viscera, thus shunting part of their flow to the muscles.[2]

The cardiac output is raised by increasing both the heart rate and the stroke volume. The heart rate rise is more marked in untrained subjects. The tachycardia is central in origin and is mediated by a decrease in vagal tone and sympathetic stimulation. This effect is potentiated by the action of carbon dioxide and acidosis on the medullary receptors. The value of the Bainbridge reflex (increased venous return leading to increase in heart rate) is very doubtful during exercise. This central tachycardia can be due to several causes: (1) psychic, as the mere anticipation of exercise will adapt the body for the excess demand; (2) impulses irradiated from the motor tracts to the cardiac centers; and (3) proprioceptive impulses from the muscles and joints.

The early physiologists thought that the increase in the stroke volume was due to the increased filling of the heart from the increased venous return (ie, Starling mechanism). However, dilatation of the heart has never been demonstrated during exercise. The increase in the stroke volume is achieved by better emptying of the blood from the left ventricle, ie, by augmenting the ejection fraction.[1] This increased ejection results from: (1) an increase in the strength of ventricular contraction from increased adrenergic activity to the heart and (2) a decrease in peripheral resistance from the vasodilatation in exercising muscles. Thus, the net effect on arterial blood pressure is a moderate rise in systolic pressure and mean pressures and a variable effect on diastolic pressure.

If the exercise intensity is increased progressively, the blood flow to splanchnic, renal, and other inactive regions is progressively reduced by active vasoconstriction. This vasoconstriction is through the sympathetic adrenergic fibers.

The venous return is increased with exercise because of (1) the vasodilatation of the active muscles, (2) the pumping effect of the contracting muscles, (3) the blood mobilized from the viscera, (4) venoconstriction, and (5) the increased pumping action of the respiratory muscles caused by hyperventilation (Table 9-1).

Temperature Regulation

Because some of the blood reaching the skin comes directly from the muscles, part of the excess heat produced in the muscles is transported directly

TABLE 9-1. Normal Cardiovascular Parameters and the Trend of Their Change with Exercise

PARAMETER	UNIT	MEAN VALUE	RANGE AT REST	EFFECT OF EXERCISE*
Pressures	mm Hg			
Brachial artery				
Systolic		130	90–140	MI
Diastolic		70	60–90	MI
Mean		85	70–105	MI, NC
Left ventricle				
Systolic		130	90–140	I
Diastolic		6	0–12	NC
Left atrium				
a wave		10	4–16	
v wave		13	6–20	
Mean		8	2–12	NC
Pulmonary wedge (capillary)		9	4–13	MI
Pulmonary artery				
Systolic		25	18–30	I
Diastolic		10	5–12	I
Mean		15	10–20	I, 10–20 mm Hg
Right ventricle				
Systolic		25	15–30	I
Diastolic		4	0–8	NC
Right atrium				
a wave		6	2–10	
c wave		5	2–10	
v wave		3	0–8	
Venous		5	3–8	NC
Flows				
Cardiac index	liters/minute/sq meter	3.2	2.8–4.2	I × 12
Stroke index	ml/beat/sq meter		30–65	I
Resistance				
Systemic	dyne/sec/cm^{-5} unit/sq meter	<35	800–1500	MD
Total pulmonary	dyne/sec/cm^{-5} unit/sq meter	<6	100–30	NC, MD
Pulmonary arteriolar	dyne/sec/cm^{-5} unit/sq meter	<5	20–100	NC, MD
Oxygen consumption	ml/minute/sq meter	130	110–150	I × 12
Minute ventilation	liters/minute/sq meter	3.3	2.0–4.5	I × 3–4
Oxygen saturation				
Systemic arterial	%	98	95–100	NC
Pulmonary arterial	%		75–80	D
AV O₂ difference	ml/100 ml	4.2	3.5–5.5	I × 3

* Abbreviations: MI, mild increase; I, increase; MD, mild decrease; D, decrease; NC, no change.

to the skin, where the heat is dissipated. Also, hyperventilation helps in the dissipation of this extra heat. Sweat secretion is also increased. The motor nerves of the sweat glands are sympathetic in origin, but they act by secretion of acetylcholine. The response of sweat glands seems to be centrally mediated, probably by the hypothalamic thermoregulatory center. The cutaneous vessels are also dilated.

Training

Trained individuals have a slower heart rate than nontrained individuals. They also have a larger stroke volume and have a tendency to have larger hearts. They increase their cardiac outputs during exercise by less acceleration of the heart. Their maximum oxygen consumptions are higher.[3]

Training improves the efficiency of work. For the same amount of work accomplished, trained people accumulate less lactic acid, consume lesser amounts of oxygen, and therefore, their increase in minute ventilation is less.

FUEL HOMEOSTASIS

The main sources of energy for the exercising muscles are:[4] (1) endogenous, from the muscle glycogen, which is an available source of carbohydrate, and (2) blood glucose or free fatty acids. The factors that determine the contribution of each one of these depends mainly on the duration and the strenuousness of the exercise.

In the first 10 minutes of mild exercise, glycogen is the main source of energy for the exercising muscle. After this initial 10 minutes, the glucose uptake by the muscle increases up to 20 times the basal values with the continuation of exercise. At about 90 minutes, glucose represents 40 percent of the fuel consumed by the muscle, whereas the remaining energy is derived from free fatty acid (40 percent) and endogenous sources, such as muscle glycogen and intramuscular lipids. With the prolongation of mild exercise, the contribution of free fatty acids increases and might represent 70 percent of the total energy consumed in about 4 hours of exercise.

In contrast to mild exercise, strenuous exercise depletes muscle glycogen stores faster, the point of exhaustion coinciding with the depletion of muscle glycogen. At this point, no significant changes in blood pressure, heart rate, blood glucose and lactate levels, or muscle electrolytes can be noted.[5] The cause of this glycogen depletion with fatigue, despite the presence of appreciable amounts of glucose and free fatty acids in circulation, is not clear.

MAXIMAL OXYGEN UPTAKE

If a person is asked to exercise at a progressively greater workload, his oxygen consumption increases linearly with the increased workload. However, a point is reached where even if he exercises at a higher load, his oxygen uptake remains the same. The amount of oxygen consumed at this peak is known as maximal oxygen uptake ($VO_{2\,max}$) (Fig. 9-1). At submaximal levels of exercise, the blood lactate concentration rises slightly. However, when the point of maximal oxygen uptake is reached and passed, then the blood lactate concentration rises markedly.[3] This level is stable and highly characteristic of the individual. In normal sedentary males, it ranges from 30 to 45 ml per kg per minute and can reach 85 ml per kg per minute in endurance athletes. These values are lower in women than in men, and in both males and females they decline with age and with cardiovascular disease.[6] The maximal oxygen consumption is increased by physical conditioning and is decreased by inactivity.

Thus, the maximal oxygen uptake is a function of the maximal cardiac output and the arteriovenous oxygen difference. In turn, the maximal cardiac output depends on the maximal heart rate and stroke volume. The maximum heart rate achieved decreases with age. In children, it can rise up to 200 beats per minute, while in adults it rarely reaches 195 and declines to 160 in old age. The arteriovenous oxygen difference depends on the maximal oxygen content in arterial blood and the minimal oxygen content in venous blood. Thus, it declines in situations in which large decreases in blood volume occur or

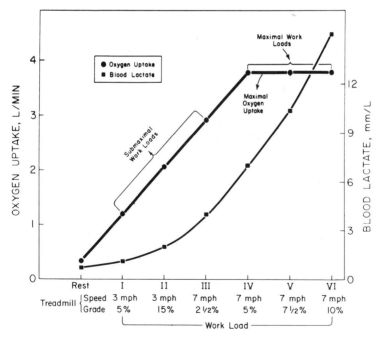

FIG. 9-1: Determination of maximal oxygen uptake on a treadmill. (Reproduced with permission from Mitchell and Blomqvist.[3])

whenever there is diminution in arterial oxygen content, which can result either from anemia or from pulmonary dysfunction. The fact that the arterial oxygen tension does not drop during strenuous exercise indicates that pulmonary factors are not the ones that limit the maximal oxygen consumption in the normal individual.

The average person who is standing at rest increases his oxygen consumption about 12-fold at the point of maximal oxygen uptake. He accomplishes this by quadrupling his cardiac output while increasing the arteriovenous oxygen difference threefold. The cardiac output is increased by doubling the stroke volume and by more than doubling the heart rate (Fig. 9-2). In the supine position, the stroke volume is higher than it is in the sitting position. Thus, the increase in stroke volume is less marked if the values are compared with those for the supine position. Also, the pulmonary minute ventilation is increased about 12-fold. This is achieved by tripling the respiratory rate and by quadrupling the tidal volume.

In contrast to the other organs, the arteriovenous oxygen difference across the heart during rest is relatively high, about 14 ml per 100 ml of blood. Thus, the heart can compensate for the increased demand only by coronary vasodilatation. At the point of maximal oxygen uptake the coronary flow increases fourfold, whereas the arteriovenous oxygen difference increases very little.

The blood flow to the abdominal organs, such as the kidney, liver, and gastrointestinal tract or the nonactive muscles, decreases markedly from vasoconstriction during heavy exercise. This diminution of blood flow is compensated by an increase in the arteriovenous oxygen difference.

Variation in Maximal Oxygen Uptake

The peak of maximal oxygen uptake is attained between the ages of 15 and 20 years, then declines gradually with age. At the age of 60, it is about two-thirds that of age 20. In children from 6 to 12 years of age there are no differences based on sex, but beyond adolescence, girls lag behind boys. Several factors contribute to these sex differences: (1) habits, (2) muscle mass presents a lower fraction in women than men, and (3) the mean concentration of hemoglobin is lower in women. Thus, the oxygen-carrying capacity is diminished.

Physical conditioning raises the maximum oxygen uptake mainly by augmenting the stroke volume, and also by increasing the arteriovenous oxygen difference. The latter is partly caused by the effect of acidosis and temperature on the oxygen dissociation curve. Also, some undetermined factors that seem to be present in these trained individuals allow the muscle to function at a lower venous oxygen tension. Conversely, bed rest leads to a diminution in mean oxygen uptake; a decrease of 20 to 25 percent has been reported after 6 weeks

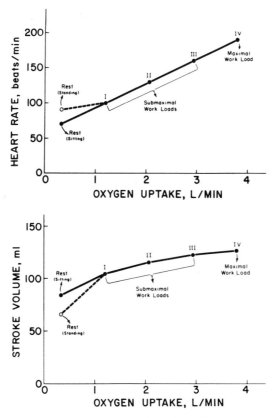

FIG. 9-2: Response of the heart rate and stroke volume to increasing levels of workload and oxygen uptake. (Reproduced with permission from Mitchell and Blomquist.[3])

of bed rest in young people. Endurance athletes have a maximum uptake of 75 to 80 ml per kg per minute (normal, 55 ml per kg per minute). These values tend to diminish with age. However, in these people, it remains higher than in the average population.

Pathologic conditions can affect the maximum oxygen uptake at the various stages of the oxygen transfer. Pulmonary diseases can confine the oxygenation of the blood during exercise. Cardiac diseases restrict the amount of oxygen that can be carried to the tissues. Anemias limit the oxygen-carrying capacity of blood.

What sets up the limit of maximum oxygen consumption in healthy people is not well defined. Pulmonary factors do not impose any limitations on the normal man, as can be seen by the fact that the arterial oxygen tension does not drop at the maximum oxygen uptake level. It is assumed that the limiting factor is from the muscles. However, if oxygen is added to inspired air, during the maximal level of oxygen consumption, the oxygen uptake is increased, ie, the muscle metabolism increases. In all probability, it is the result of a composite factor that depends on the interrelationships between maximal arteriovenous oxygen difference, blood pressure, and peripheral resistance.[2]

REFERENCES

1. Rushmer RF, Smith OA: Cardiac control. Physiol Rev 39:41, 1959
2. Rowell LB: Human cardiovascular adjustments to exercise and thermal stress. Physiol Rev 54:75, 1974
3. Mitchell JH, Blomqvist G: Maximal oxygen uptake. N Engl J Med 284:1018, 1971
4. Felig P, Wahren J: Fuel homeostasis in exercise. N Engl J Med 293:1078, 1975
5. Hultman E: Studies on muscle metabolism of glycogen and active phosphate in man with special reference to exercise and diet. Scand J Clin Lab Invest 19 (Suppl 94):1, 1967
6. Bruce RA, Kusumi F, Hosmer D: Maximal oxygen intake and nomographic assessment of functional aerobic impairment in cardiovascular disease. Am Heart J 85:546, 1973

chapter 10

Heart Failure

Almost all cardiac diseases end in heart failure.[1] The principal defect is the inability of the myocardium to utilize the energy available to it for contraction. This lack of energy depresses the force of contraction of the ventricles. If expressed in force–velocity terms, the maximal isovolumetric tension (P_0) and maximal velocity of shortening (V_{max}) are both diminished. The weakened myocardium is thus unable to pump the blood available to it. The pressure behind the heart increases, and the ventricular end-diastolic pressure rises. In the early stages of the disease, it rises on exercise; with the progression of the disease, the end-diastolic pressure becomes elevated even at rest. In left ventricular failure, the end-diastolic pressure may rise from the normal, which is less than 10 to 20 mm Hg.

As the myocardial fiber becomes weaker, the ventricles start dilating. The residual volume of the ventricle increases, stretching the myocardial muscles and, according to Starling's law, raising its output. In the early states, this compensates for the inadequacy of the ventricles to empty efficiently. However, as the intraventricular diameter increases, the tension that has to be developed by the ventricular muscle to achieve the same intraventricular pressure increases (Laplace's law). Finally, a point is reached where further increases in the myocardial fiber length do not produce any more hemodynamic advantage, and the force of contraction of myocardial fiber drops, further aggravating the heart failure.

Inasmuch as the ventricles are unable to circulate effectively all the blood reaching the heart, the pressure in the atria rises and this pressure is reflected in the pulmonary and peripheral venous systems. The increase in venous pressure will raise the intracapillary pressure whereby fluid is retained in the extracellular spaces. Tissue edema manifests when its interstitial pressure rises above that of atmospheric pressure. At this stage, the intercellular gel cannot hold any more fluid and, as a result, fluid appears in a free state between the cells.[2] If the rise of pressure is predominantly in the left atrium, the edema is mostly localized in the lungs. Then the heart failure is described as left-sided, and the principal complaint of the patient is dyspnea. At the early stages, the dyspnea will be on exertion only. With the progression of the disease, the dyspnea appears when lying flat and is relieved by sitting up (orthopnea). The reason for the appearance of dyspnea when the patient is supine is that about 400 ml of blood is shifted from the peripheral veins to the pulmonary circulation. At the terminal stage of the disease, the fluid exudates in the alveoli and pulmonary edema appears. Left ventricular failure is characterized by a diminution in stroke volume and a rise in the left ventricular end-diastolic, left atrial, and pulmonary capillary wedge pressures.

If the edema appears predominantly in the right side of the heart, the heart failure is described as right-sided, or congestive heart failure, and the prominent signs and symptoms are distension of neck veins, hepatomegaly, edema of the lower limbs starting at the ankles, and, in the later stages, ascites.

PATHOPHYSIOLOGY

This distinction between right- and left-sided failure is trivial because the fundamental disturbance in heart failure is sodium and water retention in the extracellular spaces.

This sodium and water retention in the interstitial spaces is actively mediated by the kidneys. It is an effort by the body to raise the filling pressure of the circulation and to enhance the venous return. At the early stages of the disease, this compensation by increasing the distension of the heart through Starling's mechanism improves the contraction. However, at the advanced stages of the disease, this mechanism backfires because the overdistension depresses further the myocardial performance. Also, the fluid retention in the lungs prevents gas exchange, leading to hypoxemia.

The exact mechanism whereby sodium and water are retained in the early stages of the disease is still undetermined. Probably, an acute episode of reduction in the cardiac output, which may have happened during exercise, will lead to a diminution in the glomerular filtration rate. The decrease of the sodium load that reaches the macula densa of the renal tissue activates a trigger response. That releases renin by the juxtaglomerular cells. A second theory put forward is that the diminution in the stretch of the renal afferent arterioles during this period of hypoperfusion is the stimulus of renin release from these highly differentiated juxtaglomerular cells.[3]

Once in the peripheral circulation, renin activates angiotensinogen, which is an α_2-globulin, leading to the formation of angiotensin I. Angiotensin I has a tetradecapeptide chain, which is converted in the lung to an octapeptide, leading to the formation of angiotensin II. Angiotensin II, by itself, has a pressor effect on the peripheral arterioles. However, its main mechanism of action is through the adrenal cortex, where it stimulates aldosterone secretion, which leads to sodium retention.

In patients with congestive heart failure, the daily secretion of aldosterone may vary from normal to 50 times higher values. Several other factors affect aldosterone production, eg, low sodium intake can by itself induce aldosterone hypersecretion. The metabolism of aldosterone is extremely slow in patients with heart failure, as a result of the diminution of hepatic blood flow consequent to reduced cardiac output.

LENGTH–FORCE–VELOCITY RELATIONSHIPS

The adjustment of the contractile performance of the heart to normal and abnormal situations is mediated through control systems that have to operate within the myocardial cells. This is in marked contrast to the skeletal muscles in which the control is extrinsic, and increased force is achieved by recruiting a greater number of motor units. The heart muscle functionally acts as a syncytium and the number of active muscle fibers cannot be altered. The only way to vary the force developed is by changing the intensity of its activity.[4]

The Frank–Starling curve, which describes the interrelationship between the ventricular end-diastolic volume and the cardiac output, is similar to the length–tension curve of the myocardial muscle (Fig. 10-1). Normally, the ventricles operate on the ascending limb of the curve, where an increase in the end-diastolic pressure results in an increase in the stroke volume up to a maximum limit. Further stretching of the myocardium beyond this point leads to a diminution in the stroke volume. In the force–velocity relationship, this increase of the initial muscle length leads to an increase in the force developed (P_0) without any change in the extrapolated maximum velocity of shortening (V_{max}) (Fig. 10-2). In the failing heart, the decrease in contractility is signified by a downward shift of the entire curve. Increase in the end-diastolic volume shifts the lower portion of the curve upward, and the intercept with the horizontal axis (P_0) is moved to the right without alternating V_{max},[5,6] ie, the tension produced is increased, whereas the velocity of contraction is not affected.

Conversely, inotropic stimulation with digitalis, calcium, and norepinephrine shifts the entire curve to the right (both V_{max} and P_0) so that the myocardium becomes faster and stronger in compensating any load.

The ultrastructural basis for the Frank–Starling mechanism is explained in that the increase of the myocardial fiber length leads to a diminution of the overlap of the actin filaments at the center of the sarcomere; thus, a greater number of contractile sites are available between actin and myosin. Stretching of the muscle increases the number of active contractile sites that generate force without any change in the maximal rate of reaction at these sites (hence, one gets a constant V_{max} but an increased P_0). However, with further stretch, the

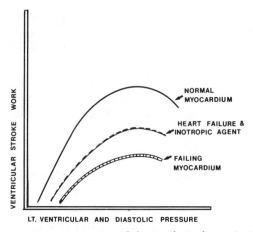

FIG. 10-1: Diagrammatic representation of the Frank–Starling principle as it applies to the normal and failing myocardium and also to the heart stimulated by inotropic agents.

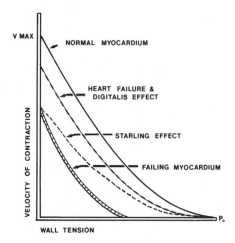

FIG. 10-2: Force–velocity relationships of the normal and failing myocardium. Note the shift of P_0 without any change at V_{max} from the Starling effect. Also note that digitalis improves the V_{max}, but it does not return to normal levels.

myofilaments become disengaged and less tension is produced (descending limb of the Starling curve). Alternatively, a change in contractility results from changes in the maximal rate of reaction at the contractile sites with or without any changes in their number.[7] This mechanism is probably due to the variation in the calcium delivery to the contractile proteins. The rate of calcium uptake by the failing heart is slower than the normal heart despite the fact that the total uptake is the same in both. In situations of increased contractility, the quantity of calcium delivered for binding to troponin C is increased. Conversely, it is diminished in conditions of decreased contractility.[4]

CLASSIFICATION OF CARDIAC PATIENTS

The following classification of cardiac patients originally was developed by the New York Heart Association and is based on the ability of the patient to perform certain physical activities.

Class I Ventricular Hypertrophy Without Heart Failure

Ordinary physical activity does not cause undue fatigue, dyspnea, palpitation, or angina. In this group of patients, the hypertrophied ventricular muscles are capable of maintaining cardiac output. However, with heavy exercise the cardiac output does not increase to the same extent as the normal heart with the same increase of the end-diastolic tension.

Class II Compensated Congestive Heart Failure

Myocardial function is mildly depressed, but the resting cardiac output is preserved at normal levels by baroreceptor-induced tachycardia and as a result of the Frank–Starling mechanism. There is moderate elevation of systemic and pulmonary venous pressures. There is also a slight limitation of physical activity, but the patient is comfortable at rest. However, ordinary physical activity results in fatigue, palpitation, dyspnea, or angina. The early fatigue is due to the inability of the myocardium to keep up with the increased oxygen demands of the tissues. The exertional angina results from the inability of the coronary arteries to cope with the increased oxygen demand of the hypertrophied myocardium.

Class III Compensated Congestive Heart Failure

There is more depressed myocardial function in this condition. Resting cardiac output is preserved with excessive elevation of systemic and pulmonary venous pressures. There is a marked limitation of physical activity. Less than ordinary activity leads to marked symptoms, such as severe palpitation and sweating from the excessive sympathetic discharge. However, these patients are comfortable at rest.

Class IV   **Decompensated Congestive Heart Failure**

The heart is unable to maintain normal cardiac output in the basal state due to marked depression of its contractile state. Patients are unable to carry on any physical activity without discomfort. Angina or symptoms of congestive heart failure are present at rest, and in the final stages there are signs of peripheral hypoperfusion, severe weakness, cachexia, mental deterioration, oliguria, and hypotension. In cardiogenic shock, cardiac output is extremely diminished, the cardiac index might be less than 1.5 liters per minute per sq meter, and the pulmonary capillary wedge pressure is more than 20 mm Hg.[8]

REFERENCES

1. Ramirez A, Abelmann WH: Cardiac decompensation. N Engl J Med 290:499, 1974
2. Moran Campbell EJ, Dickinson DJ, Slater JD: Clinical Physiology. Oxford, Blackwell, 1974, p 60
3. Davis JO: Mechanisms of salt and water retention in cardiac failure. In Braunwald E (ed): The Myocardium: Failure and Infarction. New York, H.P. Publishing, 1974, p 80
4. Katz AK: Congestive heart failure: role of altered myocardial cellular control. N Engl J Med 293:1184, 1975
5. Sonnenblick EH, Parmley WW, Urschel CW: The contractile state of the heart as expressed by force–velocity relations. Am J Cardiol 23:488, 1969
6. Mason DT, Spann J, Zelis R: New developments in the understanding of the actions of the digitalis glycosides. Prog Cardiovasc Dis 11:443, 1969
7. Sonnenblick EH, Parmley WW, Urschel CW, et al: Ventricular function: evaluation of myocardial contractility in health and disease. In Friedberg CK (ed): Congestive Heart Failure. New York, Grune, 1970, p 137
8. Buchbinder N, Ganz W: Hemodynamic monitoring invasive techniques. Anesthesiology 45:146, 1976

Respiration

chapter 11

Physical and Mechanical Aspects of Ventilation

ANATOMY

The different levels of the lower respiratory tract are usually described as generations, the trachea being the first generation, the main bronchi the second, and so on down to 23 generations, the alveolar sacs being the last.

Trachea

The trachea is a tubular structure that starts at the lower border of the cricoid cartilage opposite the level of the sixth cervical vertebra, extends vertically downward with a slight tilt to the right, and bifurcates at the carina opposite the level of the fifth thoracic vertebra. It is about 11 cm in length and has an inside diameter of 12 mm; it is narrower in females than in males. In its walls are embedded U-shaped cartilages that are joined posteriorly by smooth muscle fibers. The mucosal lining of the trachea is composed of ciliated columnar epithelium containing a large number of goblet cells that secrete mucous. The cilia beat in a manner similar to that of the upper respiratory tract, but here the direction of the stream of mucous is upward toward the pharynx. The human trachea has a capacity of 30 ml, constituting 20 percent of the anatomic dead space. Its caliber can be changed either passively by compression from outside or actively by the contraction of its smooth muscles.

Bronchi (Generations 1 to 11)

The bifurcation of the trachea at the carina is not symmetric; the right bronchus is wider and more in line with the trachea. Thus, foreign bodies, endotracheal tubes, or suction catheters are more likely to go into the right side than the left. Similar to the tracheal epithelium, the bronchial epithelium is columnar ciliated. However, the height of the epithelial cells diminishes as they approach the peripheral bronchi until they become cuboidal in the bronchioles. During forced expiration, the larger bronchi (generations 1 to 4) are liable to collapse when the intrathoracic pressure exceeds 50 cm H_2O above the intraluminar pressure, thus limiting the maximum expiratory flow rates. The bronchi are more likely to be compressed in emphysematous people, which produces the characteristic brassy cough heard in these subjects.

Bronchioles (Generations 12 to 16)

A characteristic feature of the bronchioles is the absence of cartilages and the well-developed helical muscular bands in the walls. The diameter of the air passage is about 1 mm at this level. By losing the cartilage layer, they are more inclined to be compressed. However, this is prevented by the fact that they are embedded in lung parenchyma, and the elastic recoil of the alveolar septa keeps them open. Therefore, the caliber of the bronchioles is directly related to the lung volumes, and they are not much influenced by intrathoracic pressures as are the larger bronchi. Until the 16th generation of air passages, the bronchi are supplied by the systemic vascular tree via the bronchial circulation. Beyond this level the respiratory passages are nourished by the pulmonary circulation. Also up to this level, the main function of the respiratory passages is conduction of air and humidification; beyond this point, gas exchange can occur.

Respiratory Bronchioles (Generations 17 to 19)

Respiratory bronchioles are the transitional zones between the bronchioles and the alveolar ducts. The epithelium of the early generations is cuboidal, becomes flatter, and eventually is similar to alveolar epithelium in the alveolar ducts. Therefore, there is minimal exchange at these early levels, which increases down along the line.

PRIMARY LOBULE OR FUNCTIONAL UNIT

This is the area of the lung supplied by the first-order respiratory bronchiole. Each unit has a diameter of 3.5 mm and contains about 2000 alveoli. These are probably the areas of the lung which pop open when a collapsed lung is inflated during thoracotomy.[1]

Alveolar Ducts (Generations 20 to 22) and Alveolar Sacs (Generation 23)

There is no functional difference between the alveolar ducts and alveolar sacs. Both are lined by alveolar epithelium. Across the length of the alveolar duct there are a series of rings made from the alveolar septa. These septa contain smooth muscle cells and can contract, leading to diminution of duct lumen. The only difference between alveolar sacs and ducts is that the former are blind[1] (Fig. 11-1). Half of the alveoli arise from the ducts and the other half from the sacs.

Alveoli

In man, the alveoli are about 0.2 mm in diameter. They are larger in the upper portions of the lung than the lower parts because of the effect of gravity.[2] The alveolar wall between two contiguous alveoli is made up of two layers of alveolar epithelium, each on a separate basement membrane enclosing the capillary vascular network. These capillaries are embedded between the elastic and collagen fibers and between the smooth muscles and nerves. Therefore, a gas molecule passing from inside the alveoli to the blood has to cross the following layers (Fig. 11-2):

1. A single layer of alveolar epithelial cells with its basement membrane.
2. A space containing elastic and collagenous connective tissue.
3. The basement membranes and endothelial cells of the capillaries.

The branching of the bronchopulmonary segments is completed in utero, and the growth of airways after birth is entirely by increase in size. However,

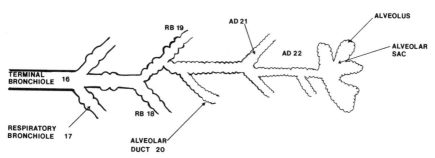

FIG. 11-1: The terminal air passages (the numbers indicate the order of generation).

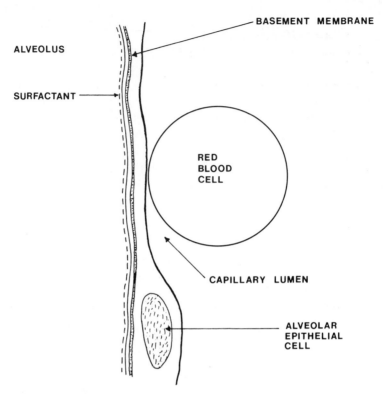

FIG. 11-2: Alveolocapillary membrane.

alveoli continue to proliferate in the first decade of life but probably not for as long as body growth continues, after which alveolar growth is mostly in size.[3]

HUMIDIFICATION AND FILTRATION OF INSPIRED GASES

The above-described respiratory passages plus the upper respiratory tract, ie, nose, pharynx, and larynx, in addition to their main function as conductive tubes, have the very important function of heating, humidifying, and filtering the inspired air. When the air reaches the alveoli, it is already at body temperature and fully saturated. This process starts at the nose whose large, highly vascular cavernous mucous membranes warm and humidify the air. Filtration of foreign particles is effected by the continuous mucous covering of the main respiratory passages. This mucous covering is very thin, elastic, and viscous and consists of two layers. The outer layer, which is more mucoid, rests on a watery serous layer in which the cilia move. Foreign particles such as dirt, pollen, and bacteria are filtered out of the air by adhering to the mucous blanket. Through the ciliary activity, this superficial layer of mucous moves toward the pharynx, where it is swallowed. Each ciliated columnar cell of the respiratory tract has about 20 cilia that produce a rapid, vigorous propulsive stroke followed by a slower, less powerful recovery stroke. These cilia beat 10 to 15 times per second. Secretions of the mucosal glands renew this mucous sheet. The direction of movement of this mucous layer is toward the pharynx, where it is swallowed with the saliva. Thus, in the upper respiratory passages, the main direction of flow is downward, while in the trachea and the bronchi the flow is upward. Its rate of movement is rather fast, eg, the entire nasal mucosa can be seen to be cleared in the pharynx within half an hour. Anesthetic agents depress the velocity of this mucous flow. It has been demonstrated that under halothane anesthesia, the velocity of the tracheal mucous flow diminishes to 7 mm per minute from a normal of 20 mm per minute.[4]

The vital function of these mucoid layers can be easily demonstrated if the upper respiratory tract is bypassed by the insertion of an endotracheal tube and by administration of dry gases. Within a short interval, hyperemia of the tracheobronchial tree can be seen with degeneration of the pseudostratified columnar and cuboidal epithelium. The dryness and the increased viscosity of the secretions lead to crust formation and obstruction of the airways, the eventual outcome being atelectasis and increased shunting of the blood at the lungs.[5,6]

THE MECHANICS OF RESPIRATION

Like water, air flows from a region of higher pressure to a region of lower pressure. In man and in all mammals, the active contraction of the inspiratory muscles creates a subatmospheric pressure inside the lungs, enlarging the bronchioles and alveoli. Thus, air at atmospheric pressure flows into the respiratory passages. In contrast to inspiration, expiration is a passive process in which the elastic recoil of the lung and chest wall creates a positive pressure inside the lung, expelling air to the atmosphere, and the lung returns to its end-expiratory position.

Inspiration

The main inspiratory muscles are the intercostals and the diaphragm, whereas the scalenes, sternomastoids, trapezius, and back muscles are the accessory ones of respiration. These accessory muscles are not active during normal quiet breathing. They show activity at high levels of ventilation (more than 50 liters per minute), and their main function is to stabilize the chest wall.

The *diaphragm* is a dome-shaped muscle separating the thoracic and the abdominal cavities and is attached around the circumference of the lower thoracic cage. It behaves like a piston. Its contractions move the abdominal contents downward and forward, creating a potential space, which is filled by the expansion of the lung. It is estimated that the diaphragm moves about 10 to 12 cm vertically during each inspiration. During quiet breathing it accounts for more than 75 percent of the change in intrathoracic volume. It may even be the only active inspiratory muscle. Under deep anesthesia, the diaphragm is the only active respiratory muscle. Occasionally, the breathing pattern at this stage is described as abdominal because the movement of the diaphragm causes outward and inward movements of the abdominal wall. The diaphragm is a voluntary muscle. For proper functioning, it requires an intact nerve supply. The main motor nerve supply of the diaphragm is the phrenic nerve, which arises chiefly from the fourth cervical nerve but also receives branches from the third and fifth cervical nerves.

With paralysis of the diaphragm, respiration can be barely adequate during quiet breathing from the action of the intercostal muscles. This paralysis can be detected by the "sniff test," in which, under fluoroscopy during rapid inspiration, the diaphragm can be seen moving upward (instead of downward) due to the decrease in intrathoracic pressure, which pulls the atonic diaphragm upward. Although the diaphragm acts like a piston, its displacement is not uniform. The posterior part moves the most because of its mechanical advantage. This is true whether the patient is standing or supine. During anesthesia with spontaneous breathing, the diaphragm is shifted about one vertebra cephalad, but the posterior (or dependent) part of the diaphragm still shows the greater displacement. However, in a paralyzed patient with controlled ventilation, the nondependent part of the diaphragm moves the most because the abdominal pressure is the least at this region.[7]

There are 11 *external intercostals* on each side. They arise from the lower border of the superior rib and are inserted into the upper border of the rib below. By contracting, they elevate the anterior end of each rib, pulling it upward and outward, thus increasing the anteroposterior diameter of the chest wall.

Expiration

In contrast to inspiration, expiration is a passive process during quiet breathing. During inspiration potential energy is stored in the elastic tissues of the lung and thoracic cage. The recoil of those stretched tissues leads to a rise in the pressure of the airways and air moves out. The expiratory muscles only become functional during heavy breathing or whenever there is an obstruction to the flow of air. The most important expiratory muscles are the abdominal and the internal intercostal muscles.

The *abdominal muscles* are the external and internal oblique and the transverse and rectus abdomines. By contracting they increase the intra-abdominal pressure, forcing the diaphragm upward. They also depress the lower ribs and flex the trunk. They are supplied by the lower six intercostal nerves and the first lumbar segment.

In normal man, a slight increase in the resistance to expiration (10 cm H_2O) leads to deeper inspiratory movements rather than actively involving the expiratory muscles. Thus, by stretching the elastic tissues more, a stronger elastic recoil is generated. However, with higher resistances the expiratory muscles contract to create a stronger expiratory pressure. They also are active during coughing, straining, vomiting, or hyperventilation.

The *internal intercostals* depress the ribs and move them downward and inward, stiffening the intercostal spaces so that they will not bulge during forced expiration.

The expiratory muscles become inactive early in anesthesia, which is not a problem in healthy people. However, it may create a problem in patients with narrowing of the airways.

The Pleura

At the resting volume of the respiratory system, the opposed recoils of the lung and chest wall tend to separate the visceral from the parietal pleura. Thus, the net intrapleural pressure should be negative, ie, subatmospheric, which is generally true. However, this pressure varies according to the region in the pleura and posture. In the sitting man at functional residual capacity (FRC), the pleural pressure is about −8 cm H_2O near the apex and −2 cm H_2O at the base. In the lateral, supine, and prone positions, it is about −6 cm H_2O to −3.5 cm H_2O at the top and about atmospheric at the bottom.[8] This diminution of transpulmonary pressure from top to bottom implies that the superior lobes of the lungs are more expanded than the lower ones, which is evidenced by the fact that alveolar size is larger in the upper lobes and the lung density is less.[9]

There is a very small amount of fluid in the pleural space, estimated to be about 2 ml. This liquid provides a lubrication system and also transmits instantaneously the pressure between the chest wall and the lung. The forces on the lung are perpendicular forces, but the presence of pleural fluid allows slide in response to shearing forces. Thus, the up and down movement of the diaphragm expands the whole lung, not just the lower lobes. For this system to function efficiently, the amount of intrapleural fluid should be kept at a minimum, which is achieved by keeping the colloid osmotic pressure of the pleural fluid at a minimum (3 to 4 cm H_2O). Thus, the net absorbing pressure toward the circulation is greater than the opposed recoil of the lung and the chest wall.[10] The parietal pleura is richly supplied with lymphatics that drain pleural liquid, proteins, and particles without any selective action. They probably are not functional under normal conditions but are an important emergency mechanism.[11]

LUNG VOLUMES (Fig. 11-3)

TIDAL VOLUME (tidal air), 500 ml*

This is the volume of air inspired or expired during each respiratory cycle.

INSPIRATORY RESERVE VOLUME (IRV) or INSPIRATORY CAPACITY (IC), 3600 ml

This is the maximum volume of air that can be inspired over and above the inspired tidal volume.

EXPIRATORY RESERVE VOLUME (ERV), 1200 ml

This is the maximal volume of air that can be expelled after the tidal volume has been allowed to escape.

VITAL CAPACITY (VC), 5 liters

This is the maximal volume of air that can be expelled from the lungs after the deepest possible inspiration. It represents the sum of tidal volume, inspiratory reserve volume, and vital capacity.

RESIDUAL VOLUME (RV), 1200 ml

This is the volume of air remaining in the lung at the end of maximal expiratory effort.

TOTAL LUNG CAPACITY (TLC), 6 liters

This is the amount of air present in the lung after a maximal inspiratory effort. It is the sum of residual volume and vital capacity.

FUNCTIONAL RESIDUAL CAPACITY (FRC), 2400 ml

This is the volume of air present in the lungs after a normal expiration. It usually increases with age and reaches about 3400 ml at age 60 years.

* *The values quoted are for males 20 to 30 years of age from Comroe JH, Jr, et al.*[12]

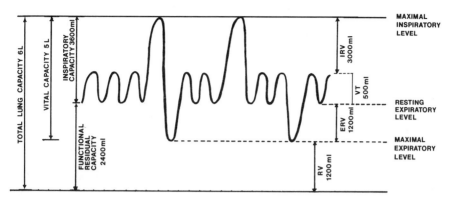

FIG. 11-3: Lung volumes and capacities in a normal young adult.

INSPIRATORY CAPACITY (IC), 3600 ml

This is the volume that can be inspired, starting at the end-expiratory level. It represents the sum of inspiratory reserve volume and tidal volume.

It should be noted that the lung volumes are single values and do not overlap, while the capacities are a combination of two or more volumes.

All these values decrease with age, except residual volume and functional residual capacity, which increase. At the age of 60 years the FRC is usually greater than 1200 ml. The lung volumes and capacities are lower in females by approximately 20 to 30 percent.

Volume Changes Per Unit Time

RESPIRATORY MINUTE VOLUME

This is the product of tidal volume and respiratory frequency per minute. At rest it is about 6 liters per minute.

MAXIMAL VOLUNTARY VENTILATION (MVV)

Maximal breathing capacity is 120 to 170 liters per minute. This is the greatest rate of pulmonary ventilation that can be sustained for approximately 20 seconds. It is also known as maximal breathing capacity.

TIMED VITAL CAPACITY (TVC)

This is the rate at which a maximal inspiration can be completely expired. It is an evaluation of muscle power and resistance to air movement. It should be at least 83 percent of the tidal volume in the first second and 97 percent at the end of the third second.

PULMONARY COMPLIANCE AND AIRWAY RESISTANCE

In the normal, resting individual, the work of breathing represents 1 to 2 percent of the total energy consumption. This work is needed to overcome two types of forces: (1) elastic resistance (static), which is mainly proportional to the changes of the lung volume and consists of the elasticity of lung parenchyma, elasticity of the chest wall, and the liquid–gas interface in the alveolus; and (2) nonelastic resistance (dynamic), which is mostly proportional to the flow rate and consists of the frictional resistance to the flow of air in the air passages, the viscous properties of the lung and chest wall, and overcoming the air inertia and providing kinetic energy to the air moved. The resistance offered by this factor is minimal and for practical purposes is ignored.

More than two-thirds of the work of quiet breathing is spent in overcoming the elastic recoil of the lungs and chest wall. However, when the respiratory rate increases or the air passages are narrowed, a higher proportion of the work is spent in overcoming the resistance to air flow.

Definitions

TRANSPULMONARY GRADIENT

This is the difference between alveolar pressure and intrapleural pressure. An increase in this gradient will lead to an increase in lung volume.

TRANSMURAL GRADIENT

The pressure difference between the pleura and the amosphere in the absence of muscle tone is the transmural gradient.

COMPLIANCE (static or elastic, liter per cm H_2O)

$$\text{Compliance} = \frac{\text{Volume change (liters)}}{\text{Change in pressure gradient (cm } H_2O)} = \frac{\Delta V}{\Delta P}$$

This is the volume change produced by a unit change of pressure. This relationship does not take into consideration the flow factor. It represents the static retractive pressure at a point when the air flow is zero.

Specific compliance

$$\text{Specific compliance} = \frac{\text{Compliance (liter per cm } H_2O)}{\text{Volume of lung at FRC}}$$

$$\text{Elastance} = \frac{1}{\text{compliance}} \text{ (not frequently used)}$$

A stiff lung has a low compliance but a high elastance.

Dynamic compliance

Dynamic compliance or resistance (cm H_2O per liter per second)

$$= \frac{\text{Pressure gradient (cm } H_2O)}{\text{Rate of volume change (liter per second)}}$$

This is the difference of pressure which is required to exchange one unit of flow.

Measurement of Compliance

STATIC COMPLIANCE

Direct measurement of the intrapleural pressure is extremely difficult, even if the patient has a chest tube. The presence of the tube distorts the physical properties of intrapleural pressure. The most convenient way to measure intrapleural pressure is to use an intraesophageal balloon positioned in the lower third of the esophagus at its intrathoracic region. In this position the esophagus is between the chest wall and the lung, and as its walls are thin, its intraluminal pressure reflects the intrapleural pressure. The peristaltic waves of the esophagus are easily identifiable.

In an awake individual, the compliance is determined by asking the person to take a breath from a spirometer and hold it until the intraesophageal pressure becomes stable and the pressure at this particular volume is recorded. This procedure is repeated at different lung volumes, and a plot is drawn. The slope of this curve is the static lung compliance in liters per cm H_2O. In the anesthetized or paralyzed person, it can be measured by inflating the lung with a known volume of air through the endotracheal (or tracheostomy) tube. By measuring the appropriate pressure gradient, the lung, chest wall, and total thoracic compliance can be determined.

DYNAMIC COMPLIANCE

The dynamic compliance of the lung is measured by recording the volume, intraesophageal pressure, and flow during spontaneous respiration. The flow is recorded by pneumotachograph and the volume by a spirometer or by integration of the flow rate. The static complicance can be obtained by relating the inspired volume to the transpulmonary pressure at the point of zero air flow at the height of inspiration (Fig. 11-4). Dynamic compliance also can be obtained by recording a series of pressure volume loops on an oscilloscope or Y-Z

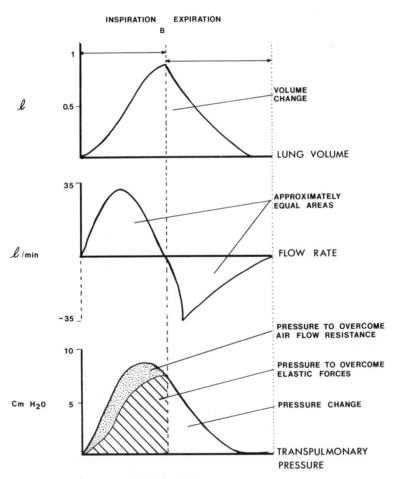

FIG. 11-4: The lung volume, flow rate, and transpulmonary pressure changes during respiration. Compliance can be computed from the change of pressure and the change of volume at the point of zero flow.

recorder. The electrical signal from a differential pressure transducer is applied on the X-axis and the volume signal from the integrated pneumotachograph on the Y-axis. From the mean slope of this curve, compliance is calculated.

Pulmonary Compliance

The two forces leading to collapse of the lung are the elasticity of the parenchymatous structure of the lung and the liquid–gas interface at the alveoli. At normal ranges of respiratory excursions, compliance of the lung is rather constant and is equal to 0.2 liter per minute. Thus, an increase in pressure of one cm H_2O can raise the lung volume by 200 ml. However, at the upper levels of chest expansion, the compliance is lower, ie, higher pressure gradients are required to expand the same lung volume, and this becomes the limiting factor in the maximum vital capacity in the normal individual.

SURFACE TENSION

Early in 1929, it was observed by Van Neergaard that the compliance of the lung was lower when inflated with fluid rather than with air. Under static conditions, the pressure required to enlarge the lung with fluid was less than half that required to inflate an air-filled lung. If the resistance to stretch is due only to elastic stretch of the lung, then changing from air to liquid should not change the compliance. Thus, the factor that the fluid eliminates is the surface tension of a material lining the liquid–gas interface of the alveoli.

The surface tension results from the attraction of the atoms and molecules of a liquid. Thus, a water molecule in the center of the liquid is attracted from all sides (Fig. 11-5). However, a water molecule at the top of a bubble is attracted only sideward and downward. This imbalance of the intermolecular forces leads to the shrinkage of the liquid to the smallest possible area. The surface tension of water is 70 dynes per cm, while that of plasma and tissue fluids is about 50 dynes per cm. However, in the lung the situation is different. If one draws pressure–volume curves of the lung with air and then with saline, the first will measure the pulmonary compliance, while the second will measure only the elastic component. The difference between the two is due to surface tension. The interesting aspect of surface tension at the alveoli is that it is much less at small lung volumes than at large lung volumes (Fig. 11-6). The surface tension of the alveolar surfactant is about 2 to 5 dynes per cm when the alveoli are small and increases to 40 to 50 dynes per cm when the alveoli are large. The surfactant is responsible for hysteresis of the loop of the pressure–volume curve, ie, the difference between the inflation and deflation curves, the latter being at the left (Fig. 11-6).

The surfactant has two very important functions: (1) It lowers the surface

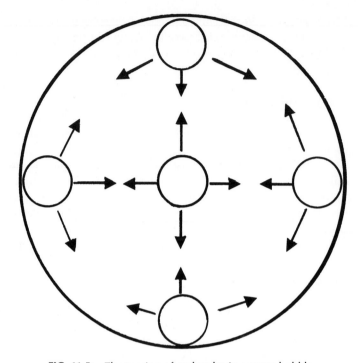

FIG. 11-5:   The tension of molecules in a water bubble.

tension, therefore diminishing the force (muscle effort) required for ventilation and aeration of the lung; and (2) because its surface tension changes with the size of the alveoli, it stabilizes them, preventing them from collapsing.

According to the law of Laplace, $P = 2T/R$, where P is the pressure inside the bubble expanding it, T is the tension in the wall tending to diminish it, and R is the radius of the sphere. If the tension is kept constant and the radius of the bubble is diminished, then the pressure in it will rise, thus emptying its content to a bigger bubble. In the absence of surfactant, all the smaller alveoli would empty into the bigger ones (Fig. 11-7). However, the pressure of surfactant lowers the surface tension as the alveolus becomes smaller in size, thus preventing it from collapsing.

The surfactant is produced by the Type II alveolar epithelial cells, which are developed as inclusion bodies and discharged by exocytosis. It is a complex lipoprotein, similar to those present in tissue membrane but has a high content of dipalmitoyl lecithin in its protein.[13] Their molecules spread apart as alveolar size increases during inspiration and move near each other during expiration, thus adjusting the surface tension during breathing.

The surfactant is deficient in the respiratory distress syndrome of the newborn. Its formation can be hastened by the administration of adrenocortical

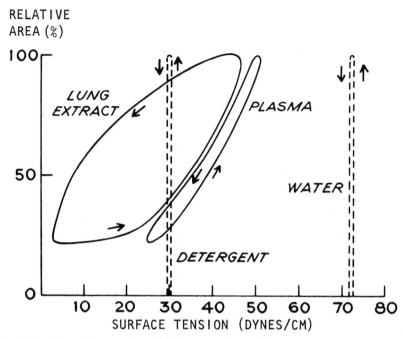

FIG. 11-6: The surface tension of the lung surfactant during compression and expansion. Note the variation of the surface tension of the lung extract from 5 dynes per cm to 45 dynes per cm, while the surface tension of the detergent and water are constant. (Reproduced with permission from Year Book.[27])

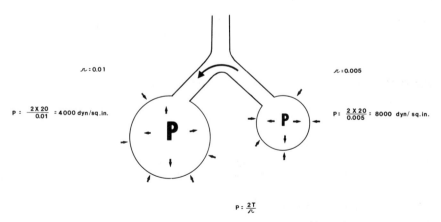

FIG. 11-7: The pressures in two alveoli of different sizes with the same surface tensions in the absence of surfactant. Note the flow from the smaller alveolus to the bigger one.

hormones during pregnancy in animals.[14,15] It also diminishes after cardiopulmonary bypass and may be deficient in lung collapse, pulmonary artery occlusion, or on inhalation of 100 percent oxygen.

Compliance of the Chest Wall

In contrast to the lung, which if not acted on by any external force contracts to an airless state, the chest wall, if not acted on by any force, enlarges to a position of about 600 ml above the resting stage. However, the two are held together by the cohesive forces of the pleural surfaces. At functional residual capacity, the chest wall is stretched *in*, whereas the lung is stretched *out* from its resting position.

In the normal range of chest expansion, the compliance of the chest wall is constant and is almost equal to that of the lungs (0.2 liter per cm H_2O). However, below the resting expiratory level the pressure–volume curve becomes skewed. At this level a unit change of pressure leads to a smaller change in volume, and this factor limits the volume of air left in the lungs after a maximal expiration (Fig. 11-8).

The reciprocal of total lung compliance is the sum of the reciprocal of the pulmonary and thoracic cage compliances. In the normal range of respiratory movements, it is:

$$\frac{1}{\text{Total compliance}} = \frac{1}{\text{pulmonary compliance}} + \frac{1}{\text{chest wall compliance}}$$

$$= \frac{1}{0.2} + \frac{1}{0.2} = \frac{2}{0.2} = \frac{10}{1}$$

or total compliance = 1/10 = 0.1 liter per cm H_2O, ie, it requires a pressure of 1 cm H_2O across the lung and chest wall to move 100 ml of air into the lung.

Factors Affecting Pulmonary Compliance

LUNG VOLUME

It is obvious that the same pressure gradient will push more air into the lungs of an adult than an infant, simply because the lung volume is greater in an adult. Therefore, compliance depends not only on the elasticity of the lung tissue, but also on the lung volume before its stretch. Because the lung compliance is most closely related to functional residual capacity,[16] the term specific compliance is used where:

$$\text{Specific compliance} = \frac{\text{Compliance (liters per cm } H_2O)}{\text{FRC (liters)}}$$

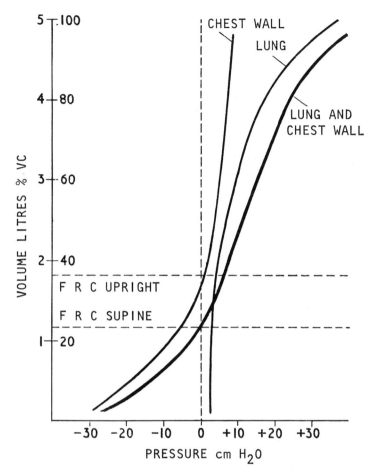

FIG. 11-8: Pressure–volume diagrams of lung, chest wall, and lung–chest wall combination in supine position. The weight of the abdominal contents causes a shift of the chest wall pressure–volume plot and a reduction in FRC. (Reproduced with permission from Heinemann.[28])

Normally, this is about 0.5 liter per cm H_2O per liter. This ratio is basically the same for adults, both men and women, as well as for children, and even for the newborn infant.

HYSTERESIS

If the lung is inflated with equal volumes and deflated in a similar fashion, it is found that the pressure required to inflate the lung at a certain volume is more than the pressure generated during deflation. This is termed hysteresis or stress relaxation. It is most probably due to recruitment of additional alveoli during expansion of the lung in addition to the effect of the surfactant.

POSTURE

At the end of expiration, the diaphragm is rather flaccid and its position is determined by the pressure gradient between the abdominal and pleural cavities. Therefore, changing from an upright position to the supine position in an awake person will cause a diminution in the FRC of about 1 liter. This reduction in lung volume will decrease the lung compliance. Also, another problem with the supine position is that measurement of intrathoracic pressure by means of an esophageal balloon becomes more difficult to interpret because of the increased pressure by the mediastinal structures over the esophagus.

PULMONARY BLOOD VOLUME

In the normal situation, pulmonary blood vessels probably have little effect on the pulmonary compliance. However, pulmonary congestion decreases the compliance. This is probably due to the increase in intrathoracic blood volume diminishing the initial lung volume.

RESTRICTION OF THE EXPANSION OF THE CHEST

Strapping of the chest reduces the FRC and also the compliance of the chest. This compliance remains reduced if the lung volume is returned to normal. However, a deep breath returns the compliance to normal values.[17] This reduction in compliance probably results from alveolar collapse and the return to normal by the deep breath is a hysteresis effect, ie, recruitment of more alveoli.

ANESTHESIA

There is no doubt that pulmonary compliance is diminished during anesthesia. The exact mechanism is not well defined; several factors probably contribute to this occurrence.

Posture. Most anesthetized patients are supine, which decreases the lung volume and consequently the compliance. In a head-down and prone position, kidney and gallbladder support further diminishes the thoracic compliance.[18]

Ventilatory pattern. Shallow regular respirations cause a progressive diminution of lung compliance in animals and man.[19] This can be returned to normal by overinflation of the lung.

Alteration of pulmonary blood flow. Alterations in the distribution of pulmonary blood flow, whether this is a separate entity or is due to shunting of blood in the collapsed alveoli, has to be determined.

Distribution of the inspired gases.   Change in the pattern of the distribution of the inspired gases during anesthesia or artificial ventilation can have an effect.

Ether and cyclopropane.   These cause a decrease in compliance probably from an increase in bronchomotor tone.[18] Similar findings can be found in stimulation at light levels of anesthesia.[20]

DISEASE STATES

Deficiency of surfactant, as seen in the respiratory distress syndrome and after the use of cardiopulmonary bypass, leads to diminution of compliance. They are further aggravated by the atelectasis from the uneven ventilation occurring in this condition. Diminution of compliance occurs in chronic inflammatory conditions of the lungs, pulmonary fibrosis, congestion of pulmonary vessels and is very marked in pulmonary edema.

Emphysema may lead to an increase in static compliance due to the destruction of septa. However, the dynamic compliance is decreased markedly from maldistribution of inspired gases. For practical purposes, the lungs of emphysematous patients are stiff.

Dynamic Compliance

The dynamic compliance or the nonelastic resistance has two main components: (1) viscous resistance of the lung and chest wall and (2) the airflow resistance. The first provides about 20 percent of the total lung nonelastic resistance in normal conditions, is a constant factor and does not vary markedly in most of the physiologic and pathologic conditions. The airflow resistance represents 70 to 80 percent of the total nonelastic resistance of the lungs and depends mainly on the characteristic of the airway, the patterns, and rate of flow.

There are three types of flow that occur in the respiratory system.

LAMINAR FLOW

Here the flow of gases is in the form of concentric cylinders sliding one over the other, with the central cylinder moving faster than the peripheral cylinder (Fig. 11-9). Laminar flow is usually silent and occurs mostly in the airways below the main bronchi. Laminar flow is governed by the Poisseuille formula (Chap. 4) according to which the pressure difference is directly proportional to the flow rate and inversely proportional to the fourth power of the diameter of the tube. The conical shape of the laminar flow has the advantage that if the tidal volume is less than the dead space of the lung,

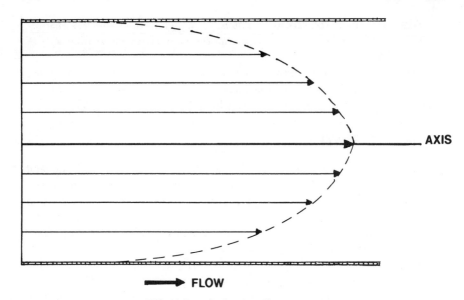

FLOW

FIG. 11-9:   The laminar flow pattern.

then some of the inspired gases (the middle of the cone) reach the alveoli. This can explain the survival of anesthetized patients with tidal volumes of as little as 100 ml.

TURBULENT FLOW

When the flow in the airway exceeds a critical velocity defined as a Reynold's number more than 2000, then the flow becomes turbulent. However, turbulence is more likely to occur when the diameter or the direction of a tube is changing or whenever branching occurs. Turbulent gas flows are usually audible. The flow in the trachea is turbulent in character. Quantitatively, turbulent flow differs from laminar flow in that the pressure gradient which is required to produce a given flow rate is proportional to the square of the gas flow rate and inversely proportional to the fifth power of the radius.

ORIFICE FLOW

This type of flow occurs at constrictions such as the larynx. In this situation, the pressure drop is also proportional to the square of flow rate, but density becomes an important factor instead of viscosity, eg, the advantage of administering a low-density gas such as helium in situations of severe respiratory obstructions.

One also must realize that the flow pattern in the airway is sinusoidal, and this characteristic flow pattern is not absolute and might change with the sequence of the respiratory cycle. With the expansion of the lung, the airways are elongated and widened. The effect of widening predominates over the elongation (fourth power against direct relationship). Thus, the airway resistance is diminished with lung expansion.

Airflow Resistance

Most of the energy used by the respiratory muscles is spent in overcoming the elastic recoil of the lungs and chest wall. In a normal man breathing at 15 times a minute, more than two-thirds of the energy spent is to overcome these elastic forces. However, the situation becomes reversed if he is breathing 50 times a minute where more than two-thirds of the work is spent in overcoming air flow resistance.[21]

During inspiration, intrapleural pressure decreases from −5 to −7.5 cm H_2O and, because the mouth pressure is atmospheric, the pulmonary resistance can be calculated from the following formula:

$$\text{Pulmonary resistance} = \frac{\text{Mouth pressure} - \text{intrapleural pressure}}{\text{Flow}}$$

The normal resistance to breathing is 0.05 to 2 cm H_2O per liter per second in adults. The total airway resistance can be affected by several factors, such as nasal breathing, head position, functional residual capacity, size of the glottic opening, and also by drugs and anesthetic agents. During oral breathing, the upper airway resistance (lips to trachea) represents about half of the total airway resistance. However, this is a very variable factor. The mere flexion of the head can double the upper airway resistance. Because of the very large number of airways smaller than 2 mm in diameter, their contribution to the pulmonary flow resistance is minimal.

VARIATIONS IN THE AIRWAY RESISTANCE

Lung volume. As the lungs are expanded, the airway resistance diminishes because the increased lung volume pulls and widens the conducting passages. The effect is partially counteracted in that the bronchi become longer with inspiration. The airway resistance is at minimum at lung volumes near the FRC, beyond which the resistance increases.[22]

At maximum inspiratory capacity, all the alveoli are open. However, during expiration with the diminution of the lung volumes, the smaller airways (0.5 to 1 mm) have a tendency to close, while the larger bronchioles and the bronchi remain open. The lung volume at which detectable small airway closure starts is known as closing volume. This airway closure occurs mostly in the dependent regions of the lung where during expiration the pleural pressure exceeds the airway pressure.

With increase in age and a progressive diminution in the elastic recoil of the lung, there is an increased tendency for airway closure, ie, an increase in closing volume.[23] Thus, in a seated person 65 years old, the closing volume exceeds the FRC. In the supine position, when the FRC decreases about 20 percent, the airway closure occurs at much smaller lung volumes.

BRONCHIAL MUSCLE TONE

Stimulation of the vagus leads to a diffuse constriction of the airway from the trachea to bronchi of about 0.5 mm in diameter, while sympathetic stimulation partially but not completely counteracts the effect of vagal stimulation.[24] Each of these components of the autonomic system can be influenced by impulses from visceral receptors, medullary centers, autonomic ganglia, and the neuroeffector junction.[25] The trachea and bronchi have cartilage in their walls. Therefore, stimulation of the bronchial muscle shortens as well as constricts them. However, the muscle fibers of the bronchioles and the alveolar ducts are well developed in comparison to their size. Thus, strong stimulation of these smooth muscle fibers can lead to an almost complete obstruction of the lumen.

Drugs can affect bronchomotor tone through several mechanisms. For example, acetylcholine causes bronchoconstriction by its action at the vagal cholinergic receptors of the bronchial smooth muscles, and this effect is blocked by atropine. Epinephrine causes bronchodilatation. This is a beta-receptor response because, if this effect is blocked by beta-blocking drugs, bronchoconstriction occurs from its alpha effect. Thus, drugs with beta-stimulating effect such as isoproterenol lead to bronchodilatation, while beta blockers such as propranolol lead to bronchoconstriction and might precipitate an asthmatic episode. Alpha activation produces the release of histamine and other humoral agents. Thus, drugs with alpha-blocking activity decrease the airway resistance.[26]

Reflex constriction of the bronchi occurs from inhalation of irritant gases, smoke, and dust that act on the subepithelial receptors that initiate the cough reflex. Histamine leads to an increase in airway resistance, and its release can be a part of antigen–antibody reaction. It can even be triggered by inhalation of cigarette smoke, and its release can be blocked by anticholinergic drugs. The source of histamine is the mast cells that also release heparin. The site of histaminergic receptors is not well defined but is probably in the bronchial smooth muscle. Similarly, microemboli injection leads to histamine release from the mast cells. The bronchi are also constricted reflexly by hypoxia and hypercapnia, mediated through the medullary and arterial chemoreceptors.

THE RESPONSE TO INCREASED AIRWAY RESISTANCE

During normal respiration, expiration is a passive process. If a resistance is added during expiration, expiration will not be complete during that time interval, leading to an increase in FRC and thus increasing the elastic recoil and causing more efficient emptying. Also, other factors come into play, such as actively using the expiratory muscle. However, too much increase in FRC puts the patient at a disadvantage because the muscles attain a position of mechanical disadvantage. Because resistance to air flow is directly related to the velocity of flow, patients with airway obstruction have a tendency to breathe slowly and deeply.

A patient usually does not experience dyspnea unless the resistance of breathing is increased to about three times, while severe dyspnea occurs when resistance is increased 5 to 15-fold.

THE EFFECT OF ANESTHESIA ON AIRWAY RESISTANCE

Anesthetics affect the bronchomotor tone.[25] Halothane produces bronchodilatation mediated by beta-receptor stimulation. Ether causes bronchodilatation through the same mechanism and also by releasing catecholamines from the adrenal medulla. Cyclopropane is the only inhalational anesthetic agent that increases the airway resistance. Atropine causes diminution in airway resistance, whereas morphine has a tendency to do the opposite. Meperidine and barbiturates have very little effect.

REFERENCES

1. Nunn JF: Applied Respiratory Physiology with Special Reference to Anaesthesia. New York, Appleton, 1960, p 6
2. Glazier JB, Hughes JM, Maloney JE, et al: Vertical gradient of alveolar size in dog lungs frozen in situ. J Physiol (London) 186:114, 1966
3. Mead J: Respiration: pulmonary mechanics. Ann Rev Physiol 35:169, 1973
4. Lichtiger M, Landa JF, Hirsch MA: Velocity of tracheal mucous in anesthetized women undergoing gynecologic surgery. Anesthesiology 42:753, 1975
5. Marfatia S, Donahoe PK, Hendren WH: Effect of dry and humidified gases on the respiratory epithelium in rabbits. J Pediatr Surg 10:583, 1975
6. Berry FA Jr, Hughes-Davies DI: Methods of increasing the humidity and temperature of the inspired gases in the infant circle system. Anesthesiology 37:456, 1972
7. Froese AB, Bryan AC: Effects of anesthesia and paralysis on diaphragmatic mechanics in man. Anesthesiology 41:242, 1974
8. Agostoni E: Mechanics of the pleural space. Physiol Rev 52:57, 1972
9. Hogg JC, Nepszy S: Regional lung volume and pleural pressure gradient estimated from lung density in dogs. J Appl Physiol 27:198, 1969

10. Agostoni E, Taglietti A, Setnikar I: Absorption force of the capillaries of the visceral pleura in determination of intrapleural pressure. Am J Physiol 191:277, 1957

11. Setnikar I, Agostoni E: Factors keeping the lung expanded in the chest. Proc Intern Union Physiol Sci 1:281, 1962

12. Comroe JH, Jr, et al: The Lung, 2nd ed. Chicago, Year Book, 1962

13. Clements JA: Pulmonary surfactant. Am Rev Resp Dis 101:984, 1970

14. Kotas RV, Avery ME: Accelerated appearance of pulmonary surfactant in the fetal rabbit. J Appl Physiol 30:358, 1971

15. Gluck L: Administration of corticosteroids to induce maturation of fetal lung. Am J Dis Child 130:976, 1976

16. Marshall R: The physical properties of the lungs in relation to the subdivision of lung volume. Clin Sci 16:507, 1957

17. Caro CG, Butler J, Dubois AB: Some effects of restriction of chest cage expansion on pulmonary function in man. J Clin Invest 39:573, 1960

18. Safar P, Aguto Escarraga L: Compliance in apneic anesthetized adults. Anesthesiology 20:283, 1959

19. Bendixen HH, Hedley-Whyte J, Laver MB: Impaired oxygenation in surgical patients during general anesthesia with controlled ventilation. N Engl J Med 269:991, 1963

20. Bromage PR: Total respiratory compliance in anaesthetized subjects and modifications produced by noxious stimuli. Clin Sci 17:217, 1958

21. Otis AB, Fenn WO, Rahm HJ: Mechanics of breathing in man. J Appl Physiol 2:592, 1950

22. West JB: Respiration. Annu Rev Physiol 34:91, 1972

23. Leblanc, P, Ruff F, Milic-Emili J: Effects of age and body position on "airway closure" in man. J Appl Physiol 28: 448, 1970

24. Nadel JA, Wolfe WG, Graf PO: Powdered tantalum as a medium for bronchography in canine and human lungs. Invest Radiol 3:229, 1968

25. Aviado DM: Regulation of bronchomotor tone during anesthesia. Anesthesiology 42:68, 1975

26. Cottrell JE, Wolfson B, Siker ES: Changes in airway resistance following droperidol, hydroxyzine and diazepam in normal volunteers. Anesth Analg (Cleve) 55:18, 1976

27. Comroe JH: Physiology of Respiration, 2nd ed. Chicago, Year Book, 1974

28. Sykes MK, Mechanics of ventilation. In Scurr C, Feldman S (eds): Scientific Foundations of Anaesthesia. Philadelphia, Davis, 1970 (originally published by Heinemann [London] 1970)

chapter 12

Regulation of Respiration

In contrast to the heart and smooth muscle, which can continue to function when completely denervated, the respiratory muscles cannot function if their central connection is severed. Another characteristic of the respiratory system is that it has a double control mechanism: (1) a voluntary system with its center in the forebrain (cerebral cortex), which sends impulses through the corticospinal tracts located in the dorsolateral part of the spinal cord, and (2) an automatic system located in the pons and medulla. The motor outflow of the latter is in the central and lateral columns of the spinal cord. The final integration of the outputs from these two centers occurs in the spinal cord.

RESPIRATORY CENTERS

Physiologists in the early part of the last century investigated respiration in animals by performing serial slices in the animal brain and watching the respiratory pattern. They found that removal of the cerebrum, cerebellum, or the midbrain had no appreciable effect on respiration.

In addition, if the upper part of the pons is transected from the brain stem, regular respiration continues. However, if the vagal nerves are cut at this stage, respiration stops at full inspiration, a phenomenon known as apneusis. This is usually followed by an apneustic pattern, ie, prolonged inspiratory spasms alternating with irregular respiratory movements. Further sectioning at the lower border of the pons leads to gasping, or irregular respirations, and, finally, transection at the lower medulla leads to complete cessation of breathing (Fig. 12-1).

With more refined techniques, such as by electrical stimulation and microelectrode recording of very small areas of the brain-stem regions, three main levels of respiratory centers have been localized, each with a different function. One of these three centers is located in the medulla, while the other

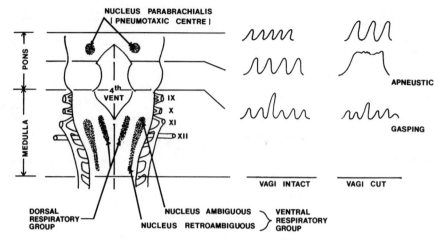

FIG. 12-1: The patterns of respiration after transection of the brain stem with vagi intact and transected. Modified after Mitchell and Berger.[1]

two are located in the pons, ie, the pneumotaxic center in the upper pons and the apneustic center in the lower pons.

Medullary Respiratory Center

The medullary respiratory center consists of three aggregations of rhythmic respiratory neurons: the dorsal respiratory grouping associated with the nucleus of the tractus solitarius and two ventrolateral respiratory groupings associated with the nucleus ambiguous and nucleus retroambiguous.[1] The classic inspiratory and expiratory centers are not well delineated as discrete nuclei but are a poorly defined collection of cells with various components. Each neural localization seems to carry an integrative function. The dorsal group provides a source of drive to the contralateral phrenic nerves and is an integration and relay site for some of the reflexes, such as the Hering–Breuer and the sniff reflex. The motor neurons of the nucleus ambiguous innervate the ipsilateral accessory nerves, while the nucleus retroambiguous provides the rhythmic drive to the intercostal muscles (inspiratory and expiratory) and probably to the abdominal muscles. Thus, there is an anatomic and functional separation between the groups of respiratory cells in the medulla, but the mechanism by which these centers are coordinated is not well understood. One theory is that there are pacemaker cells in the respiratory center that show a rhythmic pattern of activity in the absence of inputs into the cell. However, intracellular recordings from respiratory neurons have shown no evidence of such a property.[2]

A recent theory is that inhibitory phasing occurs in the dorsal respiratory group of nuclei in the medulla. The inhibitory phasing of the inspiratory cells generates the inspiratory rhythm, and periodic inhibition of tonically active expiratory neurons results in the respiratory cycle.[1]

STIMULI AFFECTING THE RESPIRATORY CENTER

The actions of the respiratory center are modified by impulses reaching it from both its central connection and the periphery. Its central connections includes the pons, hypothalamus, reticular activating system, central chemoreceptor, and cortex. The peripheral afferents are through the vagus and the glossopharyngeal nerves, which bring information from the peripheral chemoreceptors, from the lungs and chest wall.

Pontine Respiratory Centers

The medullary nuclei can maintain a gasping, rhythmic type of respiration, but, to have a smooth transition between inspiration and expiration without any interruption, the function of the pons must be intact. The pontine centers show a continuous phasic activity with the medullary centers during the respiratory cycle. There are two collections of cells in the pons affecting the medullary centers.

THE PNEUMOTAXIC CENTER

This is located in the upper part of the pons at the region of the nucleus parabrachialis in the dorsolateral rostral pons. Its neurons do not have any intrinsic activity of their own, but its destruction leads to slowing of the respiratory rate. If the vagi are cut, respiration is held in a position of full inspiration. Stimulation of the pneumotaxic center leads to an increase in respiratory rate accompanied by hyperventilation. Its function is not well defined, but it appears that it inhibits the lower pontine center and the apneustic center from holding respiration in the inspiratory apneustic position.

THE APNEUSTIC CENTER

This is located in the upper and middle part of the pons at the level of the area vestibularis. Its stimulation leads to inspiratory spasm (apneusis), while transection below it abolishes apneusis and causes a gasping type of respiration. The apneustic center is the site of the origin of the long reticulospinal fibers. These fibers affect the membrane potential of the respiratory motorneurons of the cord. This effect is important for the fine control of respiratory movements, but their effect is of secondary importance in the hierarchic structure associated with the generation of the respiratory rhythm.[3]

CORTICAL FIBERS

Voluntary acts such as speaking, breath-holding, or hyperventilation lead to alterations in the rhythmic respiratory activity. The nerve fibers from the cortical areas travel through the reticular formation and the corticospinal fibers located in the dorsolateral part of the cord, whereas the fibers transmitting the involuntary rhythmic patterns from the pons and medulla lie in the ventral and lateral parts of the cord. The final integration of these two sets of neurons occurs at the spinal level. Thus, lesions in the motor cortex can affect voluntary respiratory acts without altering automatic breathing. Conversely, localized lesions of the nuclei at the brain stem can affect respiratory rhythm without any impairment of voluntary respiratory acts. A similar situation exists in patients with bilateral anterocervical cordotomy for pain and intact lateral corticospinal tracts. These patients are liable to stop breathing when they are asleep, but their voluntary respiration is intact (Ondine's curse).[4] A condition similar to the above has been observed with tumors compressing the medulla and in bulbar poliomyelitis. Narcotic overdose, especially with sublimaze (Fentanyl), can produce a similar situation in which patients are liable to be apneic, insensitive to carbon dioxide, but will breathe on command.

CENTRAL CHEMORECEPTORS

By definition, a chemoreceptor is a receptor that responds to a change in chemistry of the blood or fluid around it. The central chemoreceptors are located close to the ventrolateral surface of the medulla near the exit of the glossopharyngeal and vagus nerves.[5] Local application or perfusion of the cerebral ventricles with simulated cerebrospinal fluid (CSF) with high CO_2 content or high H^+ concentration stimulates breathing within a few seconds. Conversely, low CO_2 and low H^+ concentrations depress ventilation.

The central chemoreceptors are influenced more by the chemical composition of CSF than by that of the blood. The blood–brain barrier is very permeable to CO_2, while it is impermeable to H^+ and HCO_3^-. Thus, whenever there is a rise in arterial P_{CO_2}, the CO_2 diffuses readily to the CSF, liberates H^+, which stimulates the chemoreceptors, leading to hyperventilation. This hyperventilation will lead to a reduction in blood CO_2 with a consequent reduction in CSF H^+, thus bringing the situation back to normal. The reason for the rapid changes in H^+ concentration in CSF due to hypo- or hypercapnia is that the CSF lacks the buffering capacity of hemoglobin. The threshold for the central ventilatory effect of P_{CO_2} is about 30 to 40 mm Hg and the effect is linear in the physiologic range.[6] In contrast to CO_2, hypoxemia has no effect on central chemoreceptors. As a matter of fact, hypoxemia in the absence of peripheral chemoreceptors depresses respiration due to its direct effect on the respiratory center (Chap. 24). However, in chronic acidosis, the pH of CSF is maintained near normal because the blood–brain barrier adjusts CSF bicarbonate concentration to bring its pH near its normal value of 7.32. The difference in bicarbonate concentration between blood and CSF is maintained by an ion pump at the blood–brain barrier.[7] A typical example is the patient with emphysema associated with CO_2 retention. He will have a near-normal CSF pH and unexpectedly low ventilation relative to his P_{CO_2}.

MIDBRAIN

Electrical stimulation of the reticular activating system in the midbrain or spontaneous increase in its activity, ie, arousal, will lead to an increase in respiration. Conversely, natural sleep or anesthesia will lead to reduced activity of this reticular-activating system and a diminution in respiration. Ablation of this area will lead to reduction in respiration and a decreased response to CO_2.

PERIPHERAL CHEMORECEPTORS

The peripheral chemoreceptors are located mainly in two discrete areas—the *carotid bodies* and *aortic bodies*. They are very richly supplied with blood vessels. As a matter of fact, they are the part of the body with highest blood supply per gram of tissue. Their blood supply is 40 times that of brain tissue (20 ml per g). Thus, a very small amount of oxygen is extracted from the blood flowing through them. The chemoreceptors are exposed to P_{O_2}, P_{CO_2}, and pH almost identical to that of the blood flowing within the arteries. The carotid body has two types of specialized cells: (1) Type I cells or glomus cells. These are relatively large cells and contain dense cored vesicles in their cytoplasm. They have a high content of catecholamines such as dopamine and 5-hydroxytriptamine. (2) Type II cells or satellite cells. These have tentacle-like structures surrounding the Type I cells. The exact mechanism by which these cells respond to low oxygen tension is not well understood. The sensory nerve terminals surrounded by the Type II cells have a high oxygen consumption. They might be directly activated by the low P_{O_2}[7] or the low P_{O_2} may release a chemical neurotransmitter such as acetylcholine, which activates the Type I cells, which leads to the release of their dopamine content. This in turn activates the sensory nerve endings.[8]

The response of the chemoreceptors to various stimuli can be studied by recording the electrical activity of the carotid sinus nerve. Because the peripheral chemoreceptors alter the ventilatory response much faster than the central chemoreceptors during changes in inspired concentration of gases, temporal isolation of their effect is possible.

The carotid bodies have the same organization and function as the aortic bodies. However, the carotid bodies seem to produce more involved respiratory response than the aortic, eg, chemical changes at the carotid chemoreceptors will increase the respiratory rate and depth, while the aortic chemoreceptors will only increase the frequency. However, the aortic chemoreceptors have a much more prominent cardiovascular effect than the carotids.[9]

The hypoxic drive for ventilation from the peripheral chemoreceptors is a very strong one. At the advanced stages of hypoxia in which the respiratory centers are so depressed that they are no longer responsive to direct chemical stimulation, the chemoreceptors by their activity can sustain respiration. The hypoxic drive for respiration is very important in emphysematous patients with CO_2 retention. Because of the chronic nature of the disease with the associated adjustment of CSF pH, the central chemoreceptors are depressed and the only stimulus to respiration in these patients is initiated by the effect of hypoxia on the peripheral chemoreceptors. Administration of high concentrations of oxygen might lead to respiratory arrest in these patients. If the clinical condition of these patients warrants the administration of oxygen, its concentration should be adjusted carefully and slowly so that the hypoxia is mildly relieved but the respiratory drive still continues.

Although the effect of hypoxia on the activity of the carotid receptors is well known, there is controversy about the threshold for its activity, ie, the Po_2 at which no change in ventilation occurs. If 100 percent O_2 is inspired instead of room air, there will be a transient respiratory depression. This respiratory depression is due to inhibition of the activity of the chemoreceptors from the high oxygen tension. Its duration is minimal because within a short time CO_2 accumulates, and this in turn stimulates the chemoreceptors, resulting in the return of minute ventilation back to normal. This transient fall in ventilation is only seen at inspired O_2 concentrations of about 35 percent (equivalent to Po_2 of 170 mm Hg). This indicates the existence of a peripheral chemoreceptor drive at a Po_2 of less than 170 mm Hg. The contribution of this drive to ventilation in a normal man is estimated to be on the order of 10 percent.[10,11]

In addition to the sensitivity of chemoreceptors to hypoxia, they are also sensitive to CO_2 changes that stimulate the receptors by decreasing their pH. There is a positive interaction between Pco_2 and Po_2 at the peripheral chemoreceptors, ie, the effect of hypercapnia on the chemoreceptor response to hypoxia is more than additive. It has been found that the efferent activity from the chemoreceptors in response to hypercapnia is higher in the presence of hypoxia than the simple addition of each response alone.[6] Also, oscillations in Pco_2 are more effective in raising chemoreceptor drive than absolute increases in P_{CO_2}. These oscillations of P_{CO_2} can account partly for the hyperventilation seen during exercise.[12]

In humans, removal of the carotid bodies without removing the aortic bodies leads to loss of ventilatory response to hypoxia and an approximately 30 percent reduction in ventilatory response to CO_2 without any change in ventilation at rest. An interesting observation in people without carotid bodies is that they can hold their breath longer than normal persons.

PULMONARY STRETCH REFLEXES

The inflation and deflation reflexes were originally described by Hering and Breuer in 1868. In anesthetized animals, distension of the lung leads to a reduction in inspiratory efforts and, conversely, deflation of the lungs causes an increase in inspiratory efforts. Cutting of the vagi abolishes this reflex, and the animal now breathes slowly with large tidal volumes, ie, there is no reflex cutting inspiration and expiration short. The receptors of the inspiratory component of the reflexes are probably located in the smooth muscles of the bronchi and bronchioles, while the receptors of the deflation reflex are in the air ducts and alveoli. The inspiratory receptors can be stimulated by chemicals such as veratrine, leading to tachypnea, and they are blocked by low concentrations of local anesthetic agents, resulting in maximal inspiratory efforts.

It was assumed that the tachypnea induced by trichloroethylene was due to sensitization of pulmonary stretch receptors. However, it has been demonstrated that in midcollicular decerebrate cats, tachypnea induced by trichloroethylene cannot be prevented by bilateral vagotomy and carotid denervation.[13]

The exact contribution of the Hering–Breuer reflex to the normal breathing pattern is not well defined. It does not seem to be active at low tidal volumes but is present at lung volumes of 800 ml above the FRC. It might be involved in regulating the respiratory rate, and, in the absence of the pneumotaxic center, it helps to maintain a relatively normal depth of breathing, ie, termination of apneusis.[14] The normal breathing pattern of man at rest (tidal volume, 400 ml; rate, 15 per minute) is adjusted so that the work of breathing is at a minimum. If he augments his tidal volume beyond the normal 400 ml and decreases his rate, the work to overcome the elastic recoil will disproportionately increase. Conversely, if he breathes at a faster rate, the airflow resistance will disproportionately increase.

In situations in which the lungs are stiffened as in pulmonary fibrosis, the respiration becomes shallow and rapid to minimize the elastic work. The receptors of the inflation reflex are probably the ones that provide the necessary information that is needed to achieve this optimal pattern of breathing. The opposite situation occurs in patients with narrowing of airways, such as in asthmatic patients who breathe slowly and deeply.

The deflation receptors are occasionally termed J receptors because of their juxtacapillary position. They are believed to be the receptors involved in the tachypnea of pulmonary congestion, edema, and embolization and also are the receptors initiating tachypnea seen with halothane.[15]

Paradoxical Reflex of Head

Inflation of the lung produces a paradoxical effect, ie, further inspiration. This is opposite to the Hering–Breuer reflex in which inflation of the lung induces expiration. It can be produced in animals by selectively cooling the vagus nerve and is abolished by cutting the vagus. It may play a part in the physiologic mechanism of sighing in the adult by perpetuating the inspiration and in producing a deep breath. It can also be elicited in the newborn in whom it can be involved in expanding the lung.

Reflexes from the Respiratory Muscles

As in other muscle control systems, the intercostal muscles contain muscle spindles that lie parallel to the extrafusal fibers, and they constitute a muscle length-detecting feedback mechanism. During inspiration, impulses reach the main intercostal muscles through the alpha motoneurons, while the intrafusal fibers are stimulated through the efferent gamma motoneurons, leading to the contraction of both the intercostal and the intrafusal muscles (Fig. 12-2). If the contraction of the muscle is unopposed, there will be a minimal increase in the

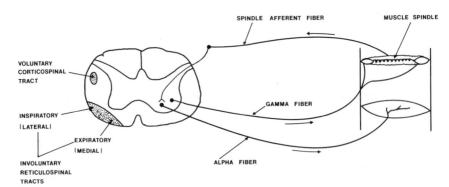

FIG. 12-2: The descending respiratory pathways in the spinal cord (left) and a diagrammatic representation of the gamma system.

tension of the stretch receptors of the spindle. However, if the muscle is contracting against a resistance (stiff chest wall), the tension in the stretch receptors in the spindle will increase. This will lead to a reflex increase in the activity of the alpha motoneurons and more muscle fibers will be activated, thus strengthening the force of contraction. Therefore, the main function of the gamma system is to adjust the force of contraction against changing resistance.[16]

In respiratory muscles, the afferents from the muscle spindles are found not to inhibit but actually excite antagonist motoneurons, ie, the gamma inspiratory motoneurons are inhibited during expiration, thus providing another mechanism by which reflex proprioceptive excitation of antagonist muscles is prevented.[1] In contrast to the intercostal nerves, the phrenic nerve seems to have very little proprioceptive activity.

Other Reflexes

There are several other reflexes that can affect respiration. The *arterial baroreceptors,* which are primarily concerned with regulation of circulation, have a respiratory component. Therefore, a sharp rise in arterial blood pressure leads to reflex hypoventilation and even apnea from the stimulation of aortic and carotid sinus baroreceptors. Conversely, hypotension leads to hyperventilation. However, the hyperventilation of shock is mostly caused by the effects of acidosis and hypoxia on the chemoreceptors. Stimulation of lung-irritant receptors located between the epithelial cells of the bronchi and bronchioles initiate the *cough reflex.* Cough starts by a deep inspiration, followed by a forced expiration against a closed glottis, then the glottis suddenly opens to expulse the contents of the airways. The air might reach a velocity of 600 mph. A *hiccup* is a sudden spasmodic contraction of the diaphragm during which the glottis closes suddenly. Hiccups involve a central mechanism largely independent of the rhythmic respiratory system.

Carbon Dioxide–Ventilation Response Curves

The most satisfactory method of defining the sensitivity of the respiratory mechanism to drugs is performed by measuring and plotting the minute ventilation at various levels of carbon dioxide tensions. The determination of the effect of a drug on the response curve is much more helpful than a single measurement of ventilation or P_{CO_2}, without any regard to the interaction of these two variables. Stimulant drugs, or any nonspecific arousal state, is associated with a shift of the CO_2 response curve to the left, while sleep shifts the response curve to the right in a somewhat parallel fashion (Fig. 12-3).

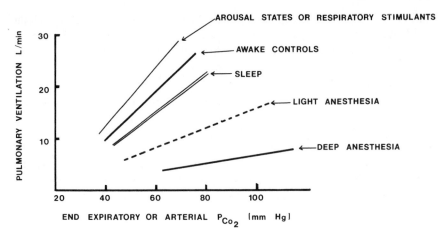

FIG. 12-3: Carbon dioxide/ventilation response curves at various states. Note the marked flattening of the curve at deep anesthetic levels.

A marked change in the slope of the respiratory response curve to carbon dioxide occurs after almost all anesthetic agents. The change in slope produced by all these dissimilar agents, such as halothane, nitrous oxide-innovar, ether, and cyclopropane, is similar when expressed at equipotent alveolar concentrations. The slope of the P_{CO_2}–ventilation curve diminishes progressively with deepening in the level of anesthesia. At high anesthetic levels it becomes flat, indicating the absence of any ventilatory response to a further rise in carbon dioxide level.[16]

In earlier studies, it was found that small doses of narcotics such as morphine and meperidine shifted the CO_2 response curve in a parallel fashion to the right. Thus, it was assumed that the respiratory centers were still as sensitive to CO_2 as in the awake state, but the threshold had been raised. However, in a recent study, it was found that 7.5 mg of morphine administered subcutaneously in normal subjects produced a substantial decrease in the slope of the CO_2 response curve.[17] In this study morphine also caused depression of hypoxic drive, indicating that there is depression in the response of the respiratory center to CO_2 in the presence of morphine, but whether this effect is at the peripheral chemoreceptors or at the level of the central nervous system is still to be determined.

REFERENCES

1. Mitchell RA, Berger AJ: Neural regulation of respiration. Am Rev Resp Dis 111:206, 1975
2. Mitchell RA, Herbert DA: Synchronized high frequency synaptic potentials in medullary respiratory neurons. Brain Res 75:350, 1974

3. Andersen P, Sears TA: Medullary activation of intercostal fusimotor and alpha motoneurons. J Physiol (Lond) 209:739, 1970
4. Severinghaus JW, Mitchell RA: Ondine's curve—failure of respiratory center automaticity while awake. Clin Res 10:122, 1962
5. Mitchell RA, Loeschke HH, Massion WH, et al: Respiratory responses mediated through superficial chemosensitive areas in the medulla. J Appl Physiol 18:523, 1963
6. Duffin J: The chemical regulation of ventilation. Anaesthesia 26:142, 1971
7. Fencl V, Miller TB, Pappenheimer JR: Studies on the respiratory response to disturbances of acid–base balance, with deductions concerning the ionic composition of cerebral interstitial fluid. Am J Physiol 210:459, 1966
8. McDonald DM, Mitchell RA: A quantitative analysis of the synaptic connections in the rat carotid body. In Purves M (ed): Chemoreceptor Mechanisms. Cambridge, Cambridge University Press, 1974
9. Comroe JH Jr, Mortimer L: The respiratory and cardiovascular responses of temporally separated aortic and carotid bodies to cyanide, nicotine, phenylguanide and serotonin. J Pharmacol Exp Ther 146:33, 1964
10. Dejours P: Chemoreflexes in breathing. Physiol Rev 42:335, 1962
11. Downes JJ, Lambertsen CJ: Dynamic characteristics of ventilatory depression in man on abrupt administration of oxygen. J Appl Physiol 21:447, 1966
12. Bhattacharyya N, Cunningham DJ, Goode RC, et al: Hypoxia, ventilation, P_{CO_2} and exercise. Resp Physiol 9:329, 1970
13. Ngai SH, Katz RL, Farhie SE: Respiratory effects of trichlorethylene, halothane and methoxyflurane in the cat. J Pharmacol Exp Ther 148:123, 1965
14. von Euler C, Herrero F, Wexler LI: Control mechanisms determining rate and depth of respiratory movements. Resp Physiol 10:93, 1970
15. Paintal AS: Vagal sensory receptors and their reflex effects. Physiol Rev 53:159, 1973
16. Dunbar BS, Ovassapian A, Smith TC: The effects of methoxyflurane on ventilation in man. Anesthesiology 28:1020, 1967
17. Weil JV, McCullough RE, Kline JS et al: Diminished ventilatory response to hypoxia and hypercapnia after morphine in normal man. N Engl J Med 292:1103, 1975

chapter 13

Pulmonary Circulation

GENERAL FEATURES

The pulmonary circulation is characteristically a low-pressure, low-resistance system, in series with the systemic circulation. It is the only arterial circuit in man that carries desaturated blood in his extrauterine life.

Anatomically, the pulmonary vessels are similar to the systemic vessels except that their walls are much thinner than the systemic vessels, and the pulmonary arterioles, unlike the systemic, have very few muscles in their walls. The pulmonary capillaries form a dense network in the walls of the 350 million alveoli and provide a gas-exchange surface of 70 sq meters. Lymphatic channels are abundantly present in the lung, but they only reach as far as the terminal bronchioles and are absent in the alveolar walls.

The mean *pulmonary arterial pressure* is 15 mm Hg, with a systolic pressure of 25 mm Hg and a diastolic pressure of 10 mm Hg. The left atrial pressure is about 7 mm Hg during diastole, so that the pressure gradient in the pulmonary bed is about 8 mm Hg. The greatest resistance to flow is in the pre-capillary vessels.

The mean *pulmonary capillary pressure* is about 10 mm Hg, whereas the plasma oncotic pressure is 25 mm Hg. Thus, a net pressure gradient of 15 mm Hg encourages the movement of fluids into the capillaries and keeps the alveoli dry.

The *pulmonary vascular resistance,* similar to the other resistances, is computed from the original Ohm's law:

$$\text{Vascular resistance} = \frac{\text{Input pressure} - \text{output pressure}}{\text{Blood flow}}$$

$$\text{Pulmonary vascular resistance} = \frac{\text{Mean pulmonary arterial pressure} - \text{left atrial pressure}}{\text{Cardiac output}}$$

$$= \frac{15 - 7}{5} = 1.6 \text{ mm Hg per liter per minute}$$
$$(100 \text{ dynes per second per cm}^{-5})$$

Therefore, the resistance offered by the pulmonary circulation to the right ventricle is less than one-tenth of the resistance offered by the systemic circulation to the left ventricle.

The *pulmonary blood volume* is about 600 ml, of which only 100 ml is present in the capillaries, while most of the remaining pulmonary blood volume is distributed in the compliant pulmonary venous system. This pulmonary blood volume can increase by 40 percent when the individual lies down, and this extra volume is shifted into the systemic circulation when standing up. This sudden shift of blood from systemic to pulmonary circulation is responsible for the decrease in vital capacity in the supine position and for the occurrence of orthopnea in heart failure.

The amount of blood present in the pulmonary circulation depends on two interacting and opposing mechanical and vasomotor effects. Under normal circumstances, the mechanical effects predominate, ie, displacement of blood by changes in posture or in the intrathoracic pressure. However, in circulatory stress, with generalized sympathetic stimulation, the vasomotor effects predominate and the pulmonary blood volume declines.

Bronchial Circulation

The blood supply of the bronchi and the parenchymatous structures of the lung are part of the systemic circulation. The bronchi receive their blood supply from the bronchial arteries, which are branches of the thoracic aorta. The capillaries of the bronchial vessels anastomose freely with the capillaries of the pulmonary circulation. A small part of the bronchial flow reaches the systemic circulation through the azygos vein; however, the greater portion drains into the pulmonary venous system. These bronchial veins emptying into the pulmonary veins and the sinusoidal veins draining the left ventricle are the main components of the "anatomic shunt."

Characteristic Features of Pulmonary Circulation

The pulmonary vessels, similar to the systemic vessels, are subject to autonomic control. The sympathetic system supplies vasoconstrictor and vasodilator fibers to the pulmonary vessels. Norepinephrine, the alpha-adrenergic stimulator, produces vasoconstriction, whereas isoproterenol, the beta-adrenergic stimulator, produces pulmonary vasodilatation.[1] The vagus supplies cholinergic parasympathetic fibers, which cause dilatation of the bronchial vessels. Despite the presence of this extensive autonomic supply, in normal resting conditions, the vasomotor tone is minimal and pulmonary vessels are almost maximally dilated.

Because the walls of the pulmonary vessels are thin, their diameter is more liable to change from variation in the intramural or transmural pressures than from changes in the contraction or relaxation of their smooth muscles. The capillaries and the very small vessels running between the alveoli are exposed to alveolar pressure. Therefore, their caliber depends mainly on the difference between their intraluminal pressure and alveolar pressure. Thus, if the pressure in the alveoli exceeds the intravascular pressure of the capillaries (during Valsalva), these capillaries collapse and the flow inside them almost ceases. The size of the moderate vessels embedded in the lung parenchyma mostly depends on the pulmonary volume. These vessels are pulled open with the expansion of the lung. Therefore, their vascular resistance is low at large lung volumes, and their resistance increases at low lung volumes.[2] Also the size of these vessels can be affected by vasoactive drugs. Serotonin, histamine, and norepinephrine increase the tone of these vessels, and these drugs are particularly effective when the lung volumes are low. The largest pulmonary vessels are located in the hilum of the lung, outside the lung parenchyma. Their caliber varies with changes in intrapleural pressure.

In the standing adult, the vessels at the apex of the lung are about 15 cm higher than the pulmonary artery, whereas those at the base are at an equal distance below it. Because the pulmonary arterial pressure is low and the distribution of blood in the pulmonary capillaries is affected by gravity, the capillaries at the apex of the lung are barely open, while those at the base are fully distended. In the supine position, the blood flow in the apical zones increases, while the flow in the basal zones remains constant. Thus, the distribution of blood flow in the supine position becomes rather uniform. If the person is suspended upside down, his apical pulmonary blood flow will be higher than his basal flow.[3] This flow distribution pattern in the lungs is reversed in patients with mitral stenosis and in patients after a myocardial infarction. Under these conditions the blood flow going to the lowest zones of the lung is reduced, while flow in the upper lobes is increased.[4] The most likely explanation is that the rise in pulmonary venous pressure leads to perivascular interstitial edema, which in turn increases the vascular resistance in the lung bases.

Clinically, segmental pulmonary blood flow can be studied by radioactive xenon (^{133}Xe), which can be injected intravenously as a saline solution while the chest is monitored by a set of radiation detectors. When the radioactive xenon reaches the pulmonary capillaries, it diffuses into the alveolar gas because of its low solubility. In the well-perfused regions of the lung, the radioactivity is detected very early, while it is delayed in the poorly diffused regions.

Hypoxic Pulmonary Vasoconstriction

A special feature of the pulmonary circulation is that alveolar hypoxia leads to pulmonary vasoconstriction, which is in marked contrast to the systemic circulation, where tissue hypoxia leads to marked vasodilatation. Whenever the oxygen tension of the alveolar gas is markedly reduced, the vascular smooth muscles supplying the arterioles in that particular region constrict, diverting the blood to a better ventilated region of the lung. This response occurs in isolated denervated lungs as well as in intact lungs. A remarkable feature of this response is that the stimulus for vasoconstriction is the alveolar oxygen tension, not the pulmonary arterial blood. Usually, the vasoconstriction occurs when the alveolar oxygen tension drops below 70 mm Hg. At oxygen tensions above 100 mm Hg, no further vasodilatation occurs. This vasoconstriction from low alveolar oxygen tension is enhanced by extracellular acidosis as well as by hypercapnia. The exact mechanism by which this vasoconstriction occurs is not well understood, but in most probability it is due to the release of a vasoconstrictor substance by the periarterial mast cells acting on the alpha receptors of the small pulmonary arteries, leading to their constriction.[5] This pulmonary vasoconstriction is very marked in the fetus with collapsed lungs. With the delivery of the fetus and the aeration of the lung, pulmonary vasoconstriction decreases, and the blood flow to the lungs increases. In the newborn infant, this reflex seems to be more active than in the adult because a short exposure of the infant to hypoxia can lead to a marked increase in pulmonary vascular resistance. Because of the patent ductus arteriosus, the pulmonary circulation will be diverted to the systemic circulation, further aggravating the hypoxia.

In addition to this regional effect of hypoxia on the pulmonary vessels, systemic hypoxia, by reflexes mediated through the chemoreceptors, can increase the pulmonary arterial and right ventricular pressures without changing the pulmonary capillary pressure. In situations of generalized hypoxia, such as in inhabitants of high altitudes, pulmonary hypertension develops, which is reversible in the early stages by oxygen breathing or returning to low altitudes.

Acetylcholine, which has no appreciable effect on the intact pulmonary circulation, reverses this pulmonary pressure response to hypoxia by relaxing the vasoconstricted pulmonary vascular smooth muscles, presumably by a direct effect.

Effects of Respiration

During inspiration, the flow to the right side of the heart increases for two reasons: (1) The drop in intrapleural pressure distends the intrathoracic portions of the venae cavae, increasing the venous return into these veins. (2) The contraction of the diaphragm and the abdominal muscles raises the intraabdominal pressure, which also increases the gradient from the intraabdominal portion of the inferior vena cava to its intrathoracic portion. This augmented blood flow to the right atrium increases the right ventricular stroke volume.[6] The left ventricular output also increases in phase with the right ventricular output, but to a lesser extent because part of this excess blood is retained in the pulmonary vascular bed, which is also distended from the increased negative intrapleural pressure. These changes in flow pattern are accentuated during deep breathing and in chronic lung disease.

During inspiration the increased capacity of the pulmonary vascular bed leads to a reduction of the blood flow in the left atrium. Thus, the output of the left ventricle falls, and consequently the aortic pressure drops. After a few beats of the right ventricle, the pulmonary vessels become filled and the pressure in the left side of the heart increases, as do the aortic pressures.

If an individual expires against a resistance such as a closed glottis in a Valsalva maneuver, the intraalveolar and intrapleural pressures rise, and the pulmonary arterial pressure rises momentarily from compression of the pulmonary arteries. However, this last effect is transient because the high intrathoracic pressure impedes the flow in the venae cavae. Thus, the venous return to the right heart is diminished and the right ventricular output falls, leading to a drop in pulmonary artery pressure. This in turn is followed by a fall in left ventricular output and systemic arterial pressure. A prolonged rise in intrapleural pressure of more than 100 mm Hg can lead to a loss of consciousness.

In contrast to spontaneous respiration, during positive pressure breathing the pulmonary vessels are compressed with each inflation, leading to a rise in pulmonary vascular resistance, and thus the output of the right ventricle falls with each inflation.

Pulmonary Emboli

Embolization of the small pulmonary vessels leads to a marked rise in the pulmonary arterial pressure associated with bronchoconstriction, tachypnea, and, in severe cases, hypotension and bradycardia. Bronchoconstriction and pulmonary vasoconstriction are reflex in origin. They also occur in the nonoccluded areas of the lung. Serotonin, histamine, and 5-hydroxytryptamine have been incriminated as causative factors for these generalized responses. Tachypnea is reportedly due to stimulation of the pulmonary deflator receptors, which are innervated by the vagus.

BALLOON FLOTATION CATHETERS (SWAN–GANZ)

The balloon flotation catheter (Swan–Ganz) (Fig. 13-1) is a practical instrument for bedside right-heart catheterization and provides an effective tool for monitoring the right atrial, right ventricular, pulmonary artery, and pulmonary capillary wedge pressures, and for sampling mixed venous blood.[7] The standard catheter is made of polyvinylchloride, 100 cm long, with an outside diameter of 1.6 mm. It has two lumens, one terminating at the tip of the catheter for pressure monitoring and blood sampling, and the other for inflat-

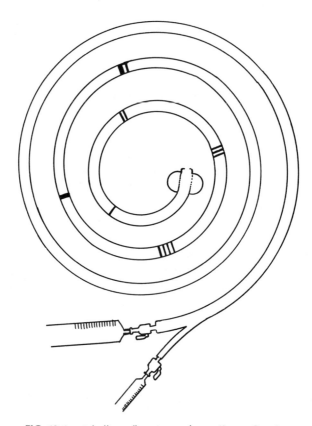

FIG. 13-1: A balloon flotation catheter (Swan–Ganz).

ing the balloon near the catheter tip. The balloon is so constructed that when inflated it does not obstruct the lumen at the catheter tip but forms a rounded end. A triple lumen catheter is also available with the third lumen terminating at 20 or 30 cm proximal to the catheter tip and is used for measuring the right atrial or right ventricular pressure simultaneously with the pulmonary pressures. Recently, a new catheter has become available with a thermistor embedded near its distal tip. Cardiac output can be measured with this catheter by recording the temperature changes in the pulmonary artery after injecting a cold (or room-air temperature) solution into the right atrium through the proximal lumen of the catheter (Chap. 3).

After filling with heparinized solution, the Swan–Ganz catheter is introduced into one of the major veins of the body—antecubital, subclavian, or jugular—either by cutdown or by percutaneous puncture. After the catheter is passed centrally for about 30 cm, it is connected to a pressure transducer. The position of the catheter is checked on the oscilloscope for pressure variations. As the catheter enters the great veins in the thoracic cavity, variations in pressures with respiration are seen. This oscillation becomes marked with coughing. At this point, the balloon is half inflated (0.8 ml) and the blood flow carries the catheter to the right atrium where the heart rate pulsations are superimposed on the respiratory pattern. As the catheter is advanced into the right ventricle, a dramatic change in the oscillatory pattern is seen. The small amplitude atrial waves are replaced by tall waves (Fig. 13-2). The normal systolic pressure in the right ventricle is about one-sixth of systemic pressure, while the diastolic is zero. As the catheter reaches the pulmonary artery a marked rise in diastolic pressure is seen.[8] Wedging the catheter by fully inflating the balloon, one can have an indirect reading of left atrial pressure. The mean values for pulmonary wedge pressures and left atrial pressures are, for practical purposes, similar. If wedging of the catheter is not possible, the pulmonary diastolic pressure is a very good approximation to it.[9]

Taking a zero reference, the midpoint between the sternum and the back of the fourth interspace at the horizontal position, the normal left atrial pressure is 6 to 8 mm Hg (always less than 12 mm Hg). However, in certain heart diseases, a left ventricular filling pressure of 14 to 18 mm Hg is optimal for cardiac performance. It seems that at this pressure the myocardial fibers are stretched to the most optimal length (Frank–Starling mechanism). At wedge pressures of 20 mm Hg, fluid starts accumulating in the lung. At 30 to 35 mm Hg, pulmonary edema is present.

The normal pulmonary artery pressure tracing is characterized by a steep rise followed by a rapid fall until the pulmonic valves close (dicrotic notch). After the dicrotic notch, this fall in pressure is more gradual. The normal pulmonary systolic pressure is about 25 mm Hg and the diastolic is 10 mm Hg.

Pulmonary hypertension can be secondary to any of the following:

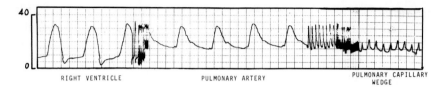

RIGHT VENTRICLE   PULMONARY ARTERY   PULMONARY CAPILLARY
                                                             WEDGE

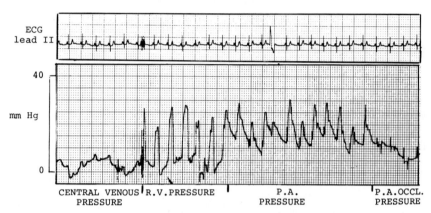

CENTRAL VENOUS   R.V.PRESSURE   P.A.   P.A.OCCL.
PRESSURE   PRESSURE   PRESSURE

FIG. 13-2: Actual recordings of right ventricular, pulmonary artery, and pulmonary wedge pressures through a Swan–Ganz catheter. (Courtesy Dr. D. G. Lappas.)

1. Intrinsic lung disease
2. Pulmonary vascular affections such as pulmonary embolism and pulmonary hypertension
3. Increased pulmonary blood flow (left-to-right shunt)
4. Raised end-diastolic pressure of the left ventricle as in left ventricular failure or of the left atrium as in mitral stenosis

ANESTHETICS AND PULMONARY CIRCULATION

The effect of anesthetics on pulmonary circulation seems to vary according to the anesthetic agent used. Halothane or halothane-nitrous oxide anesthesia does not affect the pulmonary arterial and wedge pressures nor the pulmonary vascular resistance, whereas cyclopropane almost doubles the pulmonary vascular resistance due to arteriolar constriction with a marked increase in pulmonary arterial and wedge pressures.[10] This is probably a sympathetic effect. Similarly, nitrous oxide in the presence of morphine increases the pulmonary vascular resistance and the left ventricular end-diastolic pressure in patients with coronary artery diseases.[11] Alpha-adrenergic blockers reverse these changes. Pentolinium, which is a ganglionic blocker used for hypotensive anesthesia, decreases the pulmonary vascular resistance in patients anesthetized with nitrous oxide–halothane anesthesia.[12]

NONRESPIRATORY FUNCTIONS OF THE LUNG

The anatomic location of the lung is unique such that all the blood draining from the systemic vessels must pass through its capillaries. Therefore, large-sized foreign particles are trapped in the lung. Otherwise, if these escaped into the systemic circulation they might end up in a vital artery with disastrous consequences.

Of the multitudes of nonrespiratory functions of the lung, the following seem to be the most important:[13]

Filter

In general, any foreign particles larger than the pulmonary capillaries are trapped within the lung. These include fibrin or blood clots, fat cells, bone marrow, masses of platelets, or white cells. It also clears the debris and particles that are found in intravenous solutions. This filtering of the lung is lost during cardiopulmonary bypass or whenever there is a right-to-left shunt. In these situations, an embolus in the venous system might find its way into the systemic circulation and end up in a vital artery, such as the coronary or cerebral. The pulmonary circulation also removes white cells and platelets from the blood. It is suggested that it acts as a "leukostat," maintaining a preset level of circulating white cells.

Blood Reservoir

The amount of blood present in the pulmonary circulation represents about 10 percent of the total blood volume. Occasionally, this blood volume is described as a blood store for the left ventricle, providing it with a continuous supply of blood despite the wide variation in venous return to the right. In normal physiologic conditions of rest or exercise, the pulmonary volume is rather constant even during intravenous infusion of fluids.[14] However, in chronic circulatory congestion, such as in heart failure, the pulmonary blood volume increases *pari passu* with the increase in total blood. The opposite occurs in hypovolemia and shock, in which it is diminished.

Fluid and Solute Exchange

Under normal conditions, about 250 ml of water (equivalent to 350 kcal of heat) is lost through the respiratory tract per day. This water loss is increased during fever and hyperventilation. This is the only mechanism for heat loss in furry animals, such as the dog. Conversely, if water is deposited into the lung, it gets rapidly absorbed. This is because the pulmonary capillary pressure (8 to 10 mm Hg) is lower than the plasma oncotic pressure (25 mm Hg), which pulls fluid from the alveoli into the blood. This rapid absorption of water has a special significance in fresh water drowning, in which the large amount of absorbed water can lead to hemolysis of the red cells.

The lung is also a source of solute excretion. About 15 to 30 osmoles (Osm) of CO_2 is excreted by the lung per day in contrast to the kidney, which excretes 0.5 to 1.0 Osm of solute per day.

All metabolites of the blood that are volatile at 37 C can traverse the alveolar capillary membranes according to their partition coefficient. Metabolites that appear in breath include acetone in diabetic ketoacidosis, methyl mercaptan in hepatic failure, and ammonia in renal failure. Volatile anesthetic agents are absorbed and excreted through the lungs. Drugs intended for local use in the tracheobronchial tree are rapidly absorbed into the circulation, ie, isoproterenol and local anesthetics. They will appear in the circulation as fast as in intravenous injection.

Metabolic Functions of the Lung

Metabolic functions of the lung include:

1. Formation of surfactant by the Type II alveolar cells.
2. Regulation of the plasma concentration of vasoactive agents, 5-hydroxytryptamine, bradykinin, angiotensin, and prostaglandins. It has been proposed that the lung removes substances intended for local effect, such as norepinephrine, while hormones intended for general systemic effect pass unchanged through the pulmonary circulation.[15]
3. Intrapulmonary release of histamine and serotonin from mast cells in response to embolism, hypoxia or in anaphylactic reactions.

REFERENCES

1. Porcelli RJ, Bergofsky EH: Adrenergic receptors in pulmonary vasoconstrictor responses to gaseous and humoral agents. J Appl Physiol 34:488, 1973

2. Hughes JM, Glazier JB, Maloney JE, et al: Effect of lung volume on the distribution of pulmonary blood flow in man. Resp Physiol 4:58, 1968
3. West JB: Respiratory Physiology: The Essentials. Baltimore, Williams & Wilkins, 1975, p 43
4. Kazemi H, Parsons EF, Valenca LM, et al: Distribution of pulmonary blood flow after myocardial ischemia and infarction. Circulation 41:1025, 1970
5. Bergofsky EH: Mechanisms underlying vasomotor regulation of regional pulmonary blood flow in normal and disease states. Am J Med 57:378, 1974
6. Franklin DL, Van Citters RL, Rushmer RF: Balance between right and left ventricular output. Circ Res 10:17, 1962
7. Swan HJ: Balloon flotation catheters: their use in hemodynamic monitoring in clinical practice. JAMA 233:865, 1975
8. Gilbertson AA: Pulmonary artery catheterization and wedge pressure measurement in the general intensive therapy unit. Br J Anaesth 46:97, 1974
9. Lappas DG, Lell WA, Gabel JC et al: Indirect measurement of left-atrial pressure in surgical patients—pulmonary-capillary wedge and pulmonary-artery diastolic pressures compared with left-atrial pressure. Anesthesiology 38:394, 1973
10. Price HL, Cooperman LH, Warden JC et al: Pulmonary hemodynamics during general anesthesia in man. Anesthesiology 30:629, 1969
11. Lappas DG, Buckley MJ, Laver MB, et al: Left ventricular performance and pulmonary circulation following addition of nitrous oxide to morphine during coronary-artery surgery. Anesthesiology 43:61, 1975
12. Fahmy NR, Selwyn AS, Patel D, et al: Pulmonary vasomotor tone during general anesthesia and deliberate hypotension in man. Anesthesiology 45:3, 1976
13. Heinemann HO, Fishman AP: Non-respiratory functions of mammalian lung. Physiol Rev 49:1, 1969
14. DeFreitas FM, Faraco EZ, DeAzevedo DF, et al: Behavior of normal pulmonary circulation during changes of total blood volume in man. J Clin Invest 44:366, 1965
15. Marshall BE: Non-respiratory functions of the lung. Anesthesiology 39:573, 1973

chapter 14

Ventilation–Perfusion Relationships

In an individual breathing spontaneously, the dependent regions of his lungs are better ventilated than the apical regions. This preferential distribution of ventilation to the dependent lung is true whether the individual is in a supine, prone, upright, or lateral position. In the erect person, intrapleural pressure is more negative at the apex of the lung than at the base. Because the intraalveolar pressure is the same in all regions of the lung, the distending pressure in the apical alveoli is higher. Thus, the apical alveoli are more expanded in the resting position than the alveoli in the basal regions. During inspiration, the smaller basal alveoli are represented on the steeply ascending part of the S-shaped pressure–volume curve. They expand much more per unit pressure change than the apical alveoli, which are on the upper flat portion of the curve. Therefore, during normal quiet breathing, the inspired gases are preferentially distributed in the basal region of the lung (Fig. 14-1).

At low lung volumes (at residual volume), the intrapleural pressure at the lower region of the lung will exceed atmospheric pressure. With shallow breathing, these lower portions of the lung will have less tendency to expand and the result will be a preferential ventilation of the apical alveoli. The basal regions of the lung will start ventilating only when the intrapleural pressure in their region is less than atmospheric. Similarly, if the dependent alveoli are closed for any reason at the start of inspiration, the inspired air will preferentially distribute itself to the upper lobes because the distending pressure of these alveoli is far less than the critical opening pressure of these closed airways.[1]

AIRWAY CLOSURE

In the awake, normal man airway closure practically is nonexistent at the end of inspiration (ie, all the regions of the lung are open). However, during

169

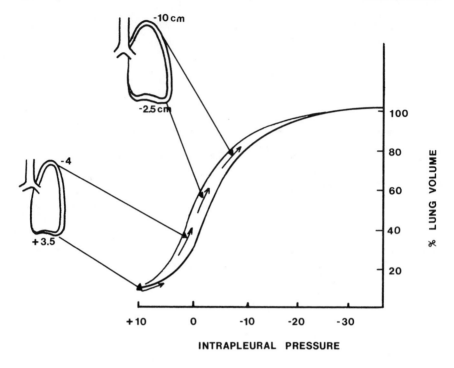

FIG. 14-1: Effect of lung volumes on regional distribution of ventilation. Note that at the larger lung volumes (above FRC) ventilation is preferentially distributed to the dependent portions of the lung as they are on the steep ascending part of the curve, whereas at residual volume most of the ventilation is at the apical region because now the apical region is on the ascending steep portion of the curve.

expiration the smaller airways show a progressive tendency to close, while the larger ones are open.[2] Closing volume is defined as the volume of the lung at which a detectable amount of airway closure begins. It is usually measured by radioactive or tracer gas methods and is expressed as a proportion of total lung capacity, functional residual capacity (FRC), or vital capacity.[3]

With an increase in age of the individual, the tendency to airway closure is increased, and thus the closing volume is raised. This is probably caused by progressive diminution in elastic recoil of the lung. In a standing person at 20 years of age, airway closure occurs at lung volumes 1.5 liters below FRC, whereas at the age of 65 FRC and closing volumes are similar. Therefore, in an upright subject less than 65 years airway closure cannot be detected. However, in the supine position in which the FRC is diminished by 20 percent, airway closure can be demonstrated at the age of 44 (Fig. 14-2).

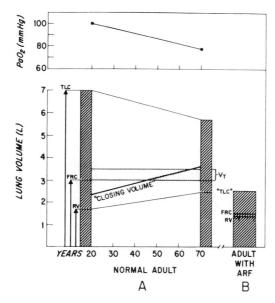

FIG. 14-2: Changes in Po₂ and lung volumes with age in normal adults in the supine position (FRC, functional residual capacity; RV, residual volume; TLC, total lung capacity; and Vᴛ, tidal volume). (Reproduced with permission from Pontoppidan et al.[3])

REGIONAL DISTRIBUTION OF PULMONARY BLOOD FLOW

Similar to the regional differences of pulmonary ventilation, the pulmonary blood flow shows the same tendency, ie, the pulmonary blood flow per unit of lung tissue increases from the apex of the lung to the base in the standing position. This is expected because the pulmonary arterial and arteriolar pressure is low. By the mere effect of gravity, the blood will preferentially go to the lower segments. This situation can be reversed if the individual is suspended upside down.

In the supine position, the blood flow in the apical regions increases, while the flow in the basal regions does not change. Therefore, the distribution of blood becomes almost uniform at this position.

A unique feature of the pulmonary circulation is that its capillaries are separated from the alveoli by a very thin, delicate membrane. Thus, for practical purposes they are exposed to alveolar (atmospheric) pressures.

Therefore, the caliber of the small blood vessels in the lung depend on pulmonary arterial pressure, alveolar pressure, and pulmonary venous pressure. To explain the relative importance of these three factors, the lung is conveniently divided into three zones[4] (Fig. 14-3).

Zone I

This is the area containing the apical or upper zones where the pulmonary arterial pressure is less than the atmospheric alveolar pressure, and where the pulmonary capillaries are compressed. The reason for this compression is that the alveolar pressure is transmitted to the thin capillaries leading to their closure and collapse, creating a dead space effect, ie, alveoli ventilated without any flow. Under normal conditions, the pressure in the pulmonary artery is just sufficient to raise blood to the apex of the lung, and zone I type of flow does not occur. It can occur if the pulmonary artery pressure is diminished as in severe hemorrhage or when the alveolar pressure is increased, eg, positive pressure ventilation.

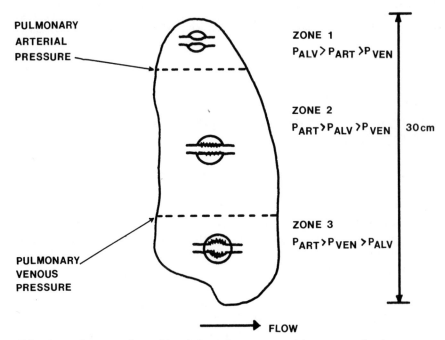

PULMONARY ARTERIAL PRESSURE

PULMONARY VENOUS PRESSURE

ZONE 1
$P_{ALV} > P_{ART} > P_{VEN}$

ZONE 2
$P_{ART} > P_{ALV} > P_{VEN}$

ZONE 3
$P_{ART} > P_{VEN} > P_{ALV}$

30 cm

FLOW

FIG. 14-3: The interrelationship of the pulmonary arterial pressure, alveolar pressure (atmospheric), and pulmonary venous pressure on the caliber of the small blood vessels in the lung.

Zone II

This is the midzone. This is the ideal situation, in which the pulmonary arterial pressure exceeds the alveolar atmospheric pressure, which in turn exceeds the pulmonary venous pressure. Because the venous pressure in this region of the lung is very low, the blood flow depends mainly on the difference between arterial and alveolar pressure.

Zone III

The basal areas are included in this zone. In these areas, the venous pressure exceeds the alveolar pressure, the main determinant of flow being the arteriovenous pressure difference.

REGIONAL DIFFERENCES IN VENTILATION–PERFUSION RATIOS

Because the situation in the lung is not a static but a dynamic one, the gas tension in the alveoli is not determined by ventilation or perfusion alone, but by the ratio of ventilation and perfusion ($\dot{V}_A / \dot{Q}$). This ratio can vary from zero to infinity. With zero ventilation–perfusion ratio, there is perfusion but no ventilation, and the gas tensions in the effluent blood are similar to those of mixed venous blood (shunt effect). On the other end of the spectrum (infinite ratio), there is ventilation without any perfusion, ie, dead space effect.

Because the gases in the capillaries are in equilibrium with alveolar gases, the sum of partial pressure of all the gases in alveoli as well as the capillaries is equal to barometric pressure.

Moving from top to bottom of the vertical lung, we find that the $\dot{V}_A / \dot{Q}$ ratio is higher at the apex that at the base, the main reason being that the rate of increase in blood flow from top to bottom is faster than the rate of increase in ventilation. This fact has been used by West to divide the lung into nine imaginary horizontal slices[5] (Fig. 14-4). The figure depicts approximately a 40-mm Hg difference between the alveolar oxygen tension at the apex of the lung and the base of the lung. The higher ventilation–perfusion ratio leads to a higher alveolar oxygen tension at the apex. Thus, a larger amount of oxygen is added by ventilation at the apex than the base. Similarly, a difference of about 15 mm Hg exists for carbon dioxide from the top to the base of the lung, with the apical venous blood having a lower CO_2 tension than the basal ones. One must

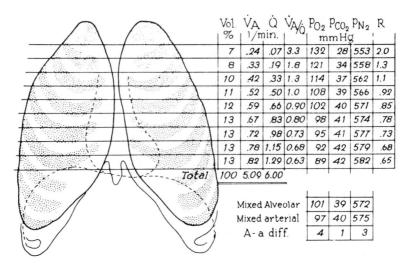

Vol. %	$\dot{V}_A$ 1/min.	$\dot{Q}$	$\dot{V}_A/\dot{Q}$	P_{O_2}	P_{CO_2} mmHg	P_{N_2}	R
7	.24	.07	3.3	132	28	553	2.0
8	.33	.19	1.8	121	34	558	1.3
10	.42	.33	1.3	114	37	562	1.1
11	.52	.50	1.0	108	39	566	.92
12	.59	.66	0.90	102	40	571	.85
13	.67	.83	0.80	98	41	574	.78
13	.72	.98	0.73	95	41	577	.73
13	.78	1.15	0.68	92	42	579	.68
13	.82	1.29	0.63	89	42	582	.65
Total 100	5.09	6.00					

Mixed Alveolar	101	39	572
Mixed arterial	97	40	575
A- a diff.	4	1	3

FIG. 14-4: Regional differences in gas exchange down the normal upright lung result-ing from the differences in the ventilation/perfusion ratio. (Reproduced with permission from West.[5])

take into consideration that the contribution of the apex to gas exchange is rela-tively small because it is the base that receives most of the blood flow to the lung. The mixed pulmonary venous blood (which contains arterialized blood) has a lower O_2 tension than the mixed alveolar air. The main reason for this dif-ference is the shape of the oxygen dissociation curve. In the apical regions where the alveolar oxygen tension is high (132 mm Hg), the oxygen-carrying capacity of blood cannot be increased any further because the hemoglobin is already fully saturated with oxygen, being on the flat part of the oxyhemo-globin dissociation curve. This is in contrast to the carbon dioxide level, which corresponds very well to mixed alveolar CO_2. The reason for this difference is due to the straight shape of the CO_2 dissociation curve.

The effect of this uneven ventilation/perfusion ratio in the total gas exchange is practically insignificant. The arterial oxygen tension is reduced by a few millimeters of mercury with a slight effect on oxygen saturation, while the effect on arterial carbon dioxide tension is minimal (1 mm Hg). The CO_2 tension is adjusted mainly through the chemoreceptors of the respiratory centers. Therefore, this small P_{CO_2} change is compensated by an increase in ventilation. With aging and lung disease, this discrepancy between ventilation/ perfusion ratios is exaggerated.[6] The rise of arterial carbon dioxide is com-pensated for by an increase in ventilation. However, this increase in ventilation cannot raise the oxygen content because of the shape of the oxygen dissociation curve. Thus, the arterial oxygen tension drops.

Physiologic Shunt (Venous Admixture, Wasted Blood Flow)

By definition, this is the part of cardiac output that does not contribute to pulmonary blood gas exchange and is returned unoxygenated to the arterial blood. In the normal man at rest, the physiologic shunt varies between 2 and 5 percent of the cardiac output depending on the age of the individual and has two main components.

ANATOMIC SHUNT

This is the portion of cardiac output that bypasses the pulmonary capillaries. This represents less than 2 percent of cardiac output and mostly is due to bronchial veins draining into pulmonary veins and thebesian and anterior cardiac veins draining into the left side of the heart (Fig. 14-5).

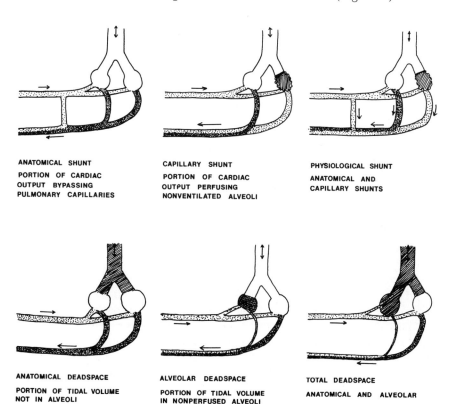

ANATOMICAL SHUNT

PORTION OF CARDIAC OUTPUT BYPASSING PULMONARY CAPILLARIES

CAPILLARY SHUNT

PORTION OF CARDIAC OUTPUT PERFUSING NONVENTILATED ALVEOLI

PHYSIOLOGICAL SHUNT

ANATOMICAL AND CAPILLARY SHUNTS

ANATOMICAL DEADSPACE

PORTION OF TIDAL VOLUME NOT IN ALVEOLI

ALVEOLAR DEADSPACE

PORTION OF TIDAL VOLUME IN NONPERFUSED ALVEOLI

TOTAL DEADSPACE

ANATOMICAL AND ALVEOLAR

FIG. 14-5: Subdivisions of the physiologic shunt (top) and the dead space. (Modified after Bendixen, et al.[26])

CAPILLARY SHUNT

This is the portion of cardiac output perfusing nonventilated alveoli, which is mostly due to uneven ventilation perfusion relationships or atelectasis, or it may be due to a diffusion gradient.

The mere measurement of arterial oxygen tension without knowing the alveolar oxygen tension is of little value. Thus, the efficiency of oxygen exchange is better stated as alveoloarterial oxygen difference $P_{(A-a DO_2)}$. The physiologic shunt, which is expressed as the percentage of cardiac output, can be derived from the following formula:

$$\frac{QS}{QT} = \frac{0.0031 \times \text{alveoloarterial oxygen gradient}}{\left(\begin{array}{c}0.0031 \times \text{alveoarterial} \\ \text{oxygen gradient}\end{array}\right) + \text{arteriovenous O}_2\text{ difference}} \times 100$$

where 0.0031 is the factor derived from the Bunsen solubility coefficient for oxygen at 37 C. It converts partial pressure of oxygen to content. For this formula to be correct, the arterial oxygen tension should be more than 150 mm Hg, a level high enough to ensure full saturation of hemoglobin. At an arterial oxygen lower than 150 mm Hg the original shunt equation is used:

$$\frac{Qs}{Qt} = \frac{O_2 \text{ content of end-capillary blood} - O_2 \text{ content of arterial blood}}{O_2 \text{ content of end-capillary blood} - O_2 \text{ content of mixed venous blood}}$$

This formula is based on the principle that the amount of oxygen present in the arterial blood equals the sum of the oxygen carried in the pulmonary capillary blood and in the shunted blood. The oxygen content of end-capillary blood can be computed from the alveolar oxygen tension and the oxygen dissociation curve. The alveolar oxygen tension can be determined by obtaining an end-expired alveolar sample. If the patient is breathing 100 percent oxygen, the alveolar oxygen equals the barometric pressure minus the water vapor and carbon dioxide pressures. A mixed venous sample ideally should be obtained from a catheter in the pulmonary artery.

During breathing of 100 percent oxygen, the oxygen tension in all the ventilated alveoli of the lung becomes approximately equal, and the factor of uneven ventilation is eliminated. Measuring the alveoloarterial oxygen gradient will be a reflection of the shunt arising from the blood flowing to nonventilated areas of the lung, ie, the areas of the lung in which the ventilation/perfusion ratio is zero. Occasionally, the shunt calculated when breathing 100 percent O_2 is termed the true shunt, while the shunt calculated while breathing air is usually known as venous admixture.

During acute respiratory failure as seen in the postsurgical patient, most of the fall in the arterial oxygen tension is due to shunting from closure of both small airways and alveoli, in contrast to patients with chronic lung disease in whom there are marked ventilation/perfusion inequalities. In the latter patients, administration of 100 percent oxygen will abolish this effect and the measured alveoloarterial oxygen difference will be low. However, if these patients are breathing a second gas, such as nitrogen, this shunt-like effect will be marked.

Effect of Cardiac Output

A decrease in cardiac output produces a decrease in arterial oxygenation.[7] This can be due to alteration of blood flow in the pulmonary capillary bed. Also, whenever the cardiac output drops, the oxygen extracted from the arterial blood at the periphery is increased because of the sluggish peripheral circulation. Therefore, the oxygen tension of mixed venous blood drops. In this situation, if the percentage of the shunted blood remains constant in the lung, as the arterialized blood is mixed with blood with a lesser oxygen content, the measured oxygen tension will be low.

Diffusion block (or alveolocapillary block) is a term that has been used to describe the shunt, presumably due to increased alveolocapillary membrane thickness. However, it has been demonstrated that the most common cause of shunting is maldistribution of ventilation relative to perfusion, whereas pure alveolocapillary block is an extremely rare phenomenon.[8]

Dead Space Ventilation

Dead space ventilation is the portion of ventilation that is not involved in gas exchange. It has two main components: anatomic dead space, which is composed of the volume of the conducting airways (nose, mouth, pharynx, larynx, trachea, bronchi, and bronchioles); and the alveolar dead space, which is the portion of tidal volume that is wasted in ventilating nonperfused alveoli. In the normal human being, the alveolar dead space is minimal, and, therefore, anatomic dead space is equivalent to total or physiologic dead space. The anatomic dead space is difficult to measure in the alive human being but can be derived easily from standard tables. It varies with body weight, age, lung volume, and tidal volume. Radford has noted that in adults the anatomic dead space in milliliters is about equal to his ideal weight in pounds (ie, 2.2 ml per kg), and it usually represents about 30 percent of the tidal volume (range, 20 to 40 percent)[9]

The most important factor affecting the value of dead space is tidal volume. At very large tidal volumes, the dead space can reach 50 percent of the tidal volume, while in very low tidal volumes it is lower than predicted values. Therefore, it is better to express dead space as a simple ratio to tidal volume, which can easily be derived from the following formula (the dead space equation):

$$\frac{V_D}{V_T} = \frac{\text{Arterial carbon dioxide tension} - \text{expired } CO_2 \text{ tension}}{\text{Arterial carbon dioxide tension}}$$

Only carbon dioxide is used in calculating dead space, since the alveoli, with an abnormally high ventilation/perfusion ratio, are the ones affecting CO_2 elimination, because the gases reaching the nonperfused alveoli will lead to a rise in P_{CO_2} and will stimulate alveolar hyperventilation by their effect on the chemoreceptors.

In terms of the ventilation/perfusion ratio, ($\dot{V}_A/\dot{Q}$), if we assume that alveolar ventilation is 51 per minute and the pulmonary blood flow is 61, the $\dot{V}_A/\dot{Q}$ ratio is about 0.85. Thus, an alveolus with a $\dot{V}_A/\dot{Q}$ ratio higher than normal will have a higher O_2 tension and a lower than normal CO_2 tension. That means it is wasting part of its ventilation, ie, dead space effect. In contrast, alveoli with a $\dot{V}_A/\dot{Q}$ ratio less than normal contribute to blood shunting because part of their perfusion is wasted. Thus, a $\dot{V}_A/\dot{Q}$ ratio of zero indicates a complete shunt.

The typical example of the dead space effect is acute pulmonary embolus, in which the ventilation of that particular segment of the lung continues while its blood supply has ceased completely (wasted ventilation). However, after a certain time, this area of the lung will collapse and most of the blood to that area of the lung will be diverted and the dead space effect will be lost. A much more common cause of increased dead space effect (V_D/V_T ratio) is hypotension. In this situation, because of the low pulmonary arterial pressure, the dependent area of the lung will be the only one perfused and the higher ones will not, resulting in an increased V_D/V_T ratio.

A rise in mean airway pressure will lead to compression of a large segment of pulmonary capillaries, leading to cessation of their blood flow, and this blood will be distributed to other areas of the lung. This effect is most marked in the presence of hypotension or hypovolemia.

The "dead space effect of shunting" is seen whenever there is a large physiologic shunt or a severe drop in cardiac output. It is caused by a greater admixture of arterial blood with mixed venous blood of high carbon dioxide content.

IMPAIRED OXYGENATION DURING ANESTHESIA

It is a well-known fact that there is impairment of pulmonary gas exchange during general anesthesia in man. The mechanism producing this defect is still not clear, but the following factors seem to be involved.

Functional Residual Capacity (FRC)

The FRC is decreased during anesthesia in man.[10] This reduction in FRC occurs during the induction of general anesthesia, does not seem to progress with time, and is most marked in elderly subjects. It occurs whether the patient is breathing spontaneously or whether his respiration is controlled in the presence of a muscle relaxant.[11] Currently, there is no obvious explanation for this substantial reduction in FRC. Miliary atelectasis or progressive absorption collapse has been suggested but not confirmed. Gas trapping and airway closure seem to be contributing factors. The reduction of FRC accompanying anesthesia might reduce the FRC below the closing volume and lead to gas trapping and venous admixture. However, the most dominant factor for this decrease in FRC is due to changes in the mechanics of the chest wall, where the pressure–volume curve of the chest wall is shifted to the right,[12] ie, the chest is stiffer.

This diminution in FRC is also seen in the postoperative stage and is more marked in patients who have undergone an upper abdominal operation.[13] This can be due to abdominal distension or to a spasm of the abdominal muscles, which prevents the full expansion of the lung.

Distribution of Ventilation

Changes in posture affect lung volume as well as the distribution of both ventilation and perfusion. For instance, in the lateral decubitus position, the majority of the blood flow is to the dependent lung, and during normal spontaneous breathing there is similar distribution of ventilation. However, in anesthetized individuals either breathing spontaneously or mechanically ventilated, the tidal volume is preferentially distributed to the nondependent lung.[14] Whereas the perfusion in the dependent lung is increased, therefore, the ventilation perfusion mismatch will increase.

A similar but less marked effect is seen in supine subjects. In the awake spontaneously breathing man, the larger portion of ventilation is distributed in the dependent portion of the lung. With anesthesia and mechanical ventilation, the distribution of ventilation becomes more uniform in the lungs.[15]

Impaired Oxygenation

In anesthetized, spontaneously breathing individuals, a progressive decrease in arterial oxygenation has been seen during ventilation with small tidal volumes, and this effect was reversed by a deep breath. It was concluded that this was due to miliary atelectasis.[16] Later, this increased alveolarterial gradient was confirmed, but was not found to be progressive and was attributed to $\dot{V}/\dot{Q}$ mismatching.[17]

Although the increased incidence of shunting has been confirmed under anesthesia, whether it is due to increased $\dot{V}/\dot{Q}$ mismatching has never been confirmed. Recently, it has been demonstrated that the FRC diminishes with anesthesia. This might displace FRC below the closing volume and cause increased trapping of gas and venous admixture.[18]

Cardiac Output

A constant shunt with decreased cardiac output will manifest as impaired arterial oxygenation. This has been suggested as a cause of hypoxemia.[19] A consistent decrease in cardiac output does not occur with all anesthetic techniques.

Dead Space Effect

The anatomic dead space may be affected during anesthesia. It can be reduced by half with tracheostomy or endotracheal intubation and increased by atropine. Extending the neck, protruding the jaw, and inserting an oral airway will increase the anatomic dead space.[20] However, if the upper airway is kept constant there is no change in the anatomic dead space with anesthesia. The alveolar dead space increases markedly during anesthesia. The arterioalveolar gradient for O_2 as well as the V_D/V_T ratio increases during halothane anesthesia. This effect is presumably due to diminution in pulmonary artery pressure under these circumstances, resulting in underperfusion of the nondependent regions of the lung.[21] A similar dead space effect is seen with hemorrhage and with ganglionic blocking agents. However, one should realize that with increased shunting, the calculated alveolar dead space is increased.

PULMONARY FUNCTION TESTS

Every anesthesiologist would like to have an ideal respiratory function test that would preoperatively identify all patients likely to develop pulmonary complications. Unfortunately, there is no single test that approaches this ideal, but the best estimate is done by combining the results of several tests.[22] No pulmonary function test can give as much valuable information as history and physical examination can provide. In the history taking, one should inquire about cough, sputum, dyspnea, and the amount of exercise tolerance. Occasionally, it becomes necessary to walk with the patient up one or two flights of stairs to determine his exercise tolerance. During the physical examination, it is essential to note the posture of the patient, the presence of cyanosis, clubbing of the finger, and auscultation of the chest. This is usually followed by observing the roentgenograms of the chest.

Although the information obtained by the clinical evaluation is invaluable, it can only detect advanced pulmonary disease. For the early detection of these diseases, one has to resort to pulmonary function tests, some of which are available for routine use in the hospital. New, more sensitive tests capable of detecting pulmonary diseases at a much earlier stage have been developed.

Vital Capacity and Forced Vital Capacity

To obtain a vital capacity measurement, the patient inhales maximally and then exhales slowly and completely. In the forced vital capacity test, he again inspires maximally and then expires as strongly and as rapidly as he can. Vital capacity is diminished in restrictive diseases and may be decreased in obstructive disease. However, the patient with obstructive diseases will have a delayed forced expiratory volume, ie, the volume of gas exhaled in the first second is less than 83 percent of the total vital capacity and at the third second, less than 97 percent of the total vital capacity. Repeating this test after the inhalation of 0.5 percent isoproterenol may relieve the obstruction due to smooth muscle contraction (asthma), but not if it is due to destructive disease such as emphysema.

Arterial Blood Gases

This is a simple test and can be performed at the bedside or just prior to the induction of anesthesia. Valuable information can be obtained if the patient is at rest and in a steady state breathing air. From the Po_2 and Pco_2 one can estimate the alveolar oxygen tension gradient, thus separating the effects of pure hypoventilation from those of ventilation–perfusion abnormalities.

Pulmonary Diffusing Capacity

In this test the patient inhales a low nontoxic concentration of carbon monoxide for 10 seconds. This is a valuable test to detect some uncommon diseases such as collagen disease, sarcoidosis, and asbestosis in which there is thickening of the alveolocapillary membrane. Pulmonary diffusing capacity is diminished in emphysema because of the loss of alveolocapillary surface area.

Radioactive Xenon

Radioactive xenon (^{133}Xe) can either be inhaled or given intravenously dissolved in saline. External detectors over the chest count the radioactivity. With the inhalation test, information can be obtained about the distribution of gas to different regions of the lung and the rate of ventilation in these regions. With the intravenous test, xenon, being insoluble in blood, is cleared from the pulmonary blood into the alveolar gas in a single circulation time. The alveoli with no perfusion will show no radioactivity. Also, the rate of disappearance of xenon from the lung reflects the ventilation characteristics of that portion of the lung.

Tagged Albumin

Microaggregates of radioactive iodinated serum albumin are given intravenously and radioactivity is observed over the chest. Being larger than the pulmonary capillaries, these aggregates lodge in patent pulmonary capillaries. Very small amounts of microaggregates are required. Thus, the number of obstructed pulmonary arteries is minimal. This test is helpful in detecting a pulmonary embolus. Recently, radioactive technetium has been used.[23]

Tests for the Detection of Peripheral Airway Diseases

As the tracheobronchial tree divides, the total cross-sectional area of the periphral airway rapidly becomes quite large. Therefore, the contribution of these peripheral airways to the total pulmonary resistance is rather small, accounting for only about 10 to 20 percent of the total resistance. If one-half of the peripheral bronchi are closed, the resistance of the airway will only increase by about 10 percent. To detect these minute abnormalities, three types of special tests have been developed.

FREQUENCY-DEPENDENT TESTS OF COMPLIANCE

These tests are based on the principle that all the alveoli of the lung fill and empty at the same time even at very rapid respiratory frequencies. Thus, the factors determining this response depend on the product of resistance of the air passages and the compliance of the air spaces. During the early stages of pulmonary disease, small airways are involved in a random and irregular fashion. During rapid breathing some of the units might be inspiring, while the narrower units will be expiring. This nonuniformity of gas distribution will be associated with reduced dynamic compliance at rapid frequencies. This is probably the most sensitive test for early detection of peripheral airway disease. However, it requires the insertion of an esophageal balloon for transpulmonary pressure measurements.

LIMITATION OF MAXIMUM EXPIRATORY FLOW

With forced exhalation, the intrapleural as well as the intraalveolar pressures increase to become markedly positive (30 to 50 cm H_2O). While this is happening, the gas flow in the airway is increased until a certain point is reached when the pressure outside the airways exceeds their intraluminal pressure and they become compressed. In normal people, this probably happens at the level of larger bronchi close to the carina. Once this narrowing occurs, the flow in these bronchi will not increase no matter how much additional effort the subject makes. This phenomenon is usually seen when the lungs have expelled about 15 percent of their volume and will continue until all the air has been expelled. Therefore, there are two components to this test: (1) effort-dependent forced expiration, which is a reflection of the force of expiratory muscles and the patency of the larger airways; and (2) effort-independent, which is a reflection of the resistance of the peripheral bronchi in the midvital capacity range.[24] Therefore, obstruction of expiratory flow characteristically causes airways to collapse at an earlier stage at a point near the alveoli. Therefore, the spirometric tests that are more useful for early detection of lung disease are those that emphasize events occurring lower in the vital capacity after the peak flow has been reached.[25] Consequently, measuring expiratory flow rates or maximum flows at 50 and 25 percent vital capacity is much more commonly used today.

CLOSING VOLUME

Closing volume is the volume at which the lung units start to close during exhalation of a deep breath and is expressed as a percentage of vital capacity. Closing capacity is the sum of closing volume and residual volume and is expressed as a percentage of total lung capacity. Closing of the alveoli occurs at an earlier stage with the advance of age and after pulmonary disease because of the loss of structural integrity of the bronchial wall during these conditions. It also occurs at an earlier stage in the supine position as well as in anesthetized patients. This is probably related to the reduction of FRC in these conditions. The test is performed by inhaling slowly 100 percent O_2 until the total lung capacity is reached, then expiring slowly while the nitrogen concentration in

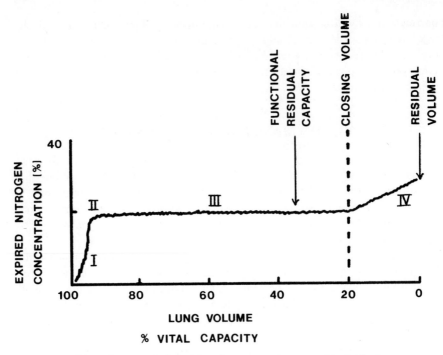

FIG. 14-6:   A typical closing volume curve in a seated individual.

the expired air is measured. Four phases can be distinguished in the curve (Fig. 14-6).

PHASE I

Nitrogen concentration is zero due to exhalation of 100 percent O_2 present in the trachea and bronchial tree.

PHASE II

Dead space and alveolar gases are mixed.

PHASE III

Known as plateau, this phase is indicative of the alveolar concentration. The nitrogen concentration progressively increases at a very slow rate as the contribution to expired gas from units in which nitrogen was less diluted progressively increases.

PHASE IV

There is a marked increase in nitrogen concentration. As the dependent airways close, their alveoli cease to empty and trace gas is contributed exclusively from nondependent (apical) alveoli. This closing volume test can be performed by using a tracer gas such as xenon.

The value of these tests is that they can detect chronic pulmonary disease at an early stage, long before spirometric tests become abnormal. They also can distinguish between asymptomatic smokers and nonsmokers.[25]

Flow–Volume Loops

This test is performed by asking the patient to perform a maximum expiratory maneuver of his vital capacity while two transducers at the mouth

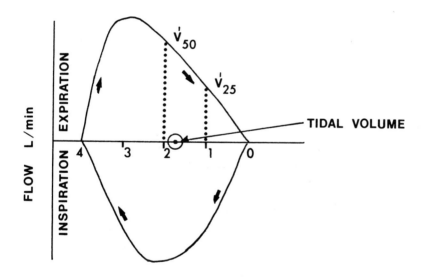

LUNG VOLUME L

VITAL CAPACITY

FIG. 14-7: Flow volume loop in a normal individual ($\dot{V}_{50}$ and $\dot{V}_{25}$ are flows at 50 percent and 25 percent of vital capacity).

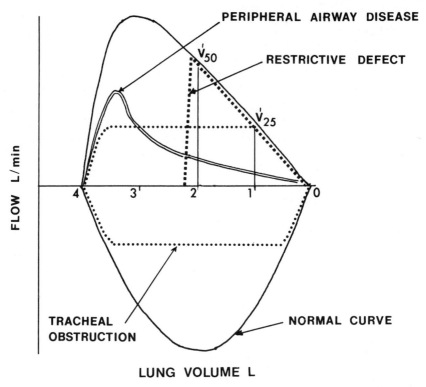

FIG. 14-8. Flow volume loops in various disease states. Note the marked diminution of flows at $\dot{V}_{50}$ and $\dot{V}_{25}$ in peripheral airway disease.

record the simultaneous changes of flow and volume. The data are recorded as an X-Y plot, the pulmonary volume being on the horizontal axis and the flow rates on the vertical axis. A maximum inspiratory effort and smaller loop indicating the tidal volume are recorded in a similar manner. From these curves the forced expiratory flow rate at 1 second (FEV_1) and the flow rates at 50 percent ($\dot{V}_{50}$) and 25 percent ($\dot{V}_{25}$) of vital capacity, ie, after exhaling 50 percent and 75 percent of the air present in the lungs are derived (Fig. 14-7). In disease states, to help define the abnormalities of pulmonary function, the patient's flow–volume loop is superimposed on the predicted curves (Fig. 14-8).

As a general rule, a diminution in flow rates will result from an obstructive lesion, whereas a reduction in vital capacity will result from restrictive defects. However, the clinical picture is more complicated; for example, with a restrictive defect the peak expiratory flow rates are also diminished because the limitation in the expansion of the lung will in turn limit the stretching of the pulmonary elastic tissue and, hence, the elastic recoil. Thus, the flow rates will decline.

During a maximum expiratory effort, the site of maximum airflow resistance varies depending on the distension of the lung. The highest resistance to airflow is in the larger airways at the beginning of vital capacity maneuver, ie, lobar and segmental bronchi, whereas at lower volumes, the site of maximum resistance is in the small airways, ie, less than 2 mm in diameter. Also, during maximum expiratory effort in the initial 25 percent of vital capacity, the flow rates are force dependent, ie, vary according to the effort of the patient, whereas in the final 75 percent of vital capacity, they are effort independent. Therefore, in a noncooperative patient, adequate information can be obtained from the shape of the last 75 percent of the loop.

In high airway obstruction such as tracheal stenosis, the flow–volume loop has a characteristic plateau shape in which the flow rises slowly and remains low during the respiratory maneuvers. In peripheral airway obstructive disease, the curve has a characteristic convex shape toward the horizontal axis with a marked diminution of the flows at 50 percent and 25 percent residual vital capacities. A pure restrictive effect will produce on attenuated curve with limited surface without any convexity (Fig. 14-8).

REFERENCES

1. Sutherland PW, Katsura T, Milic-Emili J: Previous volume history of the lung and regional distribution of gases. J Appl Physiol 25:566, 1968
2. Burger EJ, Jr, Macklem P: Airway closure: demonstration by breathing 100% oxygen at low lung volumes and by N_2 washout. J Appl Physiol 25:139, 1968
3. Pontoppidan H, Geffin B, Lowenstein E: Acute respiratory failure in the adult. N Engl J Med 287:690, 1972
4. West JB, Dollery CT, Naimark A: Distribution of blood flow in isolated lung: relation to vascular and alveolar pressures. J Appl Physiol 19:713, 1964
5. West JB: Regional differences in gas exchange in the lung of erect man. J Appl Physiol 17:893, 1962
6. West JB: New advances in pulmonary gas exchange. Anesth Analg (Cleve) 54:409, 1975
7. Philbin DM, Sullivan SF, Bowman FO, Jr, et al: Postoperative hypoxemia: contribution of the cardiac output. Anesthesiology 32:136, 1970
8. Briscoe WA, Cree EM, Filler J, et al: Lung volume alveolar ventilation and perfusion interrelationships in chronic pulmonary emphysema. J Appl Physiol 15:785, 1960
9. Radford EP, Jr, Ferris BG, Jr., Kriete BC: Clinical use of a nomogram to estimate proper ventilation during artificial respiration. N Engl J Med 251:877, 1954
10. Hewlett AM, Hulands GH, Nunn JF, et al: Functional residual capacity during anaesthesia. II. Spontaneous respiration. Br J Anaesth 46:486, 1974
11. Rehder K, Sessler AD, Marsh HM: General anesthesia and the lung. Am Rev Resp Dis 112:541, 1975
12. Rehder K, Mallow JE, Fibuch EE, et al: Effects of isoflurane anesthesia and muscle paralysis on respiratory mechaniscs in normal man. Anesthesiology 41:477, 1974

13. Alexander JI, Spence AA, Parikh RK, et al: The role of airway closure in postoperative hypoxaemia. Br J Anaesth 45:34, 1973

14. Rehder K, Sessler AD: Function of each lung in spontaneously breathing man anesthetized with thiopental-meperidine. Anesthesiology 38:320, 1973

15. Brendstrup A: The effect of artificial respiration on the regional distribution of ventilation examined with xenon 133. Acta Anaesth Scand (Suppl) 23:180, 1966

16. Bendixen HH, Hedley-Whyte J, Laver MB: Impaired oxygenation in surgical patients during general anesthesia with controlled ventilation. A concept of atelectasis. N Engl J Med 269:991, 1963

17. Nunn JF, Bergman NA, Coleman AJ: Factors influencing the arterial oxygen tension during anaesthesia with artificial ventilation. Br J Anaesth 37:898, 1965

18. Don HF, Wahba WM, Craig DB: Airway closure, gas trapping, and the functional residual capacity during anesthesia. Anesthesiology 36:533, 1972

19. Kelman GR, Nunn JF, Prys-Roberts C, et al: The influence of cardiac output on arterial oxygenation: a theoretical study. Br J Anaesth 39:450, 1967

20. Nunn JF, Campbell JM, Peckett BW: Anatomical subdivisions of the volume of respiratory dead space and effect of position of the jaw. J Appl Physiol 14:174, 1959

21. Askrog V: Changes in (a-A)CO$_2$ difference and pulmonary artery pressure in anesthetized man. J Appl Physiol 21:1299, 1966

22. Anderson WG: Respiratory aspects of the preoperative examination. Br J Anaesth 46:549, 1974

23. Comroe JH, Jr, Nadel JA: Screening tests of pulmonary function. N Engl J Med 282:1249, 1970

24. McFadden ER, Ingram RH: Peripheral airway obstruction. JAMA 235:259, 1976

25. Bergman NA: New tests of pulmonary function. Anesthesiology 44:220, 1976

26. Bendixen HH, Egbert LD, Hedley-Whyte J, Laver MB, Pontoppidan H: Respiratory care. St. Louis, Mosby 1965

chapter 15

Respiratory Failure and Artificial Respiration

No concise definition exists for what constitutes respiratory failure. A vague description would be inadequate gas exchange. The acute respiratory failure seen in the surgical patient differs markedly from the respiratory failure of the patient with pulmonary disease. In the former, the patient has little or no preexisting lung disease. However, the patient with chronic lung disease can have an acute exacerbation following trauma and surgery.

ACUTE RESPIRATORY FAILURE

Most authors consider that acute respiratory failure has occurred if the arterial tension drops below 60 mm Hg or the carbon dioxide tension rises above 49 mm Hg. The arterial oxygen tension falls with age. Taking this into consideration, Pontoppidan et al[1] have used the following definition for acute respiratory failure: "A state in which the arterial oxygen tension is below the predicted normal range for the patient's age at the prevalent barometric pressure (in the absence of intracardiac right-to-left shunting) or arterial carbon dioxide levels above 50 mm Hg (not due to respiratory compensation for metabolic alkalemia)."

The main reason for acute respiratory failure in the adult surgical patient is the accumulation of fluid in the lung. Initially it is limited to the interstitial connective tissue around the main blood vessels and bronchi ("perivascular cuffing"). With the progress of the disease, fluid accumulation occurs in the alveolar walls, leading to their "thickening" with a diminution of the alveolar diameter. With further advance of the disease process, the interstitial edema increases, leading to marked instability of the airway and fluid accumulation within the alveoli (intraalveolar edema).[2] Thus, gas exchange ceases while perfusion continues (shunt effect), leading to hypoxemia. In the initial stages, the fluid accumulation occurs in the interstitial spaces because the pulmonary capillaries are more permeable to water than the alveolar epithelium. A similar increase in extravascular water is seen in mitral stenosis. In shock or sepsis, in which there is loss of integrity of the capillary endothelium, both water and protein are found in this interstitial compartment.[3] The fluid accumulation leads to diminution of the functional residual capacity and the pulmonary compliance. The latter leads to an increase in the work of breathing several times over the normal values. Normally, the work of breathing represents only 2 to 3 percent of total oxygen consumption.

This shunt effect, ie, the nonventilation or the underventilation of the perfused alveoli, will indirectly produce a dead space effect. When the alveoli are filled with fluid or collapsed, the air that was ventilating these airways will redistribute itself to other open airways, but this redistribution is not accompanied by a similar shift in pulmonary perfusion, thus precluding any further rise in arterial oxygen content. As a general rule, significant increases in the shunt are associated with an increase in the dead space-to-tidal volume ratio.[4] Therefore, the main manifestations of acute respiratory failure are an increase in functional residual capacity with an increase in the intrapulmonary shunts and the physiologic dead space. The raised arterial shunting will lead to arterial hypoxemia, which in turn will lead to a reflex rise in minute ventilation. This hyperventilation will have a minimal effect on the arterial oxygen content but will lead to hypocapnia. In the later stages of the disease, a further increase in the work of breathing and fatigue of respiratory muscles will cause the carbon dioxide level to rise. To reverse all these changes, it is imperative that acute respiratory failure be diagnosed early by repeated arterial blood gas measurements. Oxygen administration can counteract partially the effect of shunting. It can counteract the effect of mismatched ventilation/perfusion distribution, but it is neither effective in aerating the collapsed alveoli nor in reversing the fluid accumulation in the lung. Thus, if the condition deteriorates further, it is imperative to start ventilatory support early rather than late (Table 15-1).

ACUTE EXACERBATION OF CHRONIC PULMONARY DISEASES

This includes a variety of pulmonary diseases, each one a different entity but with a few common problems. The most common ones seen are emphysema, chronic bronchitis, and bronchial asthma. A characteristic feature of these diseases is *airway obstruction,* which manifests first as obstruction to expiration. The site of this obstruction differs according to the disease process. In asthma and chronic bronchitis, the obstruction is mostly at the bronchial and bronchiolar levels. In the former disease, the spasm of the smooth muscles and

TABLE 15-1. Guidelines for Ventilatory Support in Adults with ARF*

DATA	NORMAL RANGE	TRACHEAL INTUBATION AND VENTILATION INDICATED
Mechanics		
Respiratory rate	12–20	>35
Vital capacity (ml/kg of body weight)†	65–75	<15
FEV$_1$ (ml/kg of body weight)†	50–60	<10
Inspiratory force (cm H$_2$O)	75–100	<25
Oxygenation		
Po$_2$ (mm Hg)	100–75 (air)	<70 (on mask O$_2$)
P(A-aDO$_2$)$^{1.0}$ (mm Hg)‡	25–65	>450
Ventilation		
Pco$_2$ (mm Hg)	35–45	>55§
$\dot{V}_D/\dot{V}_T$	0.25–0.40	>0.60

* The trend of values is of utmost importance. The numerical guidelines should obviously not be adopted to the exclusion of clinical judgment. For example, a vital capacity below 15 ml/kg may prove sufficient provided the patient can still cough "effectively," if hypoxemia is prevented, and if hypercapnia is not progressive. However, such a patient needs frequent blood gas analyses and must be closely observed in a well-equipped, adequately staffed recovery room or intensive-care unit. room or intensive-care unit.
† "Ideal" weight is used if weight appears grossly abnormal.
‡ After 10 minutes of 100 percent O$_2$.
§ Except in patients with chronic hypercapnia.
Reproduced with permission from Pontoppidan.[1]

the swelling of the mucous respond to bronchodilator therapy. In emphysema, the obstruction is mostly at the prealveolar level, and the changes are destructive and irreversible, since they do not respond to bronchodilator therapy. In emphysema, there is *diminished elastic recoil* of the lung from the loss of its elastic fibers. Thus, its natural recoil is partially lost. The patient tries to compensate for this loss by using his expiratory muscles. The progressive parenchymal destruction leads to a reduced gas exchange area. With the destruction of the elastic tissue in the lung, the supporting framework of the bronchioles is weakened. During an expiratory effort the rise of the pressure outside the bronchioles might exceed the intramural pressure, leading to the collapse of the bronchiole. The irony of this situation is that greater muscular effort cannot increase the flow; it causes even greater obstruction.

Patients with advanced pulmonary disease are usually in a delicate balance between their oxygen requirements and the capacity of their respiratory system. An acute exacerbation resulting from respiratory infection, anesthesia, or surgery may upset this balance and start a vicious circle with further atelectasis, further increased work of breathing, with a consequent increase in oxygen consumption and carbon dioxide production, eventually leading to fatigue of the respiratory muscles. The patient then suffers from hypoxia and hypercapnia, which can lead to coma (carbon dioxide narcosis) or right-sided heart failure.

According to the abnormality of their blood gases, patients with chronic pulmonary disease are classified into three stages.[5]

Stage I—Mild Obstructive Disease

Stage I is characterized by mild hypoxia manifested by mild drop in Po_2 (60 to 80 mm Hg). The effect of this drop in Po_2 on the oxygen saturation of hemoglobin is minimal because of the S-shaped oxygen dissociation curve (saturation, 88 to 95 percent). The mild hypoxemia leads to reflex alveolar hyperventilation (Pco_2, 32 to 38 mm Hg). The pH is well compensated for through the renal mechanism. Thus, standard bicarbonate is in the low range of normal (20 to 24 mEq per liter).

Stage II—Moderately Severe Obstructive Disease

Stage II entails moderately severe hypoxemia (Po_2, 50 to 60 mm Hg) and mild hypercapnia (45 to 55 mm Hg), indicating the start of decompensation associated with moderate acidosis (pH, 7.30 to 7.35), which is mostly caused by carbon dioxide retention. This acidosis is partially compensated for by a rise in standard bicarbonate (26 to 35 mEq per liter).

Stage III—Severe Obstructive Disease

In Stage III, the patient has severe hypoxemia, a Po_2 less than 50 mm Hg, and saturation below 75 percent. The carbon dioxide retention is severe (above 55 mm Hg, possibly reaching 80 mm Hg). This respiratory acidosis is accompanied by metabolic (lactic) acidosis from inadequate tissue oxygenation manifested by a low standard bicarbonate.

These patients are acclimatized to chronic hypoxia. They can survive at a Po_2 of 40 mm Hg, which might be fatal to another patient without such adaptation. The aim of treatment in these patients is to provide adequate oxygenation without suppression of their chemoreceptor drive to avoid hypercapnia. This can be fulfilled in most cases by gradually increasing the inspired oxygen mixture by special face masks (based on Venturi's principle) until adequate oxygenation is achieved.

In patients with emphysema, one tries to avoid intubation and artificial ventilation as much as possible because these patients, once ventilated, are extremely difficult to wean from ventilatory support. Therefore, the indications for artificial ventilation are more stringent in these patients than in patients with acute respiratory failure. Artificial ventilation in these patients is associated with a higher incidence of complications, such as tension pneumothorax and hypotension.[6]

ARTIFICIAL VENTILATION

During artificial ventilation the respirator should provide enough energy to overcome three types of forces that were previously dealt with by the respiratory muscles, ie, (1) overcoming the elastic recoil of the lung and chest wall (static compliance), (2) airflow resistance, and (3) frictional resistance of the tissue components of the lung and the chest wall. The airflow resistance is partially decreased during positive pressure ventilation mostly from bypassing the upper airway. The compliance of the chest wall can vary according to the degree of paralysis of the respiratory muscles.

Circulatory Effects

The main difference between positive pressure breathing and spontaneous breathing is that the mean intrathoracic pressure is higher during artificial ventilation. With the rise of intrathoracic pressure, the flow in the intrathoracic veins diminishes with a consequent reduction in pulmonary artery and aortic flow. With the release of airway pressure, the flow in the caval veins increases within one heart beat, pulmonary flow at the next beat, and aortic flow at the third beat. However, the peak pulmonary artery flow is not regained until late in expiration, and the peak aortic flow after another two beats.[7] The effect of this on the circulation depends mainly on the integrity of the patient's circulatory reflexes. Patients with normal reflexes compensate for the increase in intrathoracic pressure by raising venous tone.[8] This effect was investigated early in 1948 by Cournand.[9] He found that the deficit of cardiac output that occurred during the inspiratory phase is compensated for during the expiratory phase if sufficient time is given for the heart to refill during expiration, and, if expiratory time equalled inspiratory time, the effect on cardiac output was negligible.

In the clinical situation, the result of a rise of the intrathoracic pressure depends largely on the general condition of the patient. For example, a marked increase in minute ventilation and intratracheal pressure brought about by increasing the tidal volume without changing the rate does not lead to a drop in cardiac output in patients without emphysema,[6] as long as the patient can compensate for it by increasing his venous tone. However, if the patient is at a state of low blood volume or has lost his ability to increase his venous tone (eg, a patient with a transected cervical cord or on ganglionic blocking drugs) the cardiac output will diminish, resulting in hypotension. Patients with emphysema respond to the rise in intrathoracic pressure by marked diminution in cardiac output. This is probably due to inadequate emptying of the lung (air trapping) at the end of expiration. The increased functional residual capacity and intrapleural pressure will provide a much higher impedance to the flow in the pulmonary as well as in the systemic vascular bed of these patients.

The effect of positive pressure ventilation on pulmonary circulation is rather complex and varies according to the size of the vessels. The small interalveolar vessels (less than 30 mm in diameter) are affected by interstitial pressure. Increasing the lung volume will expand these vessels and diminish their resistance.[1] The pulmonary vascular resistance is least at or near the functional residual capacity. Therefore, if the initial lung volume is high, ie, near or above the FRC, further expansion of the lung will lead to a rise in pulmonary vascular resistance, a phenomenon frequently seen in emphysema. In contrast, if the initial lung volume is small, expansion of the lung will decrease the pulmonary vascular resistance as seen in postoperative patients.[10] However, there are several other factors affecting the pulmonary vascular resistance, such as acidosis, hypoxia, shock, and pulmonary edema.

To counteract the effect of a rise of intrathoracic pressure on circulation, a negative pressure phase during expiration has been suggested. However, this has found very little acceptance because it predisposes the patient to airway collapse and atelectasis, and its effect on cardiac output is rather insignificant.[10]

The application of positive end-expiratory pressure (PEEP) can improve arterial oxygenation in patients with severe respiratory failure by increasing the functional residual capacity secondary to prevention of terminal air space collapse during expiration. The effect of PEEP on the circulation is variable, but in most instances there is a 20 percent drop of cardiac output and a diminution in pulmonary shunting.[11]

The response of the patient also may depend on his arterial carbon dioxide levels. Patients retaining CO_2 will have an increased blood pressure and cardiac output from sympathetic stimulation. Institution of positive pressure ventilation and a rapid decline in P_{CO_2} might lead to a drop in cardiac output, resulting in hypotension.

In conclusion, the circulatory response of the individual patient requiring positive pressure to artificial ventilation is unpredictable. A diminution in cardiac output is expected when large tidal volumes are used in patients with emphysema and shock, while other patients are expected to tolerate it well. After the institution of artificial ventilation, and stabilization of circulation, changes in airway pressure are well tolerated.

Ventilation–Perfusion Changes

Spontaneous respiration is a much more efficient way to achieve an optimal distribution ventilation and pulmonary perfusion than positive pressure breathing. This ventilation–perfusion maldistribution pattern is usually expressed as dead space and shunt effect.

DEAD SPACE EFFECT

The dead space-to-tidal volume (V_D/V_T) ratio is usually higher in ventilated, anesthetized individuals (0.4 to 0.7) than spontaneously breathing people (0.3).[12] This V_D/V_T increases with age, and it is higher in people with abnormal pulmonary status and in those with rapid respiratory rates. The exact cause of this increased dead space effect is unknown. Probably the rise in mean airway pressure in some of the alveoli compresses the capillaries, thus causing redistribution of their blood to the other alveoli.[9] This effect is exaggerated by the fact that pulmonary blood flow is already diminished secondary to the reduced venous return. This dead space effect will be more marked if the patient is hypotensive or hypovolemic.

The patient with respiratory failure has an already elevated V_D/V_T ratio. Thus, his minute ventilatory requirement is higher than predicted by about 50 percent. However, for the individual patient, this effect will be variable, and it is preferable to put the patient on the respirator at a higher tidal volume than his predicted setting, measure his arterial blood gases, and adjust his respiratory rate accordingly.

THE ALVEOLAR–ARTERIAL OXYGEN GRADIENT

Patients ventilated with small tidal volumes will show progressive alveolar collapse demonstrated by an increase in their alveolar–arterial gradient. This trend can be reversed by frequent hyperinflations.[13] Similarly, large tidal volumes above 7 ml per kg body weight can lead to a reduction in alveolar–arterial gradient, while smaller volumes can lead to its elevation.[14]

Since airway closure occurs at low resting lung volumes, leading to increased shunting, artificial ventilation working below functional residual capacity will be less effective in oxygenating patients. In contrast, techniques that increase FRC minimize this shunting.

An inspiratory plateau, by opening more alveoli, can improve the P_{O_2} by diminishing the shunt and decreasing the V_D/V_T ratio.[15] Recently, the application of continuous positive pressure breathing was found to be effective in spontaneously breathing neonates suffering from the respiratory distress syndrome. It improved their oxygenation and their low compliance.[16] The application of continuous positive pressure during artificial respiration was found to be valuable in treating severe respiratory failure not amenable to other forms of therapy. The improvement in oxygenation is probably due to the increase in lung volume; in one study in adults, the application of 5 cm end-expiratory pressure led to an increase in the lung volume of about 350 ml with an increase in the arterial oxygen tension of 68 mm Hg.[17] The higher end-expiratory pressure will keep the lung more expanded during expiration with improvement in oxygenation. However, the incidence of complications, such as subcutaneous emphysema and pneumothorax, increases with the higher pressures. Also, in lungs with very low compliance (stiff), the application of end-expiratory pressure will lead to a lesser increase in lung volume (FRC), with little improvement in oxygenation.

The exact mechanism by which the positive pressure during expiration improves oxygenation is unknown, but it can be due to any or all of the following:

1. Prevention of airway closure. The positive pressure is transmitted from the small airway to the alveoli, thus preventing them from collapsing during expiration.
2. Prevention of gas trapping. Because the small airways are prevented from collapsing, there is less chance for gas behind these airways to be absorbed.
3. The rise of intraalveolar pressure pushes the alveolar fluid against the alveolar wall, decreasing the diffusion distance and also preventing further influx of water from the capillaries into the interstitial spaces.

Electrolyte and Water Balance

In a study in which patients received prolonged artificial ventilation, a syndrome characterized by positive water balance, gain in weight, radiographic changes suggestive of pulmonary edema, decreased pulmonary compliance, and deteriorating blood gases developed[18] in the absence of cardiac failure or a raised central venous pressure. Patients in respiratory failure are in a catabolic state. They should lose weight at a rate of approximately 400 g daily; in contrast these patients gained weight. The exact reason for this fluid retention is unknown but could be due to hypoalbuminemia, reduction of lymph flow,[19] subclinical heart failure, or inappropriate secretion of antidiuretic hormone, which is related to the presence of positive pressure during expiration. This syndrome responds satisfactorily to diuretic therapy and fluid restriction.[20]

VENTILATORS

There are several hundred types of respirators available on the market, each one claiming its superiority. They can be classified according to the source of power, such as electricity or pressure, or according to flow characteristics. However, the simplest way to classify them is through their inspiratory cycle.

Volume Cycled

In this type of respirator, the inspiratory cycle ends when a fixed volume has been delivered from the machine. The typical example is an Emerson postoperative ventilator. Its main advantage is that it has one adjustment to set the tidal volume, and the machine delivers this sinusoidal flow as long as it is in working order. Its main disadvantage is that it can develop very high pressures if obstruction occurs, or it will continue pumping even if it is disconnected. Thus, an alarm system is mandatory for this type of ventilator.

Pressure Cycled

In these, the inspiration ends when a predetermined pressure is reached, and the time taken to reach this pressure depends on the resistance offered by the patient. If the airway resistance is high, then this set pressure is reached much earlier. The typical example is the Bird ventilator, which uses a magnetic system to end the cycle. Its main drawback is that it lacks power in situations of very low compliance. It is perfectly adequate for patients with mechanical respiratory failure with normal lungs for short periods. Presently, more powerful pressure-cycled ventilators are available.

Time Cycled

In this type of respirator, the change over from inspiration to expiration occurs after a preset time and does not depend on the condition of the lung. Although they will deliver a stable tidal volume, to adjust this tidal volume one needs the interaction of three adjustments, ie, inspiratory flow, inspiratory time, and inspiration/expiration ratio. The typical examples are the Engstrom and Radcliff ventilators.

The main requirement of a ventilator is to be able to deliver a fixed tidal volume in the face of varying impedance to lung inflation, ie, it should be able to deliver a tidal volume with adequate flows to maintain a minute ventilation with an inspiratory/expiratory ratio of at least $1:1$ in the presence of high resistance to lung inflation.[21]

In conclusion. Positive pressure ventilation by mechanical means raises the mean intrathoracic pressure, which in turn leads to a diminution in dynamic lung compliance with an increase in the V_D/V_T ratio, while the airway resistance decreases. In certain conditions, it may lead to a diminution of venous return and cardiac output and an increase in physiologic shunting. The effect of a decrease in venous return is counteracted by an increase in the peripheral venous tone, which parallels the rise of intrathoracic pressure. This compensatory venoconstriction can be minimal or absent in hypovolemia and in certain other diseases or can be due to drug therapy. The application of positive pressure during the expiratory pressure accentuates these changes, except for the physiologic shunting, which is diminished.

The *optimum ventilatory pattern* is one with large tidal volumes, administered slowly, which is followed by an expiratory cycle for the same or more prolonged length of time. The carbon dioxide level is kept nearer normal by adjusting to a slow respiratory rate, and, if at this rate and setting the patient is uncomfortable, larger tidal volumes can be administered by the addition of mechanical dead space.[22] The inspired oxygen concentration should be adjusted to provide an arterial oxygen concentration in the normal range.

OXYGEN TOXICITY

Although oxygen is necessary for the production of energy and the survival of all aerobic cells, it is a universal cellular poison at high concentrations. High concentrations of oxygen interfere with cellular oxidative reactions by a number of mechanisms, among which are inactivation of sulfhydryl-dependent dehydrogenases, interference with formation of high-energy phosphate bonds, and the electron transport chain.[23]

Because the lung is the first organ exposed to the maximal concentration of oxygen, it is the first one to show the effects of oxygen damage. The first symptom of inspiring a high concentration of O_2 in the awake person is mild carinal irritation. Prolonged exposure produces the sensation of pain, which is accentuated by coughing and deep breathing. This progresses to dyspnea and paroxysmal coughing. Within 24 hours a significant decline of vital capacity and dynamic lung compliance can be demonstrated. This hyperoxia leads to an increase in systemic vascular resistance and a concomitant decline in cardiac output, the net result being unchanged systemic blood pressure.[24]

In patients ventilated with high concentrations of oxygen (90 percent), two phases can be distinguished at histologic examination: an acute oxidative phase, which starts at the capillary endothelial level and is characterized by congestion, alveolar edema, intraalveolar hemorrhage, and a fibrin exudate with the formation of prominent hyaline membranes; and a late proliferative phase, which occurs after 10 days of exposure to O_2, characterized by alveolar and intralobular septal edema and fibroblastic proliferation with early fibrous and prominent hyperplasia of the alveolar lining cells. To the naked eye, the lungs are heavy, beefy, and edematous.[25] However, one should realize that these pathologic changes are nonspecific responses to a variety of injuries of which oxygen is only one. To see the effects of pulmonary oxygen toxicity, the oxygen exposure should be prolonged at high concentrations. Exposure to oxygen (0.4 to 0.5 atm) for a very long time does not lead to any demonstrable toxic defect nor does breathing 100 percent oxygen for less than 24 hours lead to any significant toxic effect. Thus, in the operating room situation, pulmonary oxygen toxicity should not represent any problem.[24]

In any hypoxemic patient, oxygen toxicity should never be a deterrent to oxygen administration. Clinically, one can follow the assumption that an inspired oxygen concentration of 50 percent or more will lead to serious damage to the lung if used more than 48 hours. In patients with respiratory failure and a shunt of more than 30 percent, a high inspired oxygen concentration (more than 60 percent) is required to maintain near-normal arterial oxygen concentrations. In these situations, further increasing the oxygen concentration will lead to a very small improvement in oxygenation because of the large venous admixture. Therefore, in such patients one should resort to other maneuvers, such as choosing a more optimal ventilatory pattern, fluid restriction, and using a positive end-expiratory pressure in the ventilatory cycle.

The central nervous system manifestation of oxygen toxicity is usually a grand mal seizure and is only seen when oxygen is used at 2.5 atm. These occur only in the treatment of certain uncommon diseases, or in hyperbaric chambers, deep sea diving, or caisson work.

Retrolental Fibroplasia

Retrolental fibroplasia is another toxic manifestation of oxygen, which is seen only in the newborn, especially in those who are born prematurely. In contrast to pulmonary oxygen toxicity, which is due to a high concentration of oxygen in the lung, the effect on the retinal arterioles is a function of Po_2. Hyperoxia leads to vasoconstriction of the retinal vessels, which is reversible at the early stages. This has been demonstrated at an arterial oxygen level of 100 mm Hg in immature infants, while in some others 400 mm Hg has no effect. Continued exposure leads to endothelial damage of the retinal vessels, finally leading to their obliteration. After the removal of the infant to air the remaining retinal vessels overproliferate. Hemorrhage from these vessels leads to proliferation of fibrous tissue and ultimately retinal detachment and blindness in about 30 percent of these infants.

Several factors can affect these responses of the retinal vessels to hyperoxia, ie, the degree of immaturity of the infant, the duration of oxygen administration, previous hypoxia, and the rapidity of changes in oxygen concentration.[26]

Thus, whenever oxygen is used for prolonged periods in a newborn as well as in an adult, it is imperative that arterial oxygen tension be monitored closely and kept as near to normal as possible (Table 15-2).

TABLE 15-2. Normal Values for Ventilatory Function Tests*

MEASUREMENT	SYMBOL†	AVERAGE VALUE	UNIT
Lung volumes			
Tidal volume	V	500	ml
Respiratory frequency	f	12	resp/min
Minute volume	$\dot{V}$	6.000	ml/min
Respiratory dead space	$\dot{V}_D$	150	ml
Alveolar ventilation	$\dot{V}_A$	4,200	ml/min
Total lung capacity	TLC	6,000	ml
Vital capacity	VC	4,800	ml
Inspiratory capacity	IC	3,800	ml
Expiratory reserve volume	ERV	1,200	ml
Functional residual capacity	FRC	2,400	ml
Residual volume	RV	1,200	ml
Mechanics of breathing			
Total compliance, pulmonary and thoracic cage	$C_{(L+T)}$	0.1	liters/cm H_2O
Pulmonary compliance	C_L	0.2	liters/cm H_2O
Thoracic cage compliance	C_T	0.2	liters/cm H_2O
Airway resistance	RAW	1.6	cm H_2O/liters/second
Work of quiet breathing	—	0.5	kgM/min
Maximal inspiratory and expiratory pressures	—	60–100	mm Hg
Maximal voluntary ventilation	MVV	150	liters/min
Forced expiratory volume			
percent in 1 second	FEV_1	83	percent in 1 second
percent in 3 seconds	FFV_3	97	percent in 3 seconds
Maximal expiratory flow rate	MEFR	400	liters/min

* Adapted from Comroe.[27]

† Definitions for symbols (omitted for those in widest use):

Primary (capitals) denoting physical quantities: C, concentration in blood phase, also compliance; F, fractional concentration of dry gas; P, gas pressure or partial pressure; $\dot{Q}$, volume of blood per unit time; V, gas volume in general; and $\dot{V}$, volume of gas per unit time; rate of gas flow.

Secondary symbols (small capital subscripts) for gas phase, denoting location of quantity: A, alveolar gas; B, barometric (usually pressure); D, dead space gas; E, expired gas; I, inspired gas; and T, tidal gas.

REFERENCES

1. Pontoppidan H, Geffin B, Lowenstein E: Acute respiratory failure in the adult. N Engl J Med 286:690,743,799, 1972
2. Staub NC, Nagano H, Pearce ML: Pulmonary edema in dogs, especially the sequence of fluid accumulation in lungs. J Appl Physiol 22:227, 1967
3. Cothell TS, Levine OR, Senior RM, et al: Electron microscopic alteration at the alveolar level in pulmonary edema. Circ Res 21:783, 1967
4. Pontoppidan H, Laver MB, Geffin B: Acute respiratory failure in the surgical patient. Adv Surg 4:163, 1970
5. Bendixen HH, Egbert LD, Hedley-Whyte J: Respiratory Care. St. Louis, Mosby, 1965

MEASUREMENT	SYMBOL†	AVERAGE VALUE	UNIT
Arterial blood			
Oxygen tension	Po_2	100	mm Hg or Torr
Oxygen saturation	So_2	98	percent
CO_2 tension	Pco_2	40	mm Hg or Torr
Alveolar–arterial O_2 gradient (FIO$_2$ 100 percent)	$P(A\text{-}aDO_2)$	33	mm Hg or Torr
Oxygen saturation (FIO$_2$ 100 percent)	So_2	100	percent
Arterial pH	pH	7.4	
H^+ concentration of arterial blood		40	nmol/liter
Pulmonary circulation			
Pulmonary artery pressure	PA	25/10	mm Hg
Pulmonary "capillary" blood pressure (wedge)	PCWP	8	mm Hg
Pulmonary blood flow	$\dot{Q}C$	5,400	ml/min
Pulmonary capillary blood volume	$\dot{Q}C$	100	ml
Gas exchange			
O_2 consumption	$\dot{V}o_2$	240	ml/min
CO_2 output	$\dot{V}co_2$	200	,l/min
Respiratory exchange ratios (CO_2 output/O_2 uptake)	R	0.8	
Alveolar ventilation/blood flow	$\dot{V}A/\dot{V}Q$	0.8	
Physiologic shunt/cardiac output × 100		< 5	percent
Physiologic deadspace/ tidal volume × 100	(V_D/V_T)	<30	percent
CO diffusing capacity (single breath)	$D_{L\,CO}$	25	ml CO/min/mm Hg

Secondary symbols (lower case) for blood phase: a, arterial (except for arterial O_2 and CO_2 tension and O_2 saturation, for which the standard symbols Po_2, Pco_2, and So_2 have been used); b, blood in general; c, capillary; c′, end capillary; v, venous; and v′, mixed venous.

6. Hedley-Whyte J, Pontoppidan H, Morris MJ: The response of patients with respiratory failure and cardiopulmonary disease to different levels of constant volume ventilation. J Clin Invest 45:1543, 1966
7. Morgan BC, Crawford EW, Hornbein TF: Hemodynamic effects of intermittent positive pressure ventilation. Anesthesiology 27:584, 1966
8. Sharpey-Schafer EP: Venous tone. Br Med J 5267:1589, 1961
9. Cournand A, Motley HL, Werko L: Physiologic studies of the effects of intermittent positive pressure breathing on cardiac output in man. Am J Physiol 152:162, 1948
10. Grenvik A: Respiratory, circulatory and metabolic effects of respirator treatment. A clinical study in postoperative thoracil surgical patients. Acta Anaesth Scand (Suppl) 19:1, 1966

11. Kumar A, Falke KJ, Geffin B, et al: Continuous positive-pressure ventilation in acute respiratory failure. N Engl J Med 283:1430, 1970
12. Cooper EA: Physiological dead space in passive ventilation. Anaesthesia 22:90, 199, 1967
13. Laver MB, Morgan J, Bendixen HH, et al: Lung volume, compliance, and arterial oxygen tensions during controlled ventilation. J Appl Physiol 19:725, 1964
14. Hedley-Whyte J, Pontoppidan H, Laver MB, et al: Arterial oxygenation during hypothermia. Anesthesiology 26:595, 1965
15. Lyager S: Ventilation/perfusion ratio during intermittent positive pressure ventilation: importance of no flow interval during the insufflation. Acta Anaesth Scand 14:211, 1976
16. Gregory GA, Kitterman JA, Phibbs RH, et al: Treatment of the idiopathic respiratory-distress syndrome with continuous positive airway pressure. N Engl J Med 284:1333, 1971
17. Kumar A, Falke K, Geffin B: Continuous positive pressure ventilation in acute respiratory failure. N Engl J Med 283:1430, 1973
18. Sladen A, Laver MB, Pontoppidan H: Pulmonary complications and water retention in prolonged mechanical ventilation N Engl J Med 279:448, 1968
19. Pilon RN, Bittar DA: The effect of positive end-expiratory pressure on thoracic duct lymph flow during controlled ventilation in anesthetized dogs. Anesthesiology 39:607, 1973
20. Philbin DM, Baratz RA, Patterson RA: The effect of carbon dioxide on plasma antidiuretic hormone levels during intermittent positive pressure breathing. Anesthesiology 33:345, 1970
21. Cheney FW: What are the important differences in ventilation? ASA Refresher Courses in Anesthesiology, Chicago, 1975, p 209a
22. Fairley HB: Artificial respiration. In Scurr C, Feldman S (eds): Scientific Foundations of Anesthesia. Philadelphia, Davis, 1970, p 192
23. Hedley-Whyte J, Winter PM: Oxygen therapy. Clin Pharmacol Ther 8:696, 1967
24. Winter PM, Smith G: The toxicity of oxygen. Anesthesiology 37:210, 1972
25. Nash G, Blennerhassett JB, Pontoppidan H: Pulmonary lesions associated with oxygen therapy and artificial ventilation. N Engl J Med 276:368, 1967
26. Stern L: The use and misuse of oxygen in the newborn infant. Pediatr Clin North Am 20:447, 1973
27. Comroe JH, Jr, Forster RE, Dubois AB, Briscoe WA, Carlsen E: The Lung, 12th ed. Chicago, Year Book, 1962

chapter 16

The Transport of Oxygen and Carbon Dioxide by the Blood

The gases in the lung "flow downhill," ie, they diffuse from an area of higher partial pressure to an area of lower partial pressure. Because oxygen tension in the alveoli is higher than in the mixed venous blood, oxygen diffuses from the alveoli to the blood, while the opposite happens with carbon dioxide. The gases are transferred across the alveolocapillary membrane by simple diffusion. Thus, their rate of diffusion is directly proportional to the difference in tension between the two sides of the membranes. Also, the rate of diffusion is directly proportional to the solubility of the gas in blood, while it is inversely proportional to the square root of its molecular weight. The molecular weight of carbon dioxide is 44 and that of oxygen is 32. Therefore, the difference between the square root of their molecular weights is small. In contrast, CO_2 is 24 times more soluble than O_2; therefore, CO_2 diffuses 20 times faster than oxygen across the alveolocapillary membrane.

OXYGEN TRANSPORT

Oxygen is carried in the blood in two forms: in physical solution as well as in combination with hemoglobin. Because of the poor solubility of oxygen in plasma, the amount dissolved in it is very small. At a partial pressure of 100 mm Hg, the amount of oxygen dissolved in 100 ml of plasma is 0.3 ml. If a person inspires 100 percent oxygen, the oxygen dissolved in 100 ml of plasma increases to 2 ml. If this was the only way to transport O_2, the cardiac output at rest should be at least 12.5 liters per minute to satisfy the oxygen demands of the tissues (250 ml per minute) while he is breathing 100 percent oxygen, assuming also that all the oxygen is given up at the tissue level. To guard against such a high load on cardiac output, nature has provided us with a very

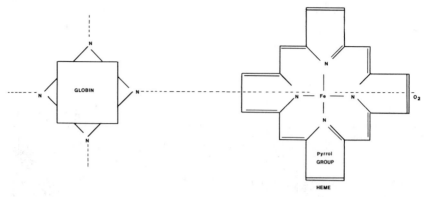

FIG. 16-1: The hemoglobin molecule.

efficient method for transfer of oxygen from the lungs to the tissues, ie, the hemoglobin.

Hemoglobin is a conjugated protein with a molecular weight of 66,700[1] (Fig. 16-1). Its protein fraction is globin, which is joined to an iron–porphyrin compound called heme. The heme molecule consists of four pyrrol groups attached to one central iron atom. Four of these heme groups are attached to the largest component of hemoglobin, the globin molecule. The linkage between the heme and the globin molecule is through the iron atom of heme to the imidazole ring of globin. The globin molecule consists of four distinct polypeptide chains of about 740 amino acids. Normal adult hemoglobin (hemoglobin A) has two identical alpha chains and two identical beta chains. The iron in hemoglobin is in the ferrous form and comprises 0.34 percent of the weight of hemoglobin. Each iron atom of the hemoglobin molecule reacts with one molecule of oxygen. Thus, 4 moles of oxygen react with 1 mole of hemoglobin, which is the equivalent of 1.39 ml of oxygen to each gram of hemoglobin.

The combination of oxygen with hemoglobin is a very loose one, varying with the oxygen tension of plasma. This reaction occurs without the intervention of any enzyme or any change in the valency of iron. Thus, this uptake of oxygen by the hemoglobin is termed oxygenation, not oxidation.

Oxyhemoglobin Dissociation Curves

The combination of hemoglobin with oxygen is accomplished in four steps, each involving a different iron atom:

$$Hb_4 \ + O_2 \rightleftharpoons Hb_4O_2$$
$$Hb_4O_2 + O_2 \rightleftharpoons Hb_4O_4$$

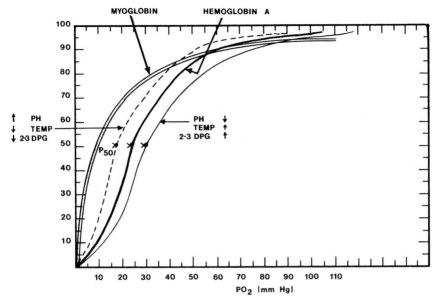

FIG. 16-2: Oxyhemoglobin dissociation curves for whole blood. Note the increase in P_{50} that occurs with shifting the curve to the right from acidosis and increasing the temperature and 2,3-DPG levels. The opposite occurs with alkalosis, drop in temperature, and 2,3-DPG levels. Note also the hyperbolic dissociation curve of myoglobin.

$$Hb_4O_4 + O_2 \rightleftharpoons Hb_4O_6$$
$$Hb_4O_6 + O_2 \rightleftharpoons Hb_4O_8.$$

Each of these reactions has a different equilibration rate (constant), and the first reaction facilitates the following reactions, thus giving the characteristic sigmoid shape to the oxyhemoglobin dissociation curves (Fig. 16-2).

On the basis of this S-shaped curve, several properties of hemoglobin can be explained:

1. At the lung, the P_{O_2} is about 100 mm Hg. Thus, hemoglobin becomes 97.5 percent saturated, each 100 ml of blood containing 19.5 ml of O_2.
2. Increasing the P_{O_2} in the lung to more than 100 mm Hg increases the O_2 content only slightly. The most it can do is to increase the oxygen dissolved in plasma to its maximum, ie, 2 ml oxygen per 100 ml blood. However, the amount is minimal when compared to the amount carried by hemoglobin.
3. At the upper flat or horizontal part of the curve, dropping the P_{O_2} from 100 to 70 mm Hg has very little effect on the oxygen content of blood (a decrease of 5 percent). Thus, a person can live at reasonably high altitudes without much diminution in his oxygen carrying capacity.

4. At the tissue level where the P_{O_2} is 20 to 40 mm Hg, the curve is very steep. Thus, large amounts of oxygen are liberated.

Factors Affecting the Shape of the Oxyhemoglobin Dissociation Curve

A convenient indicator for the position of the oxyhemoglobin dissociation curve is P_{50}, which is the partial pressure of oxygen where only 50 percent of the hemoglobin is saturated with oxygen (or 50 percent released). In the normal adult and at a pH of 7.4 and temperature of 37C, P_{50} is 27 mm Hg. With a shift to the right, P_{50} is increased, whereas with a shift to the left it is diminished (Fig. 16-2).

TEMPERATURE

A rise in body temperature shifts the dissociation curve to the right. Therefore, the affinity of hemoglobin for O_2 is decreased, allowing more oxygen to be delivered to the tissues at an equivalent partial pressure of oxygen. This is especially favorable for the actively contracting muscles, in which a local rise in temperature favors oxygen release.

pH

The effect of carbon dioxide tension and hydrogen ion (H^+) concentration on the hemoglobin dissociation curve is called the "Bohr effect." The changes produced by CO_2 on the dissociation curve are secondary to changes in H^+ within the red blood cells. Increased acidity (drop in pH), similar to a rise in temperature, shifts the curve to the right, and the opposite is true with alkalosis.

2,3-DIPHOSPHOGLYCERATE (2,3-DPG)

This is a normal product of anaerobic glycolysis via the Embden–Meyerhof pathway. It is present in erythrocytes in large amounts at a molar ratio of 1:1 with hemoglobin. Each mol of 2,3-DPG binds to 1 mol of reduced hemoglobin through the beta chain of the latter. An increase in the 2,3-DPG level enhances the oxygen release from the hemoglobin molecule. Conversely, diminution of 2,3-DPG levels leads to retention of O_2 by the hemoglobin. Several factors affect the 2,3-DPG concentration of the red cell:

1. Acidosis inhibits red cell glycolysis by decreasing the activity of phosphofructokinase, resulting in a diminution of 2,3-DPG levels. Thus, the bene-

ficial effect of acidosis in enhancing the release of oxygen from the hemoglobin molecule is of a short duration of only a few hours.[2] The decrease in
the 2,3-DPG level will shift the oxygen dissociation curve back to the left.

2. Ascent to high altitudes or chronic lung disease leads to an increase in 2,3-
    DPG levels, facilitating the release of oxygen.[3]
3. Hormones such as thyroid, growth, and androgens increase the erythrocyte
    2,3-DPG levels.
4. Most anemias are associated with an increase in 2,3-DPG levels.
5. With storage of blood there occurs a progressive decrease in red cell 2,3-
    DPG levels. After transfusion, the half recovery time for 2,3-DPG is 4
    hours, and it takes several days to reach its normal level.[4] This progressive
    decline in 2,3-DPG levels is more marked in blood stored in acid-citrated
    dextrose solution (ACD). It is better preserved in blood preserved in citrate
    phosphate dextrose (CPD) anticoagulants. However, the metabolic
    integrity as well as the respiratory function of the red cell is best main-
    tained during storage by freeze preservation when the cells are freshly
    drawn. It has been demonstrated that the addition of more organic com-
    pounds such as inosine and adenine[5] or benzoic acid derivatives can
    diminish this 2,3-DPG loss of stored blood.

TYPE OF HEMOGLOBIN

There are at least 17 varieties of human hemoglobin. They are determined
genetically and are labeled A to S. All of them except adult hemoglobin (A) and
fetal hemoglobin (F) are considered abnormal. The oxyhemoglobin dissociation curve of all these abnormal hemoglobins is to the right of adult hemoglobin.

Fetal hemoglobin has a greater affinity for oxygen than adult hemoglobin.
This is due to the failure of fetal hemoglobin to bind 2,3-DPG to the same
degree as adult hemoglobin.[6] The advantage of fetal hemoglobin is that it
facilitates the movement of oxygen in the placenta from the mother to the fetus.
However, it has the disadvantage that it does not give up the oxygen easily at
the tissues. With the growth of the newborn, the amount of fetal hemoglobin
diminishes, and the oxygen dissociation curve shifts to the right and approxi-
mates that of the infant at 4 to 6 months of age. Premature infants and infants
with the respiratory distress syndrome have a lower 2,3-DPG level. Thus, their
P_{50} values are lower and the shift toward normal is much more gradual.

Myoglobin

Myoglobin has a structural formula similar to hemoglobin, but it differs
from hemoglobin in that it binds to 1 mol of oxygen instead of 4. Thus, its

dissociation curve is a hyperbolic instead of the sigmoid curve of hemoglobin. Its main function is to assure a constant oxygen supply to the muscles, probably by facilitating the oxygen flow into the muscles.[7]

CARBON DIOXIDE TRANSPORT

The carbon dioxide produced by the cell diffuses out of the cell membrane to the capillary lumen as dissolved CO_2. The difference between the partial pressure of carbon dioxide at the tissues and the capillary lumen is rather small (1 to 2 mm Hg); however, CO_2 diffuses out of the cell easily because of its high coefficient of diffusion and solubility. After CO_2 reaches the capillary lumen, the work of its transport to the lungs is accomplished by the heart.

In the blood, carbon dioxide is carried in three forms: dissolved, bicarbonate, and as carbamino compounds. These three forms exist in plasma as well as inside the red cell at different concentrations (Fig. 16-3).

DISSOLVED

About 5 percent of the carbon dioxide in blood is present in physical solution, providing the partial pressure of carbon dioxide in blood (46 mm Hg in mixed venous blood and 40 mm Hg in arterial blood).

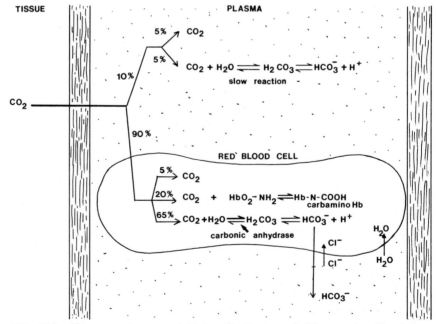

FIG. 16-3: The approximate quantitative distribution of CO_2 entering blood from tissues.

CARBAMINO COMPOUNDS

A very small amount of carbon dioxide in plasma is combined with plasma proteins, but a larger portion (21 percent) combines with the amino groups of hemoglobin to form carbamino compounds by the following reaction:

$$HbNH_2 + CO_2 \rightleftharpoons HbNHCOOH$$

BICARBONATE

Most of the carbon dioxide present in blood is in the form of bicarbonate (HCO_3^-).

$$CO_2 + H_2O \underset{}{\overset{\text{carbonic anhydrase}}{\rightleftharpoons}} H_2CO_3 \rightleftharpoons HCO_3^- + H^+$$

The first reaction, the hydration of CO_2 to carbonic acid (H_2CO_3) is a slow reaction in the plasma. However, it is a much faster one in the red blood cell because of the presence of the enzyme *carbonic anhydrase*. Carbonic anhydrase is a zinc-containing enzyme and is present in high concentrations in red blood cells, but it is practically absent in plasma. It is also present in renal and pancreatic cells, where it is involved in bicarbonate secretion and in gastric mucosa. The dissociation of carbonic acid to H^+ and bicarbonate ion is a fast one and does not need any catalyst. The bicarbonate ion, like most of the anions of the body, is a freely diffusible one through the cell membrane (in contrast to cations such as Na^+ and K^+). As the concentration of HCO_3^- rises in the cell, it diffuses out in the plasma. To keep the electrochemical neutrality inside the red cell, chloride ion (Cl^-) diffuses into the cell (the *chloride shift*). Thus, the Cl^- content of the red cell in the venous blood becomes higher than in the arterial blood. This increase in the osmotically active anions such as Cl^- and HCO_3^- in the red cell of venous blood leads to more water retention by the cell, leading to an increase in its size. That is the reason why the hematocrit of venous blood is 3 percent higher than the arterial blood.

The ratio of CO_2 in physical solution to the bicarbonate normally is $1:20$.

Hemoglobin affects the carbon dioxide transport by two mechanisms. The first is by forming carbamino compounds; the second is by accepting H^+ at the tissue level. Reduced hemoglobin is a weaker acid than oxyhemoglobin. Thus, at the tissues when the oxyhemoglobin becomes deoxygenated, the weaker acid now combines with less base. An extra base is then available to neutralize the acidity produced at the tissues (Haldane effect). It is estimated that complete deoxygenation of 1 mmol of O_2 can neutralize 0.7 mmol of hydrogen ions without any change in pH.

The net result of the 200 ml CO_2 liberated at the tissues every minute at rest is a rise in CO_2 content of blood by 4 ml per 100 ml of blood. Of this, about 5 to 10 percent stays in solution, 20 percent is transported as carbamino compound, while the remaining 70 percent is added to the HCO_3^- pool, resulting in a drop of pH from 7.40 to 7.36. This distribution of CO_2 is slightly different in arterial blood where the dissolved CO_2 and the carbamino compounds each represents less than 5 percent of the total CO_2, while the remaining 90 percent is in the form of bicarbonate. Of this bicarbonate, two-thirds is present in the plasma, whereas the remaining one-third is inside the red cell.

OXYGEN AND CARBON DIOXIDE STORES OF THE BODY

The total body stores of oxygen are minimal, equal to approximately 1500 ml. Since there is a basal metabolic requirement of 250 ml per minute, the O_2 stores cannot supply adequate tissue oxygen tension for more than 4 minutes. Most of the oxygen stores are in the arterial blood (1 liter); the lung stores of oxygen in a person breathing room air are small. If we assume that the person has a FRC of 2 liters, the amount of oxygen in the lung is about 400 ml. Because tissue function becomes impaired at an arterial pressure of approximately 40 mm Hg, this store in the lung can sustain life for only about 1 minute. However, the pulmonary storage capacity for oxygen can be increased by about tenfold if the individual breathes 100 percent oxygen. This is in contrast to the oxygen carrying capacity of blood, which can be increased very little. O_2 in 100 percent concentration raises the hemoglobin saturation from 97 to 100 percent and increases the dissolved amount by 2 ml O_2 per 100 ml plasma. Although there is a relatively large amount of oxygen bound to myoglobin, this is only available in situ. The hyperbolic curve of myoglobin "locks in" oxygen until the partial pressure drops to extremely low values.[8]

In contrast to oxygen, the carbon dioxide stores of the body are very large; the whole body can yield about 120 liters of CO_2. In an apneic individual, if oxygenation is maintained by prior ventilation with 100 percent oxygen and by providing a constant flow of oxygen (apneic oxygenation), the rate of rise of P_{CO_2} is 13 mm Hg in the first minute and subsequently the rate of rise is 3 mm Hg per minute.[9] The initial rapid rise is due to equilibration of the gas with mixed venous P_{CO_2}, while the succeeding slow rise is from the metabolic production of CO_2 divided by the available storage capacity of the body for CO_2.

HYPOXIA

For oxygen to be transferred from capillaries to tissues, a certain partial pressure gradient is required. Below this critical capillary oxygen tension, diffusion is impaired. The minimum end-capillary oxygen tension for the maintenance of adequate oxygenation is about 200 mm Hg.[10] This critical oxygen tension is variable from one tissue to another.

The capillary critical range is suggested to be between 20 and 30 mm Hg.[11] At normal pH and temperature, this represents an O_2 saturation of 35 to 55 percent. Below this level, cell metabolism becomes anaerobic, and the breakdown of glucose stops at the stage of lactic acid formation. If this inadequate oxygenation persists, the metabolic derangements finally lead to the death of the cell. The brain is the most sensitive organ. Its oxygen uptake diminishes when the venous oxygen tension falls into the 20 to 25-mm Hg range.

Cerebral Hypoxia

Cerebral hypoxia is usually manifested by impaired judgment, drowsiness, excitement, headache (effects similar to those produced by alcohol), and diminution of electroencephalographic activity. It can lead to nausea, vomiting, and Cheyne–Stokes respiration. In the early stages, ventilation is increased from stimulation of the chemoreceptor cells present in aortic and carotid areas, but in the late stages respiration is depressed from anoxia of the respiratory centers.

The kidney can tolerate moderate amounts of hypoxia. However, if its oxygen supply falls more than two-thirds of its normal flow, its sodium and urea handling becomes impaired. In severe hypoxia, tubular cell necrosis occurs with excretory failure. Splanchnic hypoxia leads to impairment of liver function tests, especially those tests that indicate release of intracellular enzymes, ie, lactic dehydrogenase (LDH) and glutamic oxalacetic transaminase (SGOT).

Clinically, hypoxia has been divided into four types: hypoxic hypoxia, anemic hypoxia, stagnant hypoxia, and histotoxic hypoxia.

HYPOXIC HYPOXIA (HYPOTONIC ANOXEMIA)

The characteristic feature of this condition is a diminution in arterial oxygen tension. It can occur in normal persons while ascending to high altitudes or from inspiring a low oxygen mixture. It is the final common pathway of almost all respiratory diseases, eg, emphysema, pneumothorax, respiratory obstruction, etc.

In a normal person ascending to a high altitude, the total barometric pressure falls. Thus, the oxygen tension in the alveoli drops, eg, at altitudes of 3000 meters above sea level, the oxygen tension in the alveoli is about 60 mm Hg. This hypoxia leads to a reflex stimulation of the respiratory centers mediated through the chemoreceptors, leading to respiratory alkalosis. At an altitude of 3700 meters, symptoms of mental irritability appear unless the individual is breathing a high concentration of oxygen. At about 14,000 meters the oxygen tension in the alveoli drops so much that even when inspiring 100 percent oxygen, consciousness is lost unless the individual is given oxygen with a high-pressure system.

In persons living in high altitudes, compensatory mechanisms appear within a few days in the body (acclimatization). The first response is an increase in 2,3-DPG levels in hemoglobin, which compensates for the shift of the oxyhemoglobin curve to the left, which has resulted from respiratory alkalosis. Therefore, the availability of oxygen to the tissues is increased. The arterial desaturation leads to an increase in erythropoietin production, resulting in polycythemia.[12] Respiratory alkalosis persists for about 3 to 4 weeks, and eventually the kidney compensates for it by increasing the excretion of the base. The tissues compensate for this constant low O_2 tension by increasing the site of oxidative reactions as manifested by an increase in the number of mitochondria. The myoglobin concentration of muscles is increased, facilitating the movement of oxygen into the muscles.

ANEMIC HYPOXIA (ISOTONIC ANOXEMIA)

In this situation, the arterial oxygen tension is normal, but the oxygen content is diminished. Thus, the oxygen carrying capacity of blood is diminished. This can be due to a decrease in the hemoglobin content of blood or to certain poisons that combine with hemoglobins, such as carbon monoxide or drugs that cause methomoglobinemia like aneline, methylene blue, and nitrophenol.

An anemic patient is usually asymptomatic at rest. However, his exercise tolerance is diminished. The basal cardiac output is affected little until the hemoglobin is below two-thirds of normal. The blood volume is unchanged because of the increase in plasma volume. The diminution in viscosity facilitates the blood flow in the vessels. The diminution in hemoglobin content decreases the buffering capacity of blood. Thus, the blood is more acidic at the venous side, which in itself facilitates the unloading of oxygen at the tissue level (shift to the right). The red cells increase their capacity to unload oxygen by increasing their 2,3-DPG levels.

A cause of severe acute "anemia" is CO poisoning. Carbon monoxide reacts directly with the hemoglobin to form carboxyhemoglobin, which has no oxygen-carrying capacity. It also shifts the dissociation curve of the remaining hemoglobin to the left, decreasing the amount of O_2 released. This is the reason that an anemic individual with 50 percent of his hemoglobin left can function satisfactorily, while, in CO poisoning with the same amount of hemoglobin available, he will be unable to compensate. The affinity for CO to hemoglobin is 210 times that of oxygen. In the treatment of CO poisoning, 100 percent oxygen is given or even hyperbaric oxygenation is used to increase the oxygen dissolved in plasma and also to help the unloading of CO from the hemoglobin molecule.

STAGNANT HYPOXIA (HYPOKINETIC ANOXIA)

Stagnant hypoxia, or diminished blood flow, can be localized from obstruction to the blood supply to that particular area or can be generalized, such as in circulatory collapse, hypotension, and heart failure. The symptoms differ according to the organ involved.

HISTOTOXIC ANOXIA

This is due to poisoning of oxidative enzymes at the tissue level. The blood, perfectly saturated, reaches the tissues, but they are unable to utilize the oxygen because the oxidative enzymes such as cytochrome oxidase are paralyzed. Cyanide is a typical poison of this kind. Cyanide poisoning is treated with nitrites and methylene blue which form methemoglobin, which in turn reacts with cyanide to form cyanmethemoglobin. In some susceptible individuals, sodium nitroprusside is transformed to sulfocyanide, which can lead to similar toxic effects.

Cyanosis

Reduced hemoglobin has a dark color in contrast to oxyhemoglobin, which has a bright red color. Cyanosis can be noticed when the concentration of hemoglobin in the capillary blood is above 5 g per 100 ml. Thus, an anemic patient with a hemoglobin concentration of less than 5 g per 100 ml of blood cannot become cyanotic. Conversely, patients with polycythemia are more liable to show cyanosis. Cyanosis is mostly evident as a bluish discoloration of the mucous membranes, nail beds, and in the areas of the body in which the skin is thin, such as earlobes, lips, and fingers.

Cyanosis can occur in the absence of generalized hypoxemia when the capillary circulation is extremely slowed. Thus, more oxygen is extracted from the blood in the capillaries. This is typically seen in exposure to moderate cold. This is sometimes termed peripheral cyanosis in contrast to that associated with hypoxemia, which is termed central cyanosis.

Although cyanosis is not an absolute sign for hypoxia, for the practicing anesthesiologist confronted with a cyanotic patient, administration of a high concentration of oxygen is mandatory unless he can prove that the cause of cyanosis is peripheral in origin.

REFERENCES

1. Hill RL, Fellows RE: Recent developments in hemoglobin structure and function. Physiol Phys 2:1, 1964

2. Finch CA, Lenfant C: Oxygen transport in man. N Engl J Med 286:407, 1972
3. Lenfant C, Torrance J, English E, et al: Effect of altitude on oxygen binding by hemoglobin and on organic phosphate levels. J Clin Invest 47:2652, 1968
4. Shappell SD, Lenfant CJ: Adaptive, genetic, and iatrogenic alterations of the oxyhemoglobin-dissociation curve. Anesthesiology 37:127, 1972
5. McConn R, Derrick JB: The respiratory function of blood: Transfusion and blood storage. Anesthesiology 36:119, 1972
6. Oski FA: Fetal hemoglobin: the neonatal red cell and 2-3-diphosphoglycerate. Pediatr Clin North Am 19:907, 1972
7. Wittenberg JB: Myoglobin-facilitated oxygen diffusion role of myoglobin in oxygen entry into muscle. Physiol Rev 50:559, 1970
8. Farhi LE: Gas stores of the body. In Fenn WD, Rahn H (eds): Handbook of Physiology, Respiration, Vol. I. Washington DC, American Physiologic Society, 1964, Chap 34
9. Eger EI, Severinghaus JW: The rate of rise of $PaCO_2$ in the apneic anesthetized patient. Anesthesiology 22:419, 1961
10. Landis EM, Pappenheimer JR: Exchange of substances through the capillary walls. In Hamilton WF (ed): Handbook of Physiology, Circulation, Vol. II. Washington, DC, American Physiological Society, 1963, Chap 29
11. Bendixen HH, Laver MB: Hypoxia in anesthesia: a review. Clin Pharmacol Ther 6:510, 1965
12. Lenfant C, Sullivan K: Adaptation to high altitude. N Engl J Med 284:1298, 1971

chapter 17

Acid–Base Regulation

One of the most important physiologic parameters that the body attempts to maintain within a narrow range is the H^+ concentration. The main reason for this is that all the enzymes of the body have an optimum pH at which the rate of their reaction is at maximum, and their activity falls off rapidly if the pH deviates from that value.

The terminology of acid–base regulation in the form of pH is slightly confusing to the practicing physician because it is the only physiologic parameter expressed on a logarithmic scale. This notation was devised by Sorensen and is based on the fact that water in neutral solution partially dissociates to form H^- and the hydroxyl ion (OH^-) according to the following formula:

$$H_2O \rightleftharpoons H^+ + OH^-$$

The concentration of each ion is 10^{-7} mol per liter at 20C. The product of the two, the ionic product of water, is a constant 10^{-14}. For the mathematical convenience in expressing these wide ranges of laboratory values and to eliminate the negative values, the negative logarithm is used where the pH is the negative logarithm of H^+, ie,

$$pH = -[\log H^+]$$

Therefore, the neutral pH is 7, which in the usual terminology would have been 0.000.000.1 mol per liter or 0.0001 mmol per liter or 100 nmol per liter (1 nmol is one thousand millionth of a mol). Increasing the H^+ concentration tenfold will drop the pH one point (pH 6 = 1000 nmol per liter) or a tenfold diminution in H^+ will increase the pH by one digit (pH 8 = 10 nmol per liter).

The normal pH of arterial blood is 7.4 (40 nmol per liter). All the buffer systems of the body are geared to keep the arterial pH as near to 7.4 as possible. However, in certain pathologic situations, these buffer systems may be exhausted and the pH may deviate markedly from the normal.

The maximum and minimum ranges of pH that are compatible with life are 7.7 (20 nmol per liter) to 7.00 (100 nmol per liter). Therefore, the body can tolerate a fivefold range in H^+ concentration. This is an extremely large variation whose conceptual effect has been minimized because of the logarithmic scale.

The amount of H^+ present in plasma is minimal compared to the other ions, eg, the concentration of sodium in plasma in 140 mmol per liter, ie, 140,000.000 nmol per liter, compared to that of H^+, which is 40 nmol per liter. There is a million-fold difference in concentration of the two ions; therefore, the effect of H^+ is omitted in calculations of the osmotic effect of blood.

ACIDS, BASES, AND BUFFERS

An acid is a substance that increases the hydrogen ion concentration in solution, while a base decreases it. The universally accepted definition of an acid is a proton or hydrogen ion donor, and a base is a proton or H^+ acceptor. Sometimes a wider definition is used for acids and bases, eg, if the substance can lead to an increase in the H^+ concentration by a certain physiologic reaction, then it is termed an acid. Hydrochloric acid (HCl), which dissociates in solution to H^+ and Cl^-, is an acid because it increases the H^+ concentration in solution. But occasionally Cl^- is termed an acidic radical because it can raise H^+ in body fluids by virtue of its physiologic properties. Similarly, Na^+ is termed a basic radical because it can increase the hydroxyl ion concentration in solution, despite the fact that it neither accepts nor donates any H^+.

The term fixed acid is used to refer to anionic radicals such as Cl^- and SO_4^{--}, which cannot be formed or destroyed in the body. The term organic acid is used for radicals that are metabolized in the body (lactate, citrate, acetoacetate). Similarly, the term fixed base applies to Na^+, K^+, Ca^{++}, Mg^{++}, because they can lead to an increase in the total amount of OH^- in the extracellular spaces.

A strong acid such as hydrochloric acid is fully dissociated to H^+ and Cl^-, whereas carbonic acid (H_2CO_3), being a weaker acid, is dissociated less completely to HCO_3^- and H^+.

$$H_2CO_3 \rightleftharpoons H^+ + HCO_3$$

At a pH of 6, carbonic acid and the bicarbonate ions are present in almost equal concentrations. However, this equilibrium can vary according to the law of mass action, which states that the velocity of a reaction is proportional to the product of the molar concentration of the reactants. For example, if a strong acid such as HCl is added to the solution, the increase in H^+ will move the reaction to the left. The number of H^+ is diminished and the H^+ are mopped up and hidden as H_2CO_3. The opposite happens when a strong base is added to the solution. This is the principle of buffers. By definition, buffers are substances that by their presence in a solution tend to ameliorate changes in pH of a solution on addition of hydrogen ions or hydroxyl ions.

In the above example, bicarbonate ion (HCO_3^-) is the conjugate base that reacts with the H^+ of the strong acid, leading to the formation of a less dissociable (weaker) acid. Obviously, a buffer system has its limitations. It can be exhausted if too much acid is added. Then a small increase in acidity will lead to a marked increase in the H^+ concentration.

REGULATION OF HYDROGEN ION CONCENTRATION

Despite the fact that the body can tolerate reasonable changes in the H^+ concentration, the body keeps it in a very narrow range. Thus, the arterial H^+ concentration rarely exceeds its narrow range of 45 to 35 nmol per liter (pH 7.35 to 7.45). This is accomplished through three main mechanisms: the buffer mechanism, respiratory adjustment, and renal regulation.

The first reaction, the fastest, is almost instantaneous, but it is an incomplete one. The other two are much slower in their time responses. The kidneys are the only organs that can definitely correct for the metabolic acid–base disorder by excreting the loading acid or base.

Buffering Action of Body Fluids

The buffers of the body fluids represent the first line of defense against any change in H^+. For example, it is estimated that the addition of 1 mmol of strong acid to 1 liter of body fluid would increase the hydrogen ion concentration by only 5 mmol per liter. Thus, out of the 1 million of H^+ radicals added only five become effective in changing the H^+, while the remainder are buffered.[1] Most of this buffering occurs in the extracellular space, and part of it occurs in the intracellular space at a much slower pace. The blood and extracellular buffers are readily available and react with the added acid or base immediately. The intracellular buffers are slower in response, occurring in several minutes, and the abundant buffering capacity of bones requires hours to days to become fully effective.

The bicarbonate buffer present in blood is the most available one. It represents about 53 percent of the total buffering capacity of blood, 35 percent being in the plasma and the remaining 18 percent in the erythrocytes. The biggest components of nonbicarbonate buffers are hemoglobin and oxyhemoglobin, which represent 35 percent of the blood-buffering capacity, whereas the remaining 12 percent is shared between the organic and inorganic phosphates (5 percent) and the plasma proteins (3 percent).[2]

The Bicarbonate Carbonic Acid Buffer System

The bicarbonate buffer system is the principal and most readily available buffer in the plasma. The bicarbonate ion diffuses relatively easily inside the erythrocyte (in contrast to body cells where it it not as freely diffusible). Therefore, the red cells share in the capacity of this buffer system; about one-third of bicarbonate buffer is present inside the red cell.

The CO_2 produced by the tissues reacts with water (hydration reaction) to form carbonic acid which in turn is dissociated to H^+ and HCO_3^-.

$$CO_2 + H_2O \rightleftharpoons H_2CO_3 \rightleftharpoons H^+ + HCO_3^-$$

The hydration of CO_2 is a slow process in the plasma. However, in the red cell because of the presence of carbonic anhydrase it is a much faster one. The second part of the reaction, the dissociation of carbonic acid to hydrogen ion and bicarbonate is a fast instantaneous reaction. In this reaction the carbonic acid is the weak acid, whereas the conjugate base is the bicarbonate ion. At equilibrium a very small part of carbonic acid is dissociated into H^+ and HCO_3^-. Out of every part of carbonic acid only 3 to 5 percent is dissociated into H^+ and HCO_3^-.

According to derivations of the law of mass action, the H^+ concentration in a buffer is proportional to the ratio of the concentration of the acid to that of its conjugate system. In the bicarbonate system this becomes:

$$[H^+] \, \alpha \, \frac{[H_2CO_3]}{[HCO_3^-]}$$

Therefore,
$$[H^+] = \frac{k\,[H_2CO_3]}{[HCO_3^-]}$$

or,
$$pH = -\log\,[H^+] = pK + \log\frac{[HCO_3^-]}{[H_2CO_3]}$$

This is known as the Henderson–Hasselbach equation.

From this equation, it can be noted that the H^+ concentration (or the pH) depends on carbonic acid concentration in blood as well as the bicarbonate concentration. The respiratory system adjusts the P_{CO_2} at 40 mm Hg. This is equivalent to an arterial CO_2 concentration of 1.2 mmol per liter (40 × CO_2 solubility coefficient of 0.03), whereas the kidneys try to fix the carbonic acid concentration at 25 mmol per liter. Therefore, the ratio of carbonic acid to bicarbonate becomes 1 : 20.

The dissociation constant (pK) of this buffer system is about 6.1. Although it is considered a constant, it can vary slightly with changes in pH of plasma, temperature, and the ionic concentration of plasma. Therefore,

$$pH = 6.1 + \log \frac{24}{1.2}$$
$$= 6.1 + \log 20$$
$$= 6.1 + 1.3 = 7.40$$

Thus, by knowing two variables in the equation, the third one can be derived.

In comparison to other buffer systems, the bicarbonate system has the unique property of being an open system, ie, the weak acid formed by the buffer reaction is excreted as CO_2 through the lung. For example, if 5 mmol of H^+ is added to 1 liter of a closed bicarbonate buffer system (P_{CO_2}, 40 mm Hg, HCO_3^-, 24 mmol per liter), the bicarbonate concentration will fall by 5 mmol to 19 mmol per liter. This 5 mmol of bicarbonate will be transformed to carbonic acid and the dissolved CO_2 will rise from 40 to 200 mm Hg (40 + 5/ 0.13). The pH according to the Henderson–Hasselbach reaction will be 6.58, an abnormally low value. However, this does not happen in the intact animal because the respiratory system excretes the excess CO_2. If we assume now that the animal has hyperventilated and dropped its P_{CO_2} to 40 mm Hg, the pH will be 7.23 (Fig. 17-1). Thus, by getting rid of the weak acid the bicarbonate buffer system is transformed from a weak system to an effective one.

The effectiveness of bicarbonate buffer system is not limited to plasma because the red cell is freely permeable to carbon dioxide and bicarbonate.

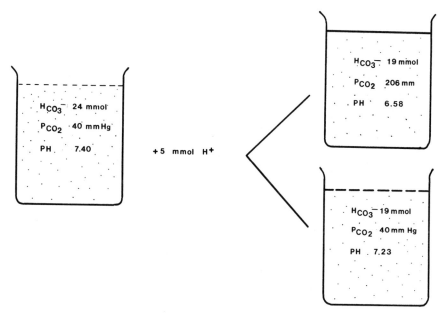

FIG. 17-1: The effect of adding 5 mmol of H^+ to 1 liter of closed or open bicarbonate buffer system.

Thus, about one-third of this reaction occurs inside the red cell where the reaction of $CO_2 + H_2O \rightleftharpoons H_2CO_3$ is facilitated by the enzyme carbonic anhydrase.

The Phosphate Buffer

$$H_2PO_4^- \rightleftharpoons H^+ + HPO_4^{--}$$

At the normal pH of blood, this buffer system is equally divided as acid and base. This system theoretically is a more effective one, but because the amount of phosphate present in the blood is very small it contributes very little (2 to 5 percent) of buffering capacity of blood. However, this system is much more effective intracellularly when phosphate is present in relatively high concentrations. In bones, phosphate is present in very high concentrations and forms a large source of available buffer. This source is not readily available, but it becomes effective within a few days. Its effect can be seen in chronic renal disturbances as in chronic renal acidosis.

The Hemoglobin and Protein Buffer System

In the slightly alkalotic pH of blood, proteins act as weak acids, and they dissociate into positively charged hydrogen ions and negatively charged proteins. Plasma proteins because of their limited quantity in blood contribute relatively little to buffering capacity of blood (7 percent). Because of its higher concentration (15 g per 100 ml) hemoglobin is a more effective buffer. It acts as weak acid like plasma protein. Also, hemoglobin has the particular advantage that its buffering capacity varies with oxygenation, reduced hemoglobin being a weaker acid than oxyhemoglobin. Therefore, at the capillaries with the deoxygenation of oxyhemoglobin, more free base becomes available to combine with the acids (carbonic acid) produced at the cells. The buffering capacity of hemoglobin is present at the imidazole group of the histidine molecules in the protein globin.

Buffering Capacity of the Body

The intracellular compartment is the first site for buffering the acids originated in the body. For instance, the H^+ produced inside the mitochondria is buffered on the spot by the local proteins,[3] but eventually this excess H^+ diffuses into the extracellular spaces.

The extracellular space is in free communication with the plasma. Thus, all of the electrolyte buffering capacity of plasma is shared with the extracellular fluid. The intracellular buffering capacity is not well understood.

It is estimated that if a strong acid is added to the body, about 15 to 20 percent is buffered by the plasma, 30 percent by the interstitial fluid, and the remaining 55 percent by the intracellular compartment.[2]

Renal Compensation

The kidney can regulate the acid–base status of the blood either by acidifying or alkalinizing the urine. The renal tubular cells can synthesize new bicarbonate from CO_2. Due to the presence of carbonic anhydrase in the renal tubular cells the hydration of CO_2 to carbonic acid is facilitated.

$$CO_2 + H_2O \underset{\text{carbonic anhydrase}}{\rightleftharpoons} H_2CO_3 \rightleftharpoons H^+ + HCO_3^-$$

Carbonic acid is dissociated into hydrogen and bicarbonate ions. The reabsorption of the bicarbonate ion into the circulation increases the available conjugate bases of the extracellular fluid, while the hydrogen ion is excreted in the urine. The H is not excreted as free H^+ but is combined with either alkaline phosphate radical to form acid phosphate or with ammonia (NH_3) to form ammonium radical (NH_4^+).

$$HPO_4^{--} + H^+ \rightleftharpoons H_2PO_4^-$$
$$NH_3 + H^+ \rightleftharpoons NH_4^+$$

Thus, for every bicarbonate ion reabsorbed into the circulation by the kidney, an equal amount of H^+ is excreted in the kidney, mostly in the form of titratable acid as acid phosphate or ammonia. The kidney can achieve acidification of urine (or retain base) by two mechanisms. The first is by reabsorption of all the filtered bicarbonate in the renal tubular system. This mechanism can only preserve the available base of the body. The second mechanism is by synthesizing new bicarbonate (Chap. 29).

The average human diet contains more acid than alkali. These acids are mostly in the form of phosphoric and sulfuric acids. These amount to 100 mmol of H^+ per day. The concentration of the acid in the body is kept constant by excretion of an equivalent amount of acid by the kidney. The amount of acid excreted by the kidney is very small compared to the amount of acid excreted by the lung (equivalent 12,500 mmol per day of H^+); however, the source of pulmonary acid load is different, since it is derived from the CO_2 produced in the tissues.

Alkalinization of the urine is relatively easy by the kidney because about 400 mmol of bicarbonate is reabsorbed by the kidney per day, and, by reabsorbing a lesser amount of this bicarbonate load, a considerable amount of base can be excreted. The alkalinizing capacity of the kidney is limited to the amount of cation (Na^+ and K^+) available to accompany the bicarbonate in the urine, eg, if sodium is reabsorbed avidly by the renal tubules cells, the bicarbonate ion will also be reabsorbed because of the absence of available cation that it needs to be excreted with. In the diet, the main source of alkali are fruits because they contain Na^+ and K^+ salts of the weak organic acids, which are metabolized to CO_2, whereas the Na^+ and K^+ are retained in the body as sodium and potassium bicarbonate. Eventually, these cations are excreted by the kidneys.

ACID–BASE DISORDERS

Terminology

The physiologic definition of acidosis and alkalosis is an abnormal condition caused by accumulation or loss of acid or base from the body fluids. This differs from the laboratory definitions of acidosis and alkalosis, which are defined from the measured change in blood pH. Therefore, according to the laboratory definition, metabolic acidosis does not exist unless the pH is diminished, but according to the physiologic term, which is the most commonly used, acidosis can exist with a normal pH if the increase in the H^+ concentration in tissues is compensated by a similar increase in base, thus keeping pH near normal values.

If the change in the acid–base status is primarily from changes in alveolar ventilation, then it is described as respiratory acidosis or alkalosis. If the basic abnormality is primarily due to changes in the metabolic component of blood, it is defined as metabolic acidosis or alkalosis. Occasionally, the terms acidemia and alkalemia are used for conditions that result in a low or high arterial pH (laboratory definition).

The term compensation is used to describe secondary physiologic processes that occur in response to the primary change of the acid–base equilibrium in an effort by the body to restore the pH back to normal. This is in contrast to correction, in which the physiologic mechanism corrects the primary abnormality, eg, if the primary condition is metabolic acidosis (addition of a strong acid), the respiratory system can only compensate for it, but the final correction must be through the kidney, which will excrete the loading acid.

The intracellular pH is different from the extracellular one. The intracellular pH of most animal tissues is about 7 under normal conditions. The cell membrane is freely permeable to CO_2, whereas it is relatively impermeable to highly ionizable acids and bases such as hydrochloric acid and sodium bicarbonate. Therefore, the effect of the latter two on intracellular pH is less marked than the effect of CO_2.

Although the intracellular concentrations of sodium, potassium, and hydrogen ions are different from those of the extracellular space, a change in the concentration of one of them is always accompanied by a relative change in the other space.[4]

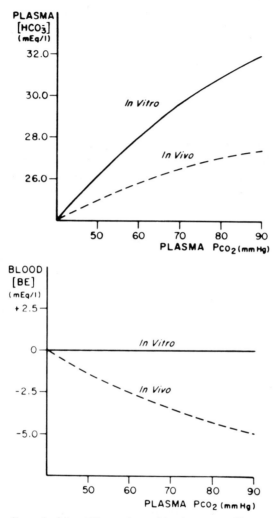

FIG. 17-2: The effect of adding CO_2 to plasma bicarbonate and base excess in vivo and in vitro. (Reproduced with permission from Little, Brown.[14])

Acidosis

Whenever there is acidosis, whatever its origin, the body will try to diminish the impact of this increased H^+ concentration by using the above-mentioned compensatory mechanism. However, if the acid load is excessive, the body will be unable to compensate for it, and significant acidemia (decrease in pH) occurs, which can be life-threatening because of its effect on the circulation and other bodily functions. An increase in H^+ concentration will lead to the depression of cerebral function. In the early stages, the patient will be confused and unresponsive, and at a higher H^+ concentration he will be unconscious. This effect is additive to the depressant effect of other drugs, such as hypnotics and narcotics. With very high H^+ concentrations, depression of vasomotor and respiratory centers occurs. The effect in the respiratory center is similar to that of morphine overdose, ie, slow, gasping respirations accompanied by a tracheal tug. At the final stage, respiratory arrest occurs. This increase in H^+ concentration will lead to a circulatory depression through several mechanisms: (1) depression of the vasomotor center, (2) direct depression of arteriolar smooth muscles, and (3) direct depression of the contractility of the cardiac muscles.

In the early stages of acidosis, this depressant effect is counteracted by a rise in catecholamine secretion, which leads to tachycardia and an increase in cardiac output, with an increased incidence of arrhythmias. The myocardial depressant of acidosis is compensated for by a concomitant increase in ionized calcium levels. This compensation is more marked with hypercapnic acidosis than in metabolic acidosis.[5] With an increase in the level of acidosis, these effects are overshadowed by the severe depressive effect of the acidosis on cardiovascular functions.

An acidotic patient manifests clinically as unconscious or semiconscious and hypotensive with warm, blue, sweaty extremities with dilated veins. Respiration is slow and gasping with a tracheal tug. Frequently, arrhythmias are present.

METABOLIC ACIDOSIS

This can be due to either accumulation of an acid other than carbonic acid in the extracellular fluid or to the loss of bicarbonate base. The acid content of blood can increase in any one of the following conditions: (1) In diabetic ketoacidosis, the levels of B-hydroxybutyric and acetoacetic acids are increased in the blood, which result in incomplete oxidation of fatty acids. (2) With tissue anoxia, the oxidation of carbohydrate is incomplete and an excessive amounts of lactic and pyruvic acids are produced. (3) Idiopathic lactic acidosis. (4) Starvation. (5) In advanced stages of renal failure, the kidney is unable to handle the excess inorganic acid produced from the normal metabolism of the diet (phosphoric and sulfuric acids), and acidosis ensues (uremic acidosis). (6) Rapid administration of ACD blood (acid citrate) leads to acidosis from citrate accumulation. (7) With infusion of acidifying salts such as ammonium chloride which dissociates into ammonia and hydrochloric acid, the ammonia is metabolized by the kidney to urea and the hydrochloric acid leads to acidosis. A similar condition occurs with infusion of lysine hydrochloride.

The second important mechanism that can cause acidosis is a loss of base (bicarbonate) from the extracellular fluid either through the kidney or the intestinal tract. All the secretions of the intestinal tract beyond the pylorus are alkaline in reaction because of their high bicarbonate concentration. Therefore, a constant loss of low intestinal secretions from a fistula, continuous intestinal suction, diarrhea, or chronic intestinal obstruction will lead to bicarbonate loss and acidosis. Also, in renal tubular acidosis, the kidneys are unable to reabsorb most of the bicarbonate present in the glomerular filtrate. The ensuing renal bicarbonate loss will lead to acidosis.

Compensatory changes in metabolic acidosis. The extra acid reacts with the bicarbonate ion and the buffer base leading to the formation of carbonic acid. The carbonic acid is dissociated into CO_2 and H_2O, and the excess is excreted through the lung by hyperventilation. Thus, hypocapnia results, with a diminution in plasma HCO_3^- and buffer base. The final correction of metabolic acidosis is slower in response and usually occurs through the kidney by excreting the offending acid. Metabolizable acids (citric and acetoacetic acids) are degraded to CO_2 in the liver and excreted by the lung. The regeneration of the buffer base occurs through the kidney, which raises its bicarbonate reabsorption as well as the H^+ excretion. The latter manifests itself as elevated titratable urinary acidity and ammonium. In almost all cases of metabolic acidosis, the urine is acidic (pH less than 5.3), the exception being situations in which the kidney is unable to secrete the H^+.

RESPIRATORY ACIDOSIS

In respiratory acidosis the primary abnormality is a rise in the carbonic acid level of blood (above 1.3 mmol per liter or P_{CO_2} above 40 mm Hg), which can either be caused by an increase in CO_2 production or a fall in alveolar ventilation. The most common cause is respiratory failure, which can affect the respiratory system at any one of the following levels:

1. Central respiratory depression arising from a head injury or drug overdose, such as anesthetics, narcotics, or barbiturates. Sleep is also associated with very mild respiratory acidosis, decreased responsiveness of the respiratory center to CO_2, and a rise of P_{CO_2} up to 44 mm Hg.
2. Pulmonary failure that can be due to a variety of pulmonary diseases including advanced emphysema, cystic fibrosis, and pulmonary edema.
3. Failure of proper functioning of the musculature of the chest wall, such as morbid obesity, abdominal distension, or severe kyphoscoliosis. Airway obstruction or increased airway resistance that can occur in anesthetized individuals can lead to respiratory acidosis.

The final outcome from all these is a rise in plasma CO_2 levels, resulting in acidosis from the accumulation of the H_2CO_3 level in blood. The first reaction of the body is to increase CO_2 excretion by hyperventilation. However, this response is inefficient because of the limited capability of the respiratory system because of its intrinsic disorder. The excess H^+ produced from the accumulation of excessive carbonic acid is buffered by the other buffer systems of plasma and other tissues by the following reaction:

$$CO_2 + H_2O \rightleftharpoons H_2CO_3 \rightleftharpoons H^+ + HCO_3^- + Buffer \rightleftharpoons H\ Buffer + HCO_3^-$$

If this reaction was limited to plasma only, the total amount of available base would not diminish, because for every molecule of buffer consumed one molecule of HCO_3^- is added.

However, in the intact animal a large amount of bicarbonate diffuses into the interstitial or extracellular spaces where there is no buffer system (the bulk of nonbicarbonate buffer system in blood being hemoglobin). Thus, the total amount of buffer base diminishes in blood (Fig. 17-2). This difference in the change of base excess during CO_2 accumulation becomes significantly important only in high P_{CO_2} levels. However, in situations in which this extracellular fluid pool is increased, such as in a newborn or in edema, an acute rise of P_{CO_2} will lead to significantly larger amounts of bicarbonate leak into the extracellular space.

Within 6 to 12 hours of respiratory acidosis, the kidney starts compensating for this extra acid load by increasing the plasma bicarbonate concentration. It accomplishes this by reabsorbing all the bicarbonate filtered in plasma and by synthesizing new bicarbonate (through the carbonic anhydrase system). Thus, the amount of bicarbonate in blood is increased. The ratio of H_2CO_3/HCO_3^- is not significantly changed. This mechanism is effective up to a P_{CO_2} of 70 mm Hg when the pH remains near the lower limit or normal of 7.35. With a higher P_{CO_2} the pH drops at a faster rate. As expected, the urine in patients with respiratory acidosis is very acid (pH 4.5) with an increase in the amount of ammonium salts in the urine.

Alkalosis

Alkalosis, similar to acidosis, can either be metabolic or respiratory in origin. Because the occurrence of acute metabolic alkalosis is extremely rare, most of the clinical effects described for alkalosis are those of respiratory alkalosis, but they also apply to metabolic alkalosis as well. The first discomfort that a hyperventilating person feels is dizziness, which can be followed by nausea and blurring of vision. Alkalosis can affect the availability of oxygen to the brain by two separate mechanisms. First, by decreasing the cerebral blood flow from an increased cerebrovascular resistance and by shifting the oxygen dissociation curve to the left (Bohr effect). Thus, less oxygen is available to the brain tissues at that particular P_{O_2}. Alkalosis also can produce cutaneous vasoconstriction. The incidence of arrhythmias increases with alkalosis. This is more marked in patients with heart disease and digitalis therapy. This probably is due to the hypokalemia associated with alkalosis from the intracellular shift of K^+ from the extracellular compartment, enhancing the toxic effects of digitalis.[6]

In patients lightly anesthetized with halothane, acute metabolic alkalosis induced by sodium bicarbonate leads to myocardial stimulation associated with peripheral vasodilatation and volume expansion. The afterload on the heart is diminished with a rise in cardiac output. With large doses of sodium bicarbonate (300 mmol) in deeply anesthetized subjects, severe hypotension with massive peripheral vasodilatation and junctional rhythms can occur.[7]

METABOLIC ALKALOSIS

The primary change in metabolic alkalosis is a rise in plasma bicarbonate levels. This can be due to any of the following: (1) excessive acid gastric juice loss during protracted vomiting; (2) renal from excessive diuretic therapy associated with K^+ depletion; (3) base gain, which occurs when a large amount of absorbable alkali such as sodium bicarbonate is ingested; and (4) salts of organic acids such as citrate, lactate, and acetate are metabolized in the liver to bicarbonate, which leads to a rise in the alkali reserve of blood. This effect is commonly seen after massive transfusion with citrated blood.[8]

In contrast to metabolic acidosis, the respiratory compensation in metabolic alkalosis is irregular and unpredictable. The reason is not well defined but probably is due to divergence between the intracellular and extracellular changes in H^+ concentration. Thus, the change in the pH is more marked in metabolic alkalosis than in metabolic acidosis.

The kidney compensates for metabolic alkalosis by increasing the reabsorption of H^+ and eliminating the excess base by increasing the excretion of basic phosphate and bicarbonate. However, this metabolic compensation is limited by the amount of sodium, potassium and chloride present in the body. For example, during protracted vomiting, there is excessive loss of chloride in association with other cations such as sodium or potassium. In these situations, the conservation of the cations takes priority over the conservation of alkali. Thus, the kidney exchanges H^+ for K^+ and Na^+. The urine becomes paradoxically acid (paradoxical aciduria). The presence of acid urine with metabolic alkalosis is a clear indication of electrolyte depletion.

RESPIRATORY ALKALOSIS

In respiratory alkalosis, the primary defect is a fall of arterial carbon dioxide level and hence the carbonic acid level (below 1.3 mmol per liter). This is seen in people living in high altitudes in whom anoxia stimulates the peripheral chemoreceptors, leading to hyperventilation. It is also seen in hysterically hyperventilating patients and with salicylate poisoning. With hyperventilation, patients start to feel headache, nausea, and vomiting. Later, twitching appears, which in severe cases leads to tetany or frank convulsions. The main reason for this tetany is that plasma protein in alkaline solution has a stronger affinity for Ca^{++} than in acidic media. Thus, this extra binding of Ca^{++} with the consequent diminution in Ca^{++} of plasma leads to a tetany. Also, normal pregnancy is associated with hyperventilation, presumably from the effect of progesterone. Patients in terminal liver failure show respiratory alkalosis.

Hyperventilation leads to a drop in the CO_2 tension and hence in the H_2CO_3 content of blood. The result is an extraavailability of HCO_3^- not in equilibrium with the H_2CO_3. This HCO_3^- reacts with the acidic buffer system of the blood by the following equation:

$$HCO_3^- + H\ Buffer \rightleftharpoons Buffer^- + H_2CO_3 \rightleftharpoons CO_2 + H_2O$$

Thus, a situation opposite to that of respiratory acidosis exists in which the plasma bicarbonate level is diminished, while the blood base remains constant (in vitro titration curve). In vivo one expects that the extracellular space will provide the extra bicarbonate ion, thus increasing the plasma buffer base. However, this usually does not happen in hyperventilating animals because of the concomitant rise of blood lactate levels, which neutralizes the effect of alkalosis.[9]

The kidney can compensate for this alkalosis by excreting bicarbonate in association with sodium and potassium. Similar to other situations the capability of the kidney to excrete this extra bicarbonate depends on the amount of cation stores of the body. This renal compensation is clearly seen in people residing in high altitudes who have near-normal pH despite their low P_{CO_2}.

Evaluation of Acid–Base Disturbances

In blood the pH and CO_2 pressures are relatively easy to measure with pH and P_{CO_2} pressure-sensitive electrodes. From the Henderson–Hasselbalch equation, the bicarbonate level can be calculated. Ideally, an arterial blood sample or a mixed venous blood sample from pulmonary artery is needed, since the acid–base content varies from one vein to another. Because of the peripheral vasodilation in anesthetized, healthy individuals, the venous P_{CO_2} and pH closely approach the values in arterial blood.[10]

To avoid extensive calculations, several momograms are available, the most frequently used being the Siggaard-Andersen curve nomogram[11,12] (Fig. 17-3). In this nomogram the log P_{CO_2} is on the vertical scale, whereas the pH

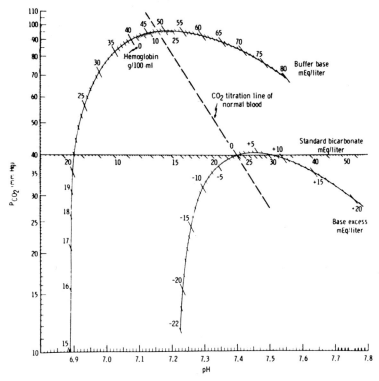

FIG. 17-3: Siggaard-Andersen curve nomogram (® Radiometer, Copenhagen.)

is on the horizontal scale. The upper curvillinear line represents the total amount of buffer base present in blood (HCO_3^-, hemoglobin$^-$, and protein$^-$). These are the anions in the blood that can accept hydrogen ions. The value in a normal individual with a hemoglobin of 15 g per 100 ml of blood is 48 m Eq per liter (mmol per liter).

The most important line on this graph is the normal buffer line passing throught the point of zero base excess (standard bicarbonate, 24 m Eq per liter) and the point hemoglobin concentration of the individual at the buffer base line. Thus, in anemic people the slope of the curve will be shifted to the left, ie, the buffering capacity is diminished. At all points along the normal buffer base line the total buffer base content is normal regardless in which direction the CO_2 tension and the pH are changing. In this graft, all the points to the left of the normal buffer line are associated with increased hydrogen ion content, and the points to the right with diminished hydrogen ion content. In both of these situations, the source of H^+ is other than carbon dioxide.

The standard bicarbonate line is the horizontal line intersecting the P_{CO_2} line at 40 mm Hg. It does not indicate the actual bicarbonate concentration of

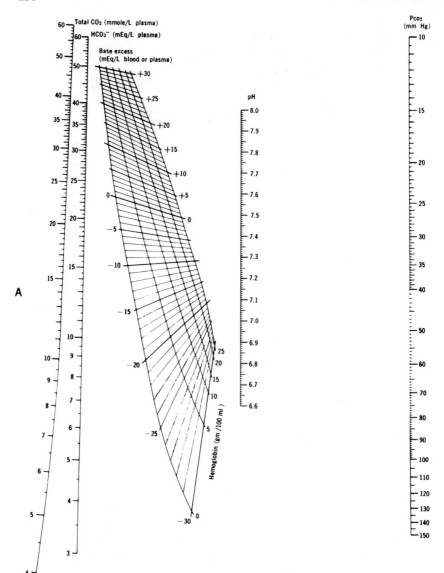

FIG. 17-4: Siggaard-Andersen alignment nomogram. (© Radiometer, Copenhagen.)

the sample, but it indicates the bicarbonate concentration after the respiratory component is eliminated. It is an indication of the alkali reserve of the blood.

The easiest way to use this graph is by plotting the point of the actual values of P_{CO_2} and pH on the graph. Then draw a line parallel to the normal buffer line (CO_2 titration line) of that particular individual. The point at which it intersects the buffer base line indicates his total buffer base available. The point intersecting the standard bicarbonate line will indicate the amount of bicarbonate he would have had if his P_{CO_2} was 40 mm Hg, indicating his alkali reserve. The point of intersection of the lower curve or the base excess is his base excess. A positive value indicates alkalosis and a negative value acidosis. This is the amount of acid or base required to restore 1 liter of blood to normal acid–base composition at a P_{CO_2} of 40 mm Hg.

In treating acid–base balance disorders, one should realize that the whole body is involved in correcting the acid–base balance, not only the blood as the nomogram indicates. In vivo advanced acute respiratory acidosis is associated with a mild metabolic acidosis. Respiratory alkalosis resulting from hyperventilation is also associated with a mild metabolic acidosis.

The contribution of the other compartments in correcting the acid–base disturbances is extremely difficult to demonstrate. In the clinical situation one estimates the base deficit from the nomogram and multiplies by 20 percent of body weight assuming that most acid–base derangement is in the extracellular space. Other authors have used a factor of 30 percent. However, in the operating room situation in which these changes are acute, it is advisable to give half of this amount of bicarbonate, measure the acid–base status again, and administer the second dose accordingly.

Beside the curved Siggaard-Andersen nomogram, there is an alignment nomogram (Fig. 17-4), which is easier to use than the curved nomogram, from which if the P_{CO_2} and pH is known, the base excess, the bicarbonate, and the total CO_2 can be derived easily.

Recently, mathematical expressions have been used for calculating acid–base variables that can be implemented on a small pocket calculator.[13]

REFERENCES

1. Campbell EJM, Dickinson CJ, Slater JDH: Clinical Physiology. Oxford, Blackwell, 1974, p 236
2. Winters RW, Dell RB: Regulation of acid–base equilibrium. In Yamamoto WS, Brobeck JR (eds): Physiological Controls and Regulation. Philadelphia, Saunders, 1965
3. Levesque PR: Acid–base disorders: application of total body carbon dioxide titration in anesthesia. Anesth Analg (Cleve) 54:299, 1975
4. Waddell WJ, Bates RG: Intracellular pH. Physiol Rev 49:285, 1969
5. Schaer H, Bachmann U: Ionized calcium in acidosis: differential effect of hypercapnia and lactic acidosis. Br J Anaesth 46:842, 1974
6. Lawson NW, Butler GH, Ray CT: Alkalosis and cardiac arrhythmias. Anesth Analg (Cleve) 52:951, 1973
7. Kaplan JA, Bush GL, Lecky JH, et al: Sodium bicarbonate and systemic hemodynamics in volunteers anesthetized with halothane. Anesthesiology 42:550, 1975

8. Barcenas CG, Fuller TJ, Knochel JP: Metabolic alkalosis after massive blood transfusion. JAMA 236:953, 1976

9. Engel K, Kildeberg P, Winters RW: Quantitative displacement of blood acid–base status in acute hypocapnia. Scand J Clin Lab Invest 23:5, 1969

10. France CJ, Eger EI, Bendixen HH: The use of peripheral venous blood for pH and carbon dioxide tension determinations during general anesthesia. Anesthesiology 40:311, 1974

11. Siggaard-Andersen O: Blood acid–base alignment nomogram scales for pH, PCO_2, base excess of whole blood of different hemoglobin concentrations, plasma bicarbonate and plasma total CO_2. Scand J Clin Lab Invest 15:211, 1963

12. Siggaard-Andersen O: The Acid–Base Status of Blood. Baltimore, Williams & Wilkins, 1964

13. Blackburn JP, Preston TD, Strickland AP: A simple method for computing acid–base states. Br J Anaesth 47:500, 1975

14. Winters RW: The Body Fluids in Pediatrics. Boston, Little, Brown, 1973

Section III

Physiology
of the Nervous System

chapter 18

Nerve Physiology: Excitability and Conductivity

ANATOMY

Nerves or nerve trunks are made up of a certain number of fibers according to their function. There are two types of fibers: *afferent,* which transmit impulses from the periphery to the spinal cord and central nervous system, and *efferent,* which transmit impulses from the spinal cord and central nervous system to the periphery.

Individual nerve fibers are covered by endoneurium. A few fibers placed together are enclosed in perineurium. The trunk is covered by epineurium. These sheaths and coverings originate from connective tissue.

Neuron

The neuron (Fig. 18-1) consists of three parts: cell body, dendrites, and axon. The axon is actually what is referred to as a nerve fiber. The axon of one neuron terminates in the cell body or the dendrites of another. The junction between two neurons is called the synapse.

The nerve fibers are covered by a myelin sheath before leaving the spinal cord. The myelin sheath is interrupted by the nodes of Ranvier. Outside the myelin sheath, the nerve fiber is covered by neurolemma. The cells of the neurolemma are called Schwann cells. Not all nerves are covered by this myelin sheath, eg, the postganglionic fibers of the autonomic nervous system.

NUTRITION

The entire nerve fiber derives its nutrition from the cell body. In the case of a complete interruption of the nerve trunk, the peripheral part undergoes

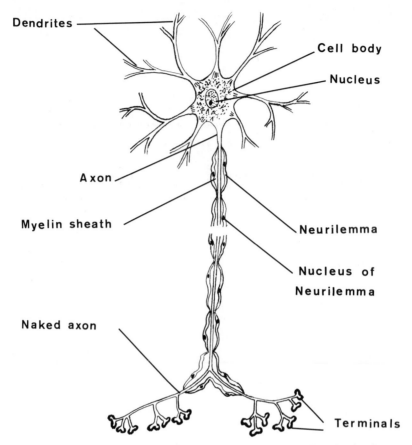

FIG. 18-1: Schematic presentation of a neuron consisting of cell body, dendrites, and axon.

degeneration, known as Wallerian degeneration. The central part, however, regenerates; the axon grows out and the Schwann cells extend. The myelin sheath also regenerates, but it is at a much slower rate. It is important to point out that lack of neurilemma prevents this type of regeneration from taking place in the brain or spinal cord.

NERVE IMPULSE

Nerves possess properties of excitability and conductivity. Functionally, the nerve membrane is the most important part of the nerve fiber. Experimentally, it has been clearly shown that the removal of the axoplasm does not significantly change the impulse conduction of the remaining membrane.

MEMBRANE POTENTIALS

The membrane is usually described as a layer consisting of lipid and protein.[1] There are multiple pores throughout the lipid framework. Both sides of the membrane are bathed in an electrolyte solution containing about 150 mEq per liter anions (negatively charged ions) and a corresponding amount of cations (positively charged ions). There is an excess of anions on the inside of the membrane and an excess of cations on the outside. This creates the membrane potential.

The concentration of potassium ions is much greater on the inside, and those of the chloride and sodium much greater on the outside of the cell membrane.[2] This imbalance is maintained by two main processes:

1. Diffusion: Potassium and chloride ions pass freely through the cell pores. The larger sodium ions have difficulty passing through. There are also large numbers of anions inside the membrane that diffuse very poorly or not at all, such as protein, sulfate, and phosphate.
2. There is an active transport of sodium from inside the cell to the outside of the cell accomplished by a *sodium pump*. The carrier is a lipoprotein most likely to be the same molecule that acts as the enzyme ATPase. This active transport occurs against a concentration gradient requiring energy.

The sodium pump decreases the concentration of sodium cations to 10 mEq per liter inside the cell and maintains a high level of 142 mEq per liter on the outside. The potassium pump on the other hand maintains a high level of potassium ions (140 mEq per liter) inside the nerve fiber and a low level (5 mEq per liter) on the outside. Potassium ions, as pointed out, diffuse through the pores very well. The existing potential, measured in many nerves, generally falls in the range of 60 to 100 mV (inside negative).

ACTION POTENTIAL

The permeability of the membrane can be changed under the influence of such factors as electrical stimulation, application of chemicals, mechanical damage, excessive heat or cold, and many others.

Depolarization and Repolarization

Under the effect of an outside stimulus, the electrical difference between the two sides of the membrane drops to 45 mV (inside negative) (Fig. 18-2). This 45 mV level is the threshold at which the membrane loses its

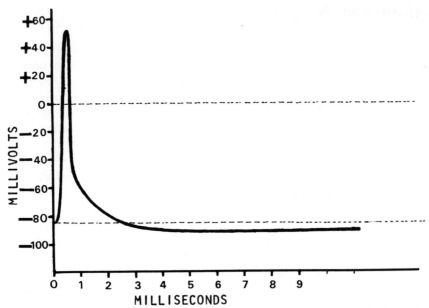

FIG. 18-2: Diagrammatic presentation of an idealized action potential. The spike potential is the portion above zero. Note how the action potential returns all the way to its resting level (–80 mV) and even becomes more negative for a short period of time.

semipermeability and the ions start passing freely from one side to the other. The influx of sodium cations through the enlarged pores not only neutralizes the membrane potential but also, for a brief period, causes reversal of the polarity. Very shortly after the motion of sodium, the potassium starts moving to the outside of the membrane.[3,4] This rapid change of the membrane voltage is called depolarization. The depolarization evokes an action potential. There is usually a change of at least 100 mV, from −60 to +40 mV on both sides of the membrane.

After the impulse has passed, the sodium cation is again excluded from the axon by the action of the sodium pump. Repolarization is accomplished by the delayed efflux of potassium cations which restores the normal polarity (60 to 100 mV) of the membrane potential.

Propagation of the Nerve Impulse

After an action potential is elicited at any point of the nerve membrane, it spreads to the adjacent areas and, thus, results in propagation of the nerve impulse.[5] Propagation occurs in both directions along a conductive fiber. The action potential increases the permeability of the membrane of the adjacent areas and enables the sodium to penetrate inside the cell.

The All-or-Nothing Law

Experiments have shown that, if the stimulus is weak, it will not produce a propagated impulse. However, a strong stimulus will create an action potential, the magnitude of which depends on the properties of the nerve fiber and is independent of the strength of the stimulus.

Propagation of Repolarization

Repolarization begins at the same area where depolarization originally started and spreads along in the direction of depolarization.

The Refractory Period

If a stimulus is applied when the membrane is still depolarized, no nerve impulse will be elicited regardless of its strength. This period of inexcitability is called the absolute refractory period. It is followed by the relative refractory period. During this period, the threshold for excitation is higher and the magnitude of the action potential is reduced. Only a strong stimulus can elicit an action potential during this period.

The refractory period is a safety factor that limits the frequency of conduction of impulses by different nerves.

SALTATORY CONDUCTION IN MYELINATED FIBERS

As pointed out, some of the nerve fibers are covered by a myelin sheath that acts as an insulator. None of the ions can flow through this myelinated sheath. At the nodes of Ranvier, however, the membrane is 500 times more permeable than are the membranes of the unmyelinated fibers. At these nodes, the nerve fibers come in contact with the extracellular fluid. The current flow spreads by jumping from node to node (saltatory) in contrast to the continuous progression in the unmyelinated nerves.

CLASSIFICATION OF PERIPHERAL NERVE FIBERS

In 1943, Gasser classified the nerve fibers according to their diameters and the conduction velocity of their nerve impulses (Table 18-1). Nerve fibers are classified as A, B, or C fibers. The A fibers have the largest diameter. They are subdivided into α, β, γ, σ, and ϵ fibers. The A and B fibers are myelinated.

TABLE 18-1. Types of Peripheral Nerve Fibers and Some of Their Properties

TERMINOLOGY	DIAMETER (μ)	CONDUCTION SPEED (mseconds)	DURATION OF ACTION POTENTIAL (mseconds)	ABSOLUTE REFRACTORY PERIOD (mseconds)
A	2–20	5–120	0.5–0.4	1.0–0.4
B	3	3–15	1.2	1.2
C	2	0.5–2	2	2

Because of saltatory-type conduction, the velocity of conduction in these fibers is much faster than in the unmyelinated C fibers.

CONDUCTION BLOCK BY LOCAL ANESTHETICS

Local anesthetics applied in sufficient concentration locally will block the conduction of impulses in nerve fibers. They have found widespread clinical application because of the reversibility of this block.

All local anesthetic drugs contain a lipophilic group, an intermediate chain, and a hydrophylic group. The intermediate chain could be an ester or an amide. The ester group is composed of procaine (Novocaine), 2-chlorprocaine (Nesacaine), and tetracaine (Pontocaine). The most commonly used amides are: lidocaine (Xylocaine), mepivicaine (Carbocaine), prilocaine (Citanest), and bupivicaine (Marcaine).

Local anesthetics, being weak bases, are kept in an acid solution, in which they form a water-soluble salt:

$$\overset{\text{base}}{NR} + HCl \rightleftharpoons \overset{\text{cation}}{NHR^+} + Cl^-$$

The base is lipid-soluble and, therefore, can penetrate through various tissue barriers. Once the local anesthetic solution has reached the nerve membrane, the cation plays an active part.[6] The concentration of base or cation in the solution depends on the pK* of the local anesthetic. The higher the pK when applied, the less concentration of base will be present in the tissues. A decrease in the amount of base will facilitate removal of the local anesthetic, thus resulting in a shorter duration of action. The pK of most local anesthetics in common use lies between 8.0 and 9.0; therefore, only 10 to 20 percent will be in the form of free base at the physiologic pH.[7]

Local anesthetics initially increase the threshold for electrical stimulation.

---

* The pK of any substance is the pH at which 50 percent of the substance is ionized.

Later, they slow the rise of action potential and propagation of impulse and, finally, establish a complete conduction block.[6] The local anesthetics exert their effect on the cell membrane by preventing its depolarization. Few theories have been put forward to explain the mode of action of the local anesthetics. They are summarized as follows:[6,8]

1. Local anesthetics block the sodium influx by occluding the pores of the membrane.
2. They inhibit the release of calcium from the cell membrane. It has been shown that calcium release precedes membrane depolarization.
3. Local anesthetics react with the phospholipids that act as ion carriers and, thus, they interfere with the transport of potassium and sodium across the cell membrane.
4. Recently, it was pointed out that there is a close relationship between the clinical potency of the local anesthetics and their ability to increase the surface tension of a monomolecular lipid layer. When local anesthetics come into contact with the membrane and decrease the surface tension, the result is a decrease in size of the pores.

Nonmyelinated fibers and the smaller fibers are affected first. The myelin sheath acts as an insulator[9] and limits the access of the local anesthetics to the membrane itself.

Sensory and autonomic fibers (those that relay pain and temperature sensation, followed by touch and deep pressure) are abolished first, followed by motor paralysis.

REFERENCES

1. Frankenhaeuser B: Nerve membranes. Proc Int Union Physiol Sci 6:105, 1968
2. Caldwell PC: Factors governing movement and distribution of inorganic ions in nerve and muscle. Physiol Rev 48:1, 1968
3. Hodgkin AL, Huxley AF: Movement of sodium and potassium ions during nervous activity. Cold Spring Harbor Symp Quant Biol 17:43, 1952
4. Huxley AF: Ion movements during nerve activity. Ann NY Acad Sci 81:221, 1959
5. Hodgkin AL: The Conduction of Nerve Impulse. Springfield, Ill, Thomas, 1963
6. Ritchie JM, Greengard P: One mode of action of local anesthetics. Ann Rev Pharmacol 6:405, 1966
7. Ritchie JM, Cohen PJ: Cocaine, procaine and other synthetic local anesthetics. In Goodman LS, Gilman A (eds): The Pharmacological Basis of Therapeutics, 5th ed. New York, MacMillan, 1975, Chap 20
8. de Jong RH, Wagman IH: Physiological mechanisms of peripheral nerve block by local anesthetics. Anesthesiology 24:684, 1963
9. Ritchie JM, Ritchie B, Greengard P: The effect of the nerve sheath on the action of local anesthetics. J Pharmacol Exp Ther 150:160, 1964

chapter 19

Synaptic Transmission and Neuromuscular Junction

The main function of the neurons is to relay information to and from the central nervous system and the periphery.

As previously mentioned, the area of transmission between two neurons is called the synapse. The area of transmission between nerve and muscle is called the neuromuscular junction.

SYNAPSE

Anatomy

As pointed out, the neuron is composed of three parts: the body cell (or soma), the dendrites (projections of the soma), and the axon (an extension of the body cell into the peripheral nerve). The axon of one neuron terminates in the cell body and the dendrites of another. The end areas of an axon are called presynaptic terminals. (Fig. 19-1).

Excitation at the Synapses

There is a gap between the presynaptic terminal and the body cell of the neuron called synaptic cleft (Fig. 19-2). The synaptic cleft has an average width of 200 Å.*

The mechanism of synaptic transmission, ie, the transmission of an impulse between two excitable neurons, has been the subject of extensive evaluation.[1-3] At the synapse, the transmission is not an "electrical" impulse as it is along the axon. It is widely accepted that it is mediated by the release of a

* The symbol Å refers to a unit of measure called an angstrom, which equals 10^{-7} millimeters.

243

Presynaptic
terminals

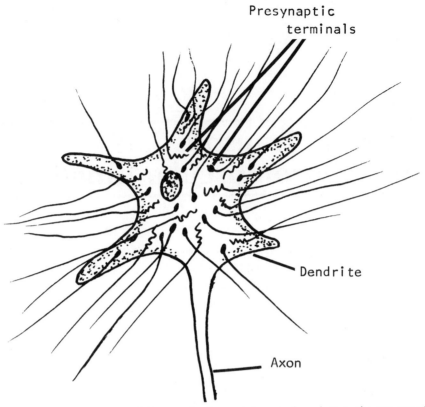

Dendrite

Axon

FIG. 19-1: Motoneuron of the anterior horn of the spinal cord. Note the presynaptic terminals (the ends of nerve fibrils from other neurons), which resemble small knobs (excitatory) and spirals (inhibitory).

transmitter substance: acetylcholine or norepinephrine. These are called excitatory transmitters. Acetylcholine is the excitatory transmitter at the synapses in the autonomic ganglia. Norepinephrine is the transmitter substance of the most sympathetic nerve endings. In the central nervous system, some of the neurons are stimulated by acetylcholine.[4] However, some of the nerve endings do not have the necessary enzymes to synthesize acetylcholine. The same applies for the norepinephrine. It is believed that other substances like serotonin and glutamic acid also act as transmitters.

When an impulse arrives at the presynaptic terminal, the transmitter is released. It crosses the synaptic cleft and acts on the neuronal membrane by changing its permeability to sodium. The normal existing membrane potential is neutralized. The newly created potential is called the *excitatory postsynaptic potential*. If this potential rises above the threshold for excitation, it creates an action potential in the neuron.

Acetylcholine

SYNTHESIS

Acetylcholine is synthesized in the presynaptic areas[5] by the enzymatic esterification of choline by acetate. Diet contains enough choline. The acetate is obtained primarily from the oxidative decarboxylation of pyruvate and from oxidation of fatty acids.

$$COA^* + acetate + ATP \rightarrow Acetyl\text{-}SCO\text{-}A + AMP + pyrophosphate \quad (1)$$

$$Acetyl\text{-}SCO\text{-}A + Choline \xrightarrow[\text{Cholinacetylase}]{} Acetylcholine + HS\text{-}CO\text{-}A \quad (2)$$

Under normal circumstances, there is an abundance of choline and cholinacetylase at the nerve endings.

STORAGE

After the acetylcholine is synthesized, it must be protected from hydrolysis. This is accomplished by its storage in the presynaptic vesicles. These vesicles, also called quantas (Fig. 19-2), are numerous; however, their size is constant. Their diameter is in the range of 650 Å. In myasthenia gravis, their size is mostly reduced, but the number of quantas is about the same or slightly less.

RELEASE

In a resting state, small quantities of acetylcholine are being continuously released. At the arrival of an impulse, numerous vesicles rupture and release the substance.

It has been shown that the presence of calcium stimulates, whereas magnesium depresses the release of acetylcholine. Also, some of the antibiotics like streptomycin, dehydrostreptomycin, neomycin, polymixin B, viomycin, and kanamycin interfere with the release of acetylcholine.[6-8]

Under normal circumstances, the stores of acetylcholine recuperate very quickly after they have been exhausted and can again respond normally.

Of interest is the fact that after the discovery of hemocholinium (a substance that blocks the transport of choline to the nerve endings), it was possible to reduce the amount of acetylcholine formed. Clinically, a similar con-

---

* *Coenzyme A.*

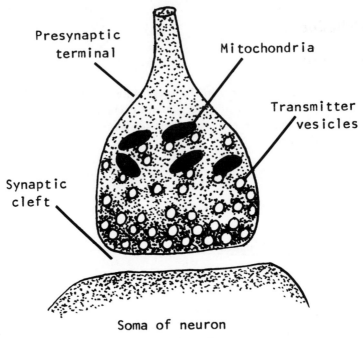

Presynaptic
terminal

Mitochondria

Transmitter
vesicles

Synaptic
cleft

Soma of neuron

FIG. 19-2:   Anatomy of synapse.

dition exists in patients with severe myasthenia gravis and possibly in premature infants under the influence of a depolarizing drug.[9, 10]

Some of the cases with bronchogenic carcinoma develop myasthenic syndrome as a result of difficulties in releasing acetylcholine.

METABOLISM

Acetylcholine is hydrolized by the enzyme acetylcholinesterase.[11] This process is extremely fast and is completed in microseconds.

Inhibition at the Synaptic Transmission

There are two different types of inhibition: presynaptic and postsynaptic. The precise structures of the inhibitory transmitters has not yet been determined. A substance, gamma aminobutyric acid, present in the cerebral cortex, has been shown to have inhibitory action. Whatever the nature of the inhibitory transmitter is, it increases the permeability of the neuronal membrane to potassium. Possibly, more small-sized pores are being opened and the potassium ions (but

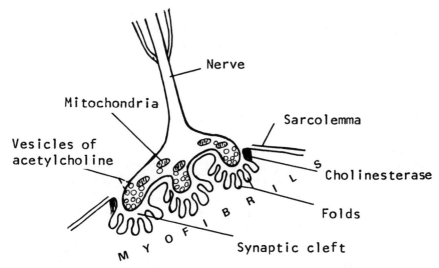

FIG. 19-3: Physiologic anatomy of the neuromuscular junction. Note the invaginations (folds) of the muscle membrane, which increase the surface area at which the transmitter can act.

not the sodium) penetrate. Once the potassium ions shift to the outside of the membrane, the negative aspect of the membrane potential rises. This is called hyperpolarization. In this state, it is more difficult for an impulse to create an action potential.

The inhibition in the central nervous system is of immense importance. Since there is continuous stimulation of the brain, this inhibitory action properly selects and transmits only the important impulses.

NEUROMUSCULAR JUNCTION

Neuromuscular junction is a term that includes the presynaptic and postsynaptic areas between the nerve ending and the muscle. The postsynaptic area is also called motor end-plate (Fig. 19-3).

The use of electron microscopy made it possible to study the micro-anatomy of the myoneural junction and the relationship between structure and function.[12] The presynaptic area, also called end-plate, is represented by the nerve ending. The nerve ending divides into a number of nonmyelinated terminal branches. The electron microscope revealed that, at the junction, the nerve ending is covered by an axoplasmastic membrane (also called the Schwann membrane). There are folds, or indentations, of this membrane toward the muscle fiber. In 1960, Waser hypothesized that these folds are actually "pores" containing the receptor sites for acetylcholine and cholinesterase.[13] The diameter of the "pores" is about 12 to 14 Å. These folds bring nerve endings and muscle fibers in close proximity with each other and increase the area at which the transmitter can act. Multiple vesicular granules (or quantas) containing acetylcholine are located at the nerve endings very close to the junction folds.[14-16]

RESTING MOTOR END-PLATE POTENTIAL

During "rest," electrical difference exists on both sides of the muscle membrane. At the neuromuscular junction, some very small changes of the resting potential can be detected. These changes are the result of small amounts of the transmitter (acetylcholine) being released from the pockets. The small amplitude of these end-plate potentials make them incapable of triggering a depolarization wave.

However, when the motor nerve is stimulated and the created action potential reaches the nerve ending, it causes simultaneous release of a large amount of acetylcholine. The acetylcholine diffuses through the synaptic cleft and acts on the postjunctional muscle membrane. The depolarization of the muscle membrane will excite the contractile elements of the striated muscle (Chap. 20).

In summary, the sequence of events taking place when the peripheral nerve is stimulated follows a similar pattern. If the stimulation is strong enough, it will create an action potential that will propagate down the nerve. At the nerve terminal, the action potential will release acetylcholine, which in turn will diffuse through the synaptic cleft. Having reached the postjunctional membrane, it activates the receptors.* The permeability of the postjunctional membrane will change. Sodium will penetrate the cell and the potassium will move to the outside. As a result, the postjunctional membrane will be depolarized. The depolarization will spread to the contractile elements of the muscle and the muscle will contract.

Depolarizing and Nondepolarizing Muscle Relaxants

The depolarizing muscle relaxants activate the receptors of the postjunctional membrane in a manner similar to acetylcholine. However, because of their longer effect, the membrane is maintained in a depolarized state and, therefore, is inexcitable.[17]

The nondepolarizing muscle relaxants occupy the receptor site of the postjunctional membrane. Thus, there are fewer receptors left on which the acetylcholine can act and the postjunctional membrane fails to depolarize to the critical level to elicit an action potential.[18]

---

* The exact nature of these receptors has not been determined.

Effect of Local anesthetics on the Myoneural Junction

Local anesthetics inhibit the release of acetylcholine at the nerve endings and have a curare-like effect on the postjunctional membrane. They can also potentiate the effect of succinylcholine and antagonize curare by inhibiting the cholinesterase at the neuromuscular junction. This shows that local anesthetics obviously have dual effects.

REFERENCES

1. Eccles J: The Physiology of Synapses. New York, Academic, 1964
2. Eccles J: The synapse. Sci Am 212:56, 1965
3. McLennan HD: Synaptic Transmission. Philadelphia, Saunders, 1963
4. Hebb C: CNS at the cellular level: identity of transmitter agents. Annu Rev Physiol 32:165, 1970
5. Hebb C: Synthesis and storage of acetylcholine considered as a special example of a synaptic transmitter. Proc Int Union Physiol Sci 6:277, 1968
6. Markalous P: Respiration and the intraperitoneal application of neomycin and meolymphin. Anaesthesia 17:427, 1962
7. Pittinger CB, Eryasa Y, Adamson R: Antibiotic-induced paralysis. Anesth Analg 49:487, 1970
8. Stanley VF, Giesecke AH, Jenkins MT: Neomycin–curare neuromuscular block and reversal in cats. Anesthesiology 31:228, 1969
9. Churchill-Davidson HC, Wise RP: The response of newborn infant to muscle relaxants. Can Anaesth Soc J 11:1, 1964
10. Churchill-Davidson HC, Richardson AT: Neuromuscular transmission in myasthenia gravis. J Physiol 122:252, 1953
11. Birks RI, Macintosh FC: Acetylcholine metabolism at nerve endings. Br Med Bull 13:157, 1957
12. De Robertis E: Ultrastructure and cytochemistry of the synaptic region. Science 156:907, 1967
13. Waser PG: The cholinergic receptor. J Pharm Pharmacol 12:577, 1960
14. Martin AR: Quantal nature of synaptic transmission. Physiol Rev 46:51, 1966
15. Martin AR: Mechanisms of transmitter release. Proc Int Union Physiol Sci 6:279, 1968
16. Katz B: Quantal mechanism of neural transmitter release. Science 173:123, 1971
17. Teshleff S: The mode of neuromuscular block caused by acetylcholine, nicotine, decamethonium and succinylcholine. Acta Physiol Scand 34:218, 1955
18. Taylor DB: The mechanism of action of muscle relaxants and their antagonists. Anesthesiology 20:439, 1959

chapter 20

Muscle Physiology

PHYSIOLOGIC ANATOMY OF SKELETAL MUSCLE

Skeletal muscles are made up of muscle fibers. Each muscle fiber contains three major components: myofibril, sacroplasm, and cell membrane.

The Myofibril

The muscle fiber is made of multiple myofibrils, which contain the contractile element. The contractile element is composed of myosin and actin filaments, which are large protein molecules. Under electron microscopy, they appear as alternating dark and light bands (Fig. 20-1). The light bands, made of actin filaments, are called I bands. The dark bands, made of myosin filaments

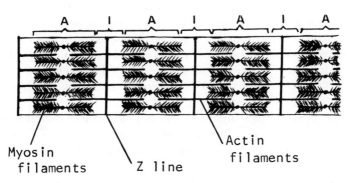

FIG. 20-1: Schematic presentation of sarcomeres. Arrangement of actin (I bands) and myosin (A bands) filaments.

251

and the part of the overlapping actin filaments, are called A bands. The combination of A and I bands makes up the sarcomere.

The line of attachment of two actin filaments is called a Z line, or Z membrane. This membrane passes all the way across the muscle fiber.

The Sarcoplasm

The sarcoplasm is a matrix around the myofibrils. It contains the nuclei, mitochondria, and fluid. The mitochondria lie in close proximity to the actin filaments. This proximity facilitates the use of adenosine triphosphate (ATP) formed in the mitochondria by the actin filaments.

The sarcoplasm also contains a very important structure called sarcoplasmic reticulum. The sarcoplasmic reticulum is composed of transverse (T) and longitudinal tubules. The T tubules extend to the cell membrane and are open to the extracellular medium. They are the channels through which the interior of the cell communicates with the exterior. The longitudinal tubules lie parallel to the myofibril. The two tubule systems are in contact with each other.

Muscle Contraction and Relaxation

When the impulse reaches the membrane, it is transmitted to the interior of the muscle fiber by way of the T-tubule system. Once the action potential reaches the terminal sacs of the sarcoplasmic reticulum, it causes a release of the calcium in the cytoplasm. The calcium stimulates the activity of ATPase and the breakdown of ATP, thus releasing energy and causing a contraction. Almost immediately, the calcium gets reabsorbed into the sarcoplasmic reticulum, and the muscle then relaxes. This reabsorption is accomplished by the calcium pump located in the sarcoplasmic reticulum membrane.[1,2]

The light filament consists of two additional proteins besides the actin. These are the proteins known as tropomyosin and troponin. Tropomyosin and troponin block the interaction of the force-generating portions of the dark filaments, with reactive sites on the actin molecules, and in this way maintain the relaxed state of the muscle cell.

Troponin has a high affinity for calcium ions. If it is saturated with calcium, the protein, which holds tropomyosin blocked in the relaxed muscle, allows it to move out of the way. Actin and myosin can then interact. Calcium ions are, therefore, the trigger substance initiating the contraction.

Chemistry of Contraction and Relaxation

Energy is required in order for the muscle to contract. The production of the necessary amount of energy involves a series of reduction and oxidation processes. ATP is the main store of energy in the muscle.[3] The energy produced in the respiratory chain is used for the oxidative phosphorylation of adenosine diphosphate (ADP) to form ATP. The process is catalyzed by the enzyme adenosinetriphosphatase in the respiratory chain. The process of oxidative phosphorylation takes place within the mitochondria, as shown in the following reaction:

$$ADP + P + \text{Energy (from the respiratory chain)} \rightleftharpoons ATP \text{ (stored energy)}.$$

Thus, the ATP produced is the main source of energy. Under the effect of the enzyme ATPase from the myosin, ATP breaks down and energy is thus released:

$$ATP + H_2O \xrightleftharpoons{\text{ATPase from the myosin}} ADP + P + \text{Energy}$$

The energy produced is used for muscle contraction. Calcium ions take an active part in the production and storage of energy. They stimulate the action of myosin ATPase and release energy. However, the excess of calcium ions causes an uncoupling of oxidative phosphorylation by depressing the activity of the ATPase in the respiratory chain. Under these circumstances, the level of ADP rises, the concentration of ATP decreases, and the energy derived from the respiratory chain is released as heat. However, ATP acts not only as a storage for energy but is necessary for the relaxation of the muscle fiber. Rigor mortis is a direct result of the uncoupling of oxidative phosphorylation.

ATP can also be produced from ADP and energy derived from creatinine phosphate. This reaction is influenced by the enzyme creatinine phosphokinase.

MALIGNANT HYPERPYREXIA

During the last few years, anesthesiologists have become exceedingly aware of a syndrome called "malignant hyperthermia."[4] It is a pharmacogenetic syndrome affecting animals and humans. The mode of inheritance is autosomal dominant.

Most of the patients appear normal before anesthesia. Some are more muscular than normal; others have diffuse muscle weakness and wasting. Spontaneous muscle cramps are quite common in these patients.

The serum creatinine phosphokinase (CPK) has been found to be elevated in about two-thirds of the patients. Similar elevations are also seen in their relatives.

Some of the more potent inhalation agents like halothane and depolarizing skeletal muscle relaxants like succinylcholine are capable of triggering this syndrome. The main feature of the hyperthermic crisis is tachycardia, fast rising temperature, skeletal muscle rigidity, hyperventilation, and metabolic disorders.

Late findings are acute heart failure, consumption coagulopathy, and acute renal failure. Mortality used to be extremely high, in the range of 70 percent; however, with knowledge, awareness of the problem, and prompt treatment, the percentage of deaths has decreased.

The etiology is not completely determined. However, there is convincing evidence that the main problem lies in the inability of some muscle cells to store calcium effectively. The elevated myoplasmic calcium level (1) activates myosin ATPase, thus accelerating the hydrolysis of ATP to ADP; (2) depresses the activation of the ATPase in the respiratory chain and, as a result, ATP synthesis is depressed and the energy is released in the form of heat; (3) inhibits troponin, thus permitting a biochemical contracture to occur.

In suspected cases, the levels of serum CPK should be predetermined. Muscle biopsies are also strongly suggested.

To administer anesthesia to a suspect patient, it will be best to avoid halothane and succinylcholine. Use of neurolept anesthesia is considered to be the best and, if muscle relaxant is necessary, curare or pancuronium should be used. Mepivicaine and lidocaine should also be avoided, since they cause release of calcium from the sacroplasmic reticulum. The local anesthetic of choice is procaine.

THE MOTOR UNIT

Each motoneuron innervates many different muscle fibers. These muscle fibers innervated by one single motor nerve fiber form a motor unit. The number of muscle fibers in each motor unit depends on the function of that particular muscle.

MUSCLE SPINDLES AND SMALL FIBER SYSTEM

Histologically, muscle spindles are elongated and encapsulated structures, lying parallel to the muscle fibers and having the same attachments. Contraction of the spindles sends stimuli back to the spinal cord along the large afferent sensory fibers.

The small fiber system consists of muscle spindle, gamma efferent fiber, and large afferent fiber synapsing with the anterior horn cell of the motor unit. The important role this system plays is in the maintenance of constant length of different muscle groups.

SINGLE MUSCLE TWITCH AND TETANUS

Single muscle twitch and tetanus can be elicited by electrically stimulating the peripheral nerve. This is actually how the neuromuscular transmission is studied. The intensity of the electrical current of supramaximal stimulation is enough to excite all nerve fibers in the bundle.

If the rate of nerve stimulation is 50 per second, or less, and the neuro-muscular transmission is normal, it will elicit well-sustained action potential in the muscle. However, if the muscle is stimulated at greater rates, a frequency is reached at which the contractions of the muscle cannot be differentiated from one another. This state is called tetanus.

EVALUATION OF DEPOLARIZING AND NONDEPOLARIZING BLOCK CAUSED BY MUSCLE RELAXANTS

The nerve is stimulated and the action potential is recorded from the muscle. Then the muscle relaxant is administered and its effect on the height of the action potential is recorded (Fig. 20-2).

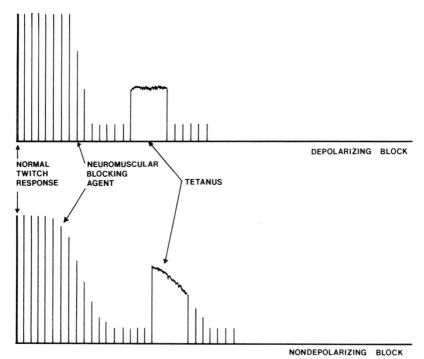

FIG. 20-2: Schematic representation of twitch and tetanus response of the thumb to a stimulus applied to the ulnar nerve. In case of depolarizing block, the tetanus is sustained and there is no posttetanic facilitation. In case of a nondepolarizing block there is a fade of twitch response, fade with tetanus, and presence of posttetanic facilitation.

Characteristics of the Depolarization Block

The characteristics of the depolarization block are:[5] (1) fasciculations observed prior to the beginning of the paralysis; (2) Well-sustained tetanic and twitch rates of nerve stimulation; and (3) absence of posttetanic potentiation.

As pointed out, the depolarizing muscle relaxants act as acetylcholine. In a partial block resulting from the depolarizing agent, the postjunctional membrane potential is closer to the critical level. This explains the second characteristic of this type of block; eg, the tetanic stimulation is well maintained. Only small additional amounts of acetylcholine are needed to drive the depolarization to a threshold level and thus elicit an action potential. Anticholinesterase agents will not antagonize this type of block because the muscle fibers are in a depolarized state, making them inexcitable.

Characteristics of the Nondepolarizing Block

The characteristics of the nondepolarizing block are: (1) no fasciculations; (2) a "fade" in both the tetanic and twitch rates of stimulation; and (3) posttetanic potentiation.

The classic representative of this group is curare. As noted, this agent interacts with the same receptor sites as that of the acetylcholine. It is a competitive type of block. Any increase in the amount of acetylcholine available for receptor activation will antagonize the block. In experiments, it has been demonstrated that the amount of acetylcholine released declines during tetanic stimulation and increases after rest. Therefore, in conditions in which partial curarization exists, the tetanic contraction will not be maintained and posttetanic potentiation will occur. The nondepolarizing block is antagonized by anticholinesterase agents. In conditions associated with low calcium and high magnesium concentration and myasthenia gravis, the amount of acetylcholine released following nerve stimulation is less than normal. It will require less nondepolarizing agent to achieve the same degree of block than in normal conditions.

"Dual" Block[6]

At times, during administration of succinylcholine (most common depolarizing agent used), "dual" block may develop. This block develops in two stages; first, it reveals characteristics of depolarizing block, followed by nondepolarizing. This type of block is also called Phase II or desensitization block. After prolonged exposure to a depolarizing muscle relaxant, the postjunctional membrane becomes less sensitive to acetylcholine and muscle contraction cannot be elicited by nerve stimulation. It has been shown that this desensitization process starts immediately with the administration of the deplarizing agent, but its magnitude depends on the amount and time of administration. Also, signs of this block develop when atypical forms of cholinesterase enzyme are present in the plasma. Since the succinylcholine cannot be hydrolyzed, it circulates in the blood for prolonged periods of time.

REFERENCES

1. Huxley HE: The mechanism of muscular contraction. Sci Am 213:18, 1965
2. Podolsky RJ: Contraction of striated muscle fibers. Proc Int Union Physiol Sci 6:89, 1968
3. Hotta K, Bowen WJ: Contraction of ATPase activity of glycerinated muscle fibers and myofibril fragments. Am J Physiol 218:332, 1970
4. Gordon RA, Britt BA, Kalow W: International Symposium on Malignant Hyperthermia. Springfield, Ill, Thomas, 1974
5. Wylie WD, Churchill-Davidson HC (eds): A Practice of Anesthesia. Chicago, Year Book, 1972, Chap 30
6. Churchill-Davidson HC, Katz RL: Dual, phase II, or desensitization block? Anesthesiology 27:536, 1966

chapter 21

Spinal Cord

ANATOMY

The spinal cord is situated in the vertebral canal and extends from the medulla oblongata to the lower border of the first lumbar vertebra. In some cases, it reaches the second lumbar vertebra. Below the spinal cord, the vertebral canal is occupied by cauda equina, which consists of the roots of the lumbar, sacral, and coccygeal nerves.

The cord is composed by gray and white matter and is divided into two parts by anterior and posterior sulci. The gray matter is located around the central canal and, in a cross section, it has the shape of the letter "H." There are anterior, lateral, and posterior horns of the gray matter (Fig. 21-1).

In the anterior horn are located:

1. Alpha motoneurons: The axons of the alpha motoneurons leave the spinal cord through the anterior roots and innervate the striated muscles. Each neuron innervates about 100 to 150 myofibrils and, together, form the motor unit (Chap. 20).
2. Gamma motoneurons: The gamma motoneurons innervate the muscle spindles. Their axons also leave the spinal cord through the anterior roots.
3. Cells of Renshaw: Functionally, the cells of Renshaw are intermediate neurons. Their axons synapse with alpha motoneurons without leaving the gray matter. There is a collateral neuron, extending from the alpha motoneuron to the cells of Renshaw, which establish a circle with a feedback mechanism. When an impulse is conducted through the motoneuron, it excites the cell of Renshaw through the collateral neuron. The cell of Renshaw, through its axon, inhibits the action of the motoneuron. Thus, an autoregulation is established, which limits the overconduction of impulses.

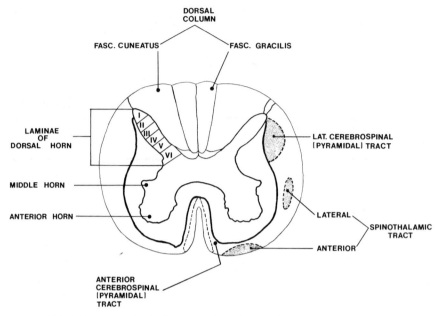

FIG. 21-1: The principal tracts in the spinal cord on transverse section.

There are numerous other nerve cells and nonmedullated nerve fibers in the anterior horn that are held together by neuroglia.

The cells of the preganglionic neurons of the sympathetic nervous system are located in the lateral horns of the thoracolumbar area.

The cells of the intermediate neurons are located in the posterior horns, which synapse with the axons of the spinal ganglia cells of the posterior roots. The intermediate neurons of substantia gelatinosa transmit tactile, pain, and temperature impulses to the spinothalamic tract.

The white matter of the spinal cord is formed by axons of the spinal ganglia cells, axons of the intermediate neurons, and the ascending and descending tracts. It is divided into dorsal, lateral, and ventral columns.

Impulses to and from various portions of the brain are carried by the tracts. The dorsal column of the spinal cord is composed of tracts that transmit touch and pressure sensation with fine graduation of intensity and location, vibratory sensation, and kinesthetic sensations.

The spinothalamic tract is composed of small and, in the main, nonmyelinated nerve fibers. It is far more crude in its transmitting of sensory impulses than is the dorsal column system. The conduction velocity of impulses by the spinothalamic tract is very slow and the fibers have poor spatial orientation. In the dorsal column, the fibers transmitting impulses from the lower parts of the body occupy the center. Those from the upper part form successive layers on the lateral side of the column. This is not the case with the spinothalamic tract, especially with the lateral one. However, specific sensations like pain, warmth, cold, and sexual sensations are transmitted only by the spinothalamic tract.

The lateral spinothalamic tract mediates pain and temperature, and, after crossing to the opposite side of the spinal cord, ascends in the lateral funiculus and reaches the thalamus. The ventral spinothalamic tract also crosses to the opposite side and ascends to the thalamus and transmits impulses of touch.

The lateral pyramidal tract arises from large cells in the precentral gyrus and carries impulses to the primary motoneuron of the opposite side.

The direct pyramidal tract arises from cells in the central area of the cortex, passes in the anterior median fissure of the same side and then crosses to the opposite side in the anterior commissure and synapses with the anterior horn cells.

Spinal Nerves

The spinal cord is composed of 31 segments. There is one pair of spinal nerves that spring from each segment. Spinal nerves are made up of fibers of the dorsal and ventral roots. The ventral roots carry efferent motor fibers. The body cells of the axons forming the ventral roots lie in the gray matter of the ventral and lateral horns.

The posterior roots are formed by axons, the body cells of which lie in the spinal ganglia. Each ganglion cell possesses a T-like nerve process with a central branch running to the spinal cord and another to the periphery. After it enters the white matter, the central branch reaches the posterior horn where it branches out. One of the branches synapses with an intermediate neuron in the gray matter, the other leaves the gray matter and enters the white, where it divides into two subbranches. The longer subbranch ascends to the central nervous system and, on the way, gives collaterals to different segments of the spinal cord. The shorter subbranch descends into the spinal cord.

Both anterior and posterior roots pierce the dura separately as they leave through the intervertebral foramina. Usually, the posterior root is thicker than the anterior. They are enclosed in a common dural sheath extending just past the spinal ganglion, where they form the spinal nerve.

Each pair of ventral and dorsal spinal roots innervates specific segments of the skin (dermatome) and muscles (myotome). The dermatomes are, in fact, more extensive than shown in Fig. 21-2. To get complete denervation of a specific dermatome, it is necessary to interrupt three consecutive nerve roots. There is considerable overlap in the areas supplied by adjacent roots.

The segmental innervation of the myotomes, with exception of the intercostal muscles, is not as well outlined as the dermatomes. Usually, one muscle group receives motor innervation from few roots.

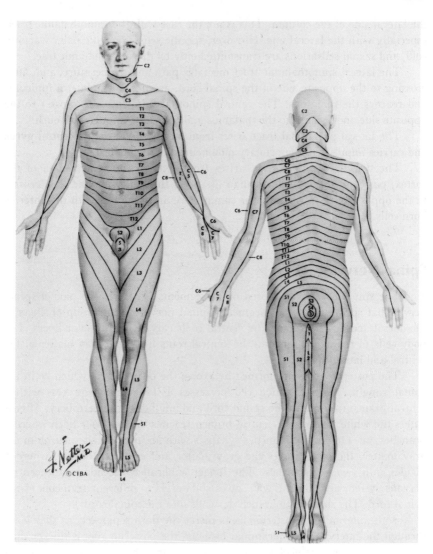

FIG. 21-2: The dermatomes, which are skin fields innervated by each spinal nerve. (© 1953, 1972 Ciba Pharmaceutical Co., Division of CIBA GEIGY Corp. Reproduced with permission from the CIBA Collection of Medical Illustrations by Frank H. Netter, M.D. All rights reserved.)

Spinal Cord Coverings

The spinal cord is enveloped by membranes, dura, arachnoid, and pia, which are direct continuations of those surrounding the brain.

The dura matter in the cranial cavity consists of two layers. The outer periosteal layer is the periosteum of the skull bones. In the spine, this periosteal layer acts as the periosteum lining of the spinal canal. The inner layer continues in the spinal canal. The epidural space is located between these two layers. The fact that the inner layer firmly adheres to the margin of the foramen magnum and blends with the periosteal layer is very important to the anesthesiologist. It means that the spinal epidural space extends to the level of the first cervical nerves. Hence, local anesthetic solutions placed in the epidural space cannot enter the cranial cavity and produce a block extending only to the first cervical nerves. The greatest width of the epidural space is in the mid-thoracic area.

The inner layer of the dura carries tubular prolongations in the form of dural cuffs that eventually blend with the perineurium of the spinal nerve. Both the arachnoid and the dura end at the second sacral vertebra.

The spinal arachnoid is a continuation of the cerebral. The pia matter is in very close contact with the spinal cord.

PAIN

Pain is one of the most extraordinary and compelling experiences man encounters. The science of anesthesia was created to alleviate surgical pain. Anesthesiologists take active part in the relief of acute and chronic pain.

Pain and Temperature Receptors

Pain receptors in the skin and various organs are free nerve endings. Receptors can be classified into three groups: mechanoreceptors, which sense touch and motion; thermoreceptors, which sense temperature changes; and nociceptors, which are stimulated by strong mechanical and temperature stimuli.

The receptors can be activated by various substances like bradykinin, histamine, or serotonin. Accumulation of large amounts of lactic acid during ischemia has also been known to cause pain. The skin receptors for temperature sensation are the bulbs of Krause for cold and the bulbs of Ruffini for warmth.

There are three major categories of painful stimuli: physical injury of mechanical and thermal origin; ischemia; and inflammation caused by toxins, infection, or various chemicals.

The Peripheral Nerve Fibers

Pricking pain signals are carried by the A-δ fibers that have a velocity of conduction between 3 and 10 meters per second. Aching and burning pain signals are conducted by C fibers at velocities of 0.5 to 2 meters per second. Hence, a painful stimulus creates a double pain perception: a fast pricking sensation and a slow burning sensation. The fibers involved with temperature sensation follow the same pathways as the fibers for pain.

The Spinal Cord

The cell bodies of A-δ fibers and C fibers are located in the dorsal root ganglia and synapse with dorsal horn neurons. Rexed[1,2] divided the dorsal horn of the spinal cord into six longitudinal laminae, Lamina I being the most posterior (Fig. 21-1). Laminae I and V contain large cells that are stimulated by high-threshold, noxious stimuli and by inputs from low-threshold thermo- and mechanoreceptors. The activity of Laminae IV and V can be modified by the descending pathways (see section to follow on descending control).

Ketamine, morphine sulfate, nitrous oxide, and hyperventilation suppress the activity of Lamina V cells and the cells of nucleus caudalis (trigeminal nerve). The suppression of Lamina V cells is important for its role in pain perception.[3-6]

Laminae II and III (substancia gelatinosa) contain small cells that are stimulated by A-α fibers and inhibited by A-δ fibers and C fibers. Melzack and Wall based their gate control theory on these findings.

The Somatic Ascending Sensory System

The fast-conducting large-diameter A-α cutaneous afferent fibers ascend in the posterior column and the medulla, and synapse in Gracile and Cuneate nuclei. The neurons originating from these nuclei cross the midline (medial lemniscus) and terminate in the ventrobasal nuclei of the thalamus. From the thalamus, impulses are relayed to the somatosensory cortex through the thalamocortical projection.

The dorsal column carries the sensation of touch position, and fine discrimination.

The slowly conducting afferent A-δ fibers and C fibers synapse in the spinal cord with dorsal horn neurons. Axons of the second neurons cross the midline and turn upward in the lateral spinothalamic tract. The tract ascends through the spinal cord, medulla, and pons, and terminates in the posterolateral nucleus of the thalamus. From there, impulses project to the postcentral gyrus of the parietal lobe.

The tracts of the ventrolateral column transmit pain and temperature. Recent evidence suggests that they also receive input from low-threshold mechanoreceptors as well.

Pain fibers from the face, cornea of the eye and mucosa of the lips, cheeks, and tongue are carried in the trigeminal nerve.

Pain Appreciation

The exact site of pain appreciation is not well defined. Painful stimuli can evoke the following changes in the nervous system

1. In the spinal cord, segmental reflex changes are evoked.
2. In the medulla and pons, the cardiac and respiratory centers can be stimulated.
3. In the hypothalamus, the pituitary hormone secretions are influenced and anger and fear may appear.
4. The midbrain and lumbic system have been implicated for the suffering of pain.
5. The frontal lobe is concerned with memory.

Crude perception of pain is experienced when the impulse reaches the thalamus. However, complete appreciation of pain stimuli is elicited only when the impulse is conducted to the parietal cortex. In this area, pain sensation is integrated with other sensory stimuli.

Descending Control

Pyramidal tract, rubrospinal tract, and reticulospinal tract stimulation inhibits the response of Lamina V cells to painful stimuli.[7]

In psychodynamic control, pain causes both reflex motor and mental reactions. It can arouse strong emotional protest such as anguish, anxiety, and crying. Pain can be considered from several perspectives with regard to its psychologic and psychiatric aspects, including the influence of personality and culture on pain tolerance and description.[8,9] However, they do not change the physiologic threshold* for pain sensation.

It has been shown that there is very little difference in the physiologic thresholds of pain in different people. What actually varies is the reaction to it.

Visceral Pain

Frequently, visceral pain is used to diagnose inflammation or disease. The parenchyma of internal organs, including the brain, has no pain receptors.

---

* *The pain threshold is the stimulus intensity at which the subjects report the pain sensation to be present with 50 percent of the stimuli.*

Peritoneum, pleura, and other viscera have sensory receptors for pain only.

Pain sensation from most of the internal organs of the body is conducted by fibers that pass along the visceral sympathetic nerves and the lateral spinothalamic tract. Pain fibers from the distal colon, rectum, and bladder enter the spinal cord through the sacral parasympathetic nerves. The ones from the pharynx, trachea, and upper esophagus are transmitted via the glossopharyngeal and the vagus nerves.

Visceral pain is diffuse in character and cannot be localized easily. Muscular rigidity is frequently associated with it. Sometimes pain is felt on a surface area of the body far away from its original source. It is called referred pain. Frequently, pain caused by coronary insufficiency is felt in the precordial chest wall area, radiating down the left arm. Pain originating in the gallbladder area may be felt over the right shoulder. The nerve fibers supplying the painful skin area enter the spinal cord at the same segment as the ones conducting pain from the visceral organ. For example, the spinal cord's first and second thoracic segments receive skin sensory fibers from the left upper extremity and from the heart.

Deep Pain

Pain may be referred from deep structures like joints, tendons, muscle, and fascia. Pain impulses from deep structures travel the same pathways as those from the skin. The periosteum has a very rich nerve supply and, therefore, is very sensitive to pain stimulation.

Deep pain endings can be stimulated chemically and mechanically. Various metabolic products can cause ischemic pain as in intermittent claudication. Muscle contractions and spasms are also frequent causes of pain.

Sensory Changes Other than Pain

Paresthesia is spontaneous sensation of prickling, tingling, or numbness. It can result from dorsal root, peripheral nerve, or central nervous system irritation. Impulses are carried all the way to the brain and a sensation is localized to an area of the body that has not been directly stimulated.

Hyperesthesia is hypersensitivity of the sensory fibers. There is no spontaneous sensation.

Tic Douloureux

Excruciating pains occurring along the sensory distribution of the fifth nerve over one side of the face is called "tic douloureux." Frequently, the pain is set off by a sensitive "trigger area" on the surface of the face, mouth, or nose. Several surgical procedures are designed to alleviate this type of pain with more or less successful results. This can be accomplished by cutting the peripheral nerve inside the cranium, where the motor and sensory roots of the fifth nerve can be separated. This type of surgery will leave the side of the face numb. The spinal tract of the fifth nerve can be cut in the medulla. This will block the pain sensation and will preserve touch and pressure.

There are two relatively new procedures for the relief of trigeminal neuralgia. One of these has been pioneered by Peter Jannetta at the University of Pittsburgh.[10] He demonstrated that a compressing arterial loop in apposition to the trigeminal nerve at its root entry zone was the cause. These vessels, usually a branch of the superior cerebellar artery, elongate with the aging process and shift into this position. Using a limited posterior fossa craniectomy, the vessel is displaced from the nerve and secured with a small plastic prosthesis to prevent reapposition to the nerve. The procedure is nondestructive and it avoids numbness, corneal anesthesia, and anesthesia dolorosa. The second procedure involves selective destruction of trigeminal nerve fibers utilizing a percutaneously placed needle electrode and radiofrequency current. The needle is introduced through the foramen ovale and stimulation is carried out to localize the appropriate trigeminal division. When a suitable low-threshold locus is obtained, sequential lesioning with a radiofrequency current is achieved.

Theories of Pain

The most popular ones include the specific theory, the pattern theory, and the gate control theory.

SPECIFIC THEORY

According to this theory, specific fibers conduct specific sensation and terminate in the central nervous system in a specific area. For instance, when pain fibers are stimulated, pain is felt, although the stimulus could be heat, electricity, or any other kind. These pain receptors are the free nerve endings of the A-δ fibers and the C fibers.

PATTERN THEORY

According to this theory, summation of stimuli, after the impulse has entered the spinal cord, is important in initiating pain sensation. Livingston emphasizes that the summation is the result of reverberating circuits in the spinal cord. There are several varieties of reverberating, or so-called oscillating, circuits in the nervous system, the simplest being presented in Fig. 21-3. In this case, the output neuron discharges a collateral nerve fiber back to its own body

Input   Output

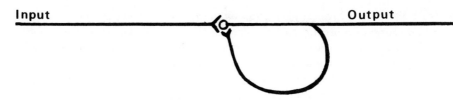

FIG. 21-3: Simple reverberatory circuit.

cell to restimulate itself. Thus, the feedback stimuli could, theoretically, keep the neuron discharging for a very long period of time. In the spinal cord, the reverberating circuits exist in the internuncial pool.*

Other pattern theories propose the absence of inhibition as a main cause for summation.

GATE CONTROL THEORY

The gate control theory (Fig. 21-4) was originated by Melzack and Wall [11,12] and has been revised on several occasions.

The authors suggest that the sensory impulse from the skin is modulated before eventual pain perception is evoked. This modulation takes place in two levels, spinal cord and brain.

In the spinal cord. The impulse from the skin is transmitted to three different systems in the spinal cord: the tracts of the dorsal column, which transmit the impulse to the brain; the central transmission cells in the dorsal horn (T); and the cells of substantia gelatinosa.

The gating cells in substancia gelatinosa exert presynaptic inhibition. These cells inhibit both the large and small fiber endings. The small fibers transmit impulses to the spinal cord without any apparent stimulation. Melzack and Wall propose that small fibers inhibit the gating cells and maintain the gate open, thus allowing conduction of impulses. Strong stimulation will elicit impulses predominantly in the large fibers. They excite the gating cells, close the gate, and thus inhibit transmission to the T cells.

Adaptation of the large fibers develops during sustained stimulation and, eventually, the activity of the small fibers will predominate. Hence, the gate will open and the outflow from the T cells will increase.

The authors point out that the brain may excite or inhibit the presynaptic transmission and can open or close the gate. This has been called the "central control trigger." Recently, new anatomic and physiologic evidence has identified visceral afferent fibers, which synapse with the T cells, which are the same cells receiving cutaneous impulses.

---

* *Internuncial neurons are located in the spinal cord between the anterior and posterior horns. Their role is to coordinate and relate impulses to the appropriate areas.*

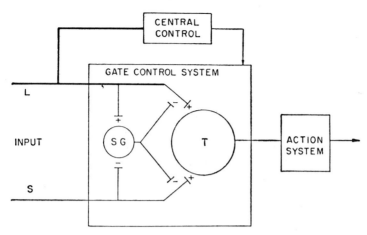

FIG. 21-4: Schematic diagram of the gate control theory of pain mechanisms (see text for explanation). (© 1965 by the American Association for the Advancement of Science. Reproduced with permission from Melzack and Wall.[36]

In the brain. The gating process, which begins at the spinal cord, is a continuous one, and filtering of the impulse occurs in every level of the conductive pathway.

Melzack further stresses the tonic inhibitory action of the reticular formation at all levels, which he calls "the central biasing mechanism."

The gate control theory successfully explains many phenomena, like intractable pain, causalgia, phantom limb pain, and others. When there is a selective degeneration of the large fibers, the unopposed activity of the small fibers will keep the gate open and so produce severe pain.

This theory also explains the alterations of an impulse by mechanical, chemical, and electrical stimulations, as well as the effect of different tranquilizers and sedatives.

Pain Relief

Relief from pain can be obtained by interfering with pain reception or interrupting pain conduction at the various sites of the pain pathway:

1. Receptor-pain relief obtained by administering aspirin is due to its effect on the receptor site.
2. Conduction in peripheral somatic nerves can be temporarily or permanently interrupted by nerve blocks or neurectomy. A-δ fibers and C fibers are affected by injection of cold hypertonic saline in the subarachnoid space.[13,14]
3. Modulation of pain impulses by stimulating Aα fibers can be accomplished

     by compresses, massage, percutaneous or implanted stimulators (gate control theory).

4. Posterior nerve roots can be anesthetized and partially destroyed by neurolytic agents such as absolute alcohol and phenol-glycerine.

5. The sympathetic nerves can be blocked by paravertebral sympathetic block or sympathectomy.[15]

6. At the spinal cord, pain conduction is interrupted by the effect of inhalation anesthetic agents and ketamine on Lamina V. Interruption of the lateral spinothalamic tract can be accomplished by tractotomy.[16] The pain and temperature perception of the contralateral side is lost. It is necessary to perform bilateral cordotomy to abolish pain from visceral organs.

7. Thalamic sensation is crude. The pain impulse is localized and the intensity determined in the sensory cortex. In individuals with severe emotional reaction to pain, a prefrontal leukotomy of a stereotactic ablation of intraluminar nuclei of the thalamus is performed. They still feel pain but do not suffer.

8. In descending inhibitory control, hypnosis or placebos[17, 18] exert the desired effect by influencing the activity of the descending cortical inhibitory mechanism. Reynolds, in 1969, found that stimulation of a group of cells in the periaqueductal periventricular gray matter can produce inhibition of pain. It is very likely that morphine produces analgesia by acting on the same group of cells.

SUBARACHNOID BLOCK

     The introduction of local anesthetics in the subarachnoid space produces subarachnoid (spinal) block. This regional technique is widely used in surgical and obstetric anesthesia and also for diagnostic and therapeutic reasons.

     Subarachnoid block can be achieved by the introduction of small amounts of local anesthetics into the subarachnoid space.[19] This is possible because the site of action of the local anesthetics is in the fibers of the dorsal and ventral roots, which are thinly covered by the pia matter. This is in contrast to the site of action of peridural block where the formed spinal nerves are enclosed in thick fibrous tissues, which make the penetration of the local anesthetics much more difficult. The onset of subarachnoid block is more rapid than peridural, and the block is more intense and longer lasting.

Sequence of Block

     The concentration of the drug declines after its introduction in the subarachnoid space because of the dilution by the cerebrospinal fluid. The preganglionic sympathetic fibers are affected first, causing a vasomotor block followed by loss of temperature, pain, touch, and pressure sensations. Finally, the somatic motor impulses are blocked and loss of proprioception takes place. Differential block, averaging two spinal segments, exists between the levels of sensory and vasomotor blockade, the latter being the higher.

Usually, the injected local anesthetic agent blocks all the sensory and motor fibers. However, due to dilution, there is an area in which only C fibers and A-δ fibers are blocked. These fibers transmit pain, pressure, touch, and temperature. The somatic motor block is about two to three segments below the level of the sensory block.

Factors Influencing the Spread of Anesthetic

The following influence the spread of anesthetic in the subarachnoid space: volume and total dose of drug; specific gravity and position of patient during, and after, block; and speed of injection and size of needle.

In pregnancy, there is an obstruction of the venous return with consequent engorgement. This decreases the size of the subarachnoid and peridural spaces and influences the spread.

Fate of the Drug

The drug is primarily removed by absorption into the capillaries. Only a small portion of it is taken up by the neural tissue.

Physiology

From a purely physiologic point of view, the most important effect of spinal anesthesia is the sympathetic blockade. Subarachnoid block affects the function of the cardiovascular and respiratory systems, as well as others, and cerebrospinal fluid.

CARDIOVASCULAR SYSTEM

Greene[19] regards arterial hypotension to be a result of preganglionic sympathetic blockage with consequent vasodilatation.

The cardiac output is not decreased unless the block involves cardiac sympathetic fibers in the upper five thoracic segments. The position of the patient has great influence on the changes of cardiac output. If placed in head-up position, the patient's cardiac output will fall due to pooling of blood. There is compensatory vasoconstriction above the level of the sympathetic blockade.[20] The degree of hypotension is related to the level of the vasomotor block.

In unmedicated normovolemic man, a block up to the tenth thoracic segment will not cause hypotension, whereas a block up to the fifth thoracic segment will reduce the mean arterial pressure 10 to 15 percent.[21,22] The condition of the patient influences the degree of hypotension. It is more pronounced in diseased states, old age, hypertension, pregnancy, and also hypovolemia.[23]

Bradycardia seen during spinal anesthesia is due to the combination of two factors: the block of cardiac accelerator fibers (T_1 to T_4) and decreased pressure in the right side of the heart and great veins associated with changes in venous return. This is mediated through the intrinsic chronotropic stretch receptors.

RESPIRATORY SYSTEM

Ventilation is not affected in the awake unmedicated subject even if the block extends to the thoracic segments. Blood gases remain essentially the same.[24 25] However, paralysis of the abdominal and the intercostal muscles will decrease the ability to cough.

Respiratory arrest can occur during high-level subarachnoid block, as a result of medullary ischemia due to a decrease in cardiac output. Phrenic paralysis can also occur, leading to respiratory arrest.

Pulmonary blood flow is essentially unchanged. The effect of sympathetic blockade on pulmonary perfusion is minimal.

OTHER ORGAN FUNCTIONS

High levels of spinal anesthesia can decrease renal plasma flow, glomerular filtration rate,[26,27] and hepatic blood flow.[28] These effects are directly related to decrease in the mean arterial blood pressure.

Sympathetic blockade results in contracted bowel, relaxed sphincters, and depressed uterine contractility.

CEREBROSPINAL FLUID

Spinal anesthesia usually causes an elevation in the albumin and sugar contents of the cerebrospinal fluid.

In summary, subarachnoid block may be regarded as a chemical sympatectomy. The effect is most pronounced shortly after the administration of the drug. "Fixing"* takes place during the first 5 to 6 minutes, during which the level of the block can change.

The local anesthetic can be mixed with vasoconstrictor drugs to prolong the duration of the subarachnoid block. Epinephrine (most used) will reduce

---

* The term "fixed" applies to the concentration of the local anesthetic that falls below the effective level due to a mixing with cerebrospinal fluid.

the absorption of the agent by constricting the vessels in the subarachnoid space and thus prolong the action of the local anesthetic.

PERIDURAL BLOCK

In the course of the last few years, peridural block has become more popular and, in many institutions, has replaced subarachnoid block for surgical and obstetric purposes.

To perform a peridural block, the local anesthetic is deposited in the space between the dura mater and the walls of the spinal canal. As pointed out, the first cervical nerve is the highest possible level of block achieved by peridural anesthesia. The local anesthetic cannot penetrate the cranium, since the spinal peridural space ends at the foramen magnum.

Larger amounts of local anesthetics have to be injected into the peridural space than in the subarachnoid to achieve the same degree of block. Local anesthetics have to overcome what Bromage calls "formidable barricades" to reach the target nerves.[29] Placed in the peridural space, the solution spreads in all directions, passing through the intervertebral foramina and into the paravertebral space.

The factors that influence the spread of anesthetic solution are:[30] (1) total volume, concentration, and penetrance of the drug; (2) age, height, and weight of the patient, and pregnancy determine the capacity of the peridural space; (3) the speed of injection; and (4) the effect of gravity.

Site of Action

There appears to be no single site of action. It has been shown that local anesthetic solutions do penetrate from the peridural into the subarachnoid space and also diffuse through the intervetebral foramina. It has also been demonstrated that in the area of the dural cuffs, substances can easily diffuse between the subarachnoid and the peridural spaces.

Absorption of drugs in the peridural space occur mainly by way of epidural vessels (Fig. 21-5).

CARDIOVASCULAR SYSTEM.[31–33]

Peridural block (like subarachnoid) blocks the sympathetic nerves; therefore, the cardiovascular effects of both are similar. The hypotension following peridural block has delayed onset and is less severe than in subarach-

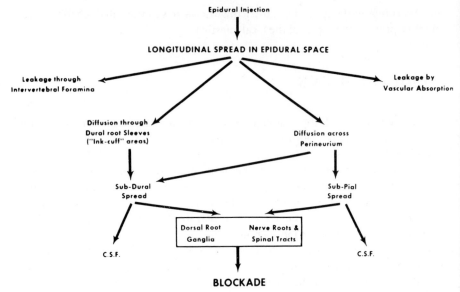

FIG. 21-5:   The fate of an epidural injection. Courtesy of Bromage: Br J Anaesth 34:176, 1962).

noid block. The compensatory mechanism in peridural block has more time to act. It is important to note that with peridural block, levels of sympathetic and sensory blockage are the same. Hence, sympathetic block with peridural is less extensive than with subarachnoid with the same degree of sensory block.

The level of motor blockade is four to five segments lower than the level of sensory blockade (pin prick). Therefore, in peridural block, muscle paralysis is less extensive.

The local anesthetic agent can influence the circulatory responses to peridural analgesia. In doses used for surgical anesthesia, lidocaine can cause cardiovascular stimulation.[32] Depression can occur by accidental intravascular injection of the local anesthetic, or when very large doses are used.

Frequently, vasoconstrictors are added to the local anesthetic agent to prolong the effect and to reduce the systemic reaction caused by absorption into the circulation. The most commonly used vasoconstrictor is epinephrine in concentrations of 1 : 200,000 to 1 : 400,000. In these concentrations, it has been shown that the epinephrine exerts predominantly beta-receptor stimulation without an alpha effect. The cardiac output is usually increased and the total peripheral resistance further decreased.

The condition of the patient is of prime importance in determining the cardiovascular responses to peridural and subarachnoid blocks. Hypovolemia, even in modest degree, predisposes to severe cardiovascular depression.[34]

As in subarachnoid block, the main compensatory mechanism counteracting the sympathetic blockade is the vasoconstriction in the unanesthetized area above the level of blockade. However, this can be easily depressed by the administration of narcotics, sedatives, and intravenous anesthetics.

RESPIRATORY SYSTEM

Respiration is barely affected in normal individuals. A continuous peridural segmental block is a very useful tool in the hands of an experienced anesthesiologist when dealing with postoperative pain. It preserves active coughing and deep breathing, and enables the patient to maintain his preoperative respiratory function.[35]

REFERENCES

1. Rexed B: The cytoarchitectonic organization of the spinal cord of the cat. J Comp Neurol 96:415, 1956
2. Rexed B: A cytoarchitectonic atlas of the spinal cord in the cat. J Comp Neurol 100:297, 1954
3. Taub A, Hoffert M, Kitahata LM: Lamina-specific suppression and acceleration of dorsal-horn unit activity by nitrous oxide. Anesthesiology 42:24, 1974
4. Kitahata LM, Kosaka Y, Taub A, et al: Lamina-specific suppression of dorsal-horn unit activity by morphine sulfate. Anesthesiology 41:39, 1974
5. Kitahata LM, Taub A, Sato I: Lamina-specific suppression of dorsal horn unit activity by nitrous oxide and by hyperventilation. J Pharmacol Exp Ther 176:101, 1971
6. Kitahata LM, Taub A, Kosaka Y: Lamina-specific suppression of dorsal horn unit activity by ketamine hydrochloride. Anesthesiology 38:4, 1973
7. Wall PD: The laminar oganization of dorsal horn and effects of descending impulses. J Physiol (Lond) 188:403, 1967
8. Bobey MJ, Davidson PO: Psychological factors affecting pain tolerance. Psychosom Res 14:371, 1970
9. Schalling D: Tolerance for experimentally induced pain as related to personality. Scand J Psychol 12:271, 1971
10. Jannetta P: The cause of hemifacial spasm: definitive microsurgical treatment at the brainstem in 31 patients. Presented at the 79th Annual Meeting of the American Academy of Ophthalmology and Otolaryngology, Dallas, Texas, October 6–10, 1974
11. Melzack R, Wall PD: Gate control theory of pain. In Soulaizac A, Cahn J, Carpentier J (eds): Pain. New York, Academic, 1968, pp 11–31
12. Melzack R: The Puzzle of Pain. New York, Basic, 1973
13. King JS, Jowett D, Sundberg HR: Differential blockage of dorsal C fibers by various chloride solutions. Presented at the Annual Meeting of the Association of Neurological Surgeons, Houston, Texas, 1971
14. Squire AW, Calvillo O, Bromage PR: Painless intrathecal hypertonic saline. Can Anaesth Soc J 21:308, 1974

15. Bergan JJ, Conn J, Jr: Sympathectomy for pain relief. Med Clin North Am 52:147, 1968
16. Lipton S: Percutaneous electrical cordotomy in relief of intractable pain. Br Med J 2:210, 1968
17. Clark WC: Sensory decision theory analysis of the placebo effect on the criterion for pain and thermal sensitivity (d'). J Abnorm Psychol 74:363, 1969
18. McGlashaw TH, Evans FJ, Orne MT: The nature of hypnotic analgesia and placebo responses to experimental pain. Psychosom Med 31:227, 1969
19. Greene NM: Physiology of Spinal Anesthesia, 2nd ed. Baltimore, Williams & Wilkins, 1969
20. Neumann C, Foster A Jr, Rovenstine EA: The importance of compensatory vasoconstriction in unanesthetized areas in the maintenance of blood pressure during spinal anesthesia. J Clin Invest 24:345, 1945
21. Berges PU: Effects of various levels of subarachnoid block on hemodynamics and ventilation. In Proceedings of the Annual Meeting of the American Society of Anesthesiology, 1970, p 58
22. Ward RJ, Bonica JJ, Freund FG, et al: Epidural and subarachnoid anesthesia. Cardiovascular and respiratory effects. JAMA 191:275, 1965
23. Kennedy WF, Jr, Bonica JJ, Akamatsu TJ, et al: Cardiovascular and respiratory effects of subarachnoid block in the presence of acute blood loss. Anesthesiology 29:29, 1968
24. Freund FG, Bonica JJ, Ward RJ, et al: Ventilatory reserve and level of motor block during high spinal and epidural anesthesia. Anesthesiology 28:834, 1967
25. Freund FG: Respiratory effects of subarachnoid and epidural block. Clin Anesth 2:97, 1969
26. Kennedy WF, Jr, Sawyer TK, Gerbershagen HU, et al: Simultaneous systemic cardiovascular and renal hemodynamic measurements during high spinal ancsthesia in normal man. Acta Anaesth Scand (Suppl) 37:163, 1970
27. Kennedy WF, Jr: Effects of spinal and peridural blocks on renal and hepatic functions. Clin Anesth 2:109, 1969.
28. Kennedy WF, Jr, Everett GB, Cobb LA, et al: Simultaneous systemic and hepatic hemodynamic measurements during high spinal anesthesia in normal man. Anesth Analg 49:1016, 1970
29. Bromage PR: Physiology and pharmacology of epidural analgesia. Anesthesiology 28:592, 1967
30. Bromage PR: The physiology and pharmacology of epidural blockade. Clin Anesth 2:45, 1969
31. Bonica JJ, Berges PU, Morikawa K: Circulatory effects of peridural block. I. Effects of level of analgesia and dose of lidocaine. Anesthesiology 33:619, 1970
32. Bonica JJ: Cardiovascular effects of peridural block. Clin Anesth 2:63, 1969
33. Bonica JJ, Akamatsu TJ, Berges PU, et al: Circulatory effects of peridural block. II. Effects of epinephrine. Anesthesiology 34:514, 1971
34. Bonica JJ, Kennedy WF, Jr, Akamatsu TJ, et al: Circulatory effects of peridural block. III. Effects of acute blood loss. Anesthesiology 36:219, 1972
35. Bromage PR: Extradural Analgesia for pain relief. Br J Anaesth 39:721, 1967
36. Melzack R, Wall PD: Pain mechanisms: A new theory. Science 150:975, 1965

chapter 22

The Autonomic Nervous System

The autonomic nervous system controls the visceral function of the body. It consists of sympathetic and parasympathetic components (Fig. 22-1).

ANATOMY OF THE SYMPATHETIC NERVOUS SYSTEM

The sympathetic nerves originate in the spinal cord between the first thoracic and second lumbar segments. The cell bodies of the preganglionic fibers lie in the lateral horn and their fibers join the spinal nerve through an anterior root. Shortly thereafter, they leave the mixed spinal nerve as white rami and synapse with the postganglionic neuron in the lateral or paravertebral ganglia. The paravertebral ganglia, 22 in pairs, are connected by intervening fibers forming the sympathetic chain on each side of the spinal column (Fig. 22-2).

Some of the lateral horn neurons do not synapse in the lateral ganglia but in a second group called collateral sympathetic ganglia. Such are the celiac, superior, and inferior mesenteric neurons. The postganglionic fibers end in vessels and visceral organs and control their activity.

Some of the fibers of the postganglionic neurons (C type) rejoin the mixed spinal nerve via the gray rami to continue their course as part of that nerve.

ANATOMY OF THE PARASYMPATHETIC NERVOUS SYSTEM

The parasympathetic nervous system consists of two parts: the cranial and the sacral. The cranial part consists of parasympathetic fibers carried by the vagus, the third, the seventh, and the ninth cranial nerves. The sacral part consists of the second and the third sacral nerves, and, occasionally, the first

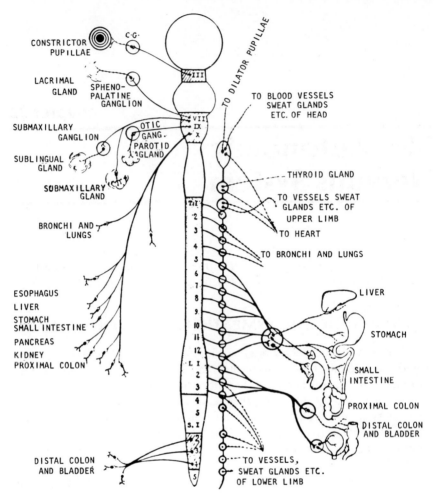

FIG. 22-1: Showing plan of autonomic nervous system from a functional viewpoint. CG, ciliary ganglion. The celiac, inferior mesenteric, and hypogastric ganglia are represented in this order from top to bottom by the circles in the lower right portion of the diagram. (Reproduced with permission from Williams & Wilkins.[1])

and the fourth sacral nerves. The sacral nerves form the sacral plexus on each side of the spinal cord and vertebrae and innervate the descending colon, rectum, bladder, and part of the ureters.

The major part of the parasympathetic fibers run in the vagus nerves. They innervate the heart, the lungs, the esophagus, the stomach, the liver, the pancreas, the gallbladder, the jejunum and the ileum, the upper parts of the colon, and the ureters.

The parasympathetic ganglia lie in very close proximity to the organs. Their postganglionic fibers are very short.

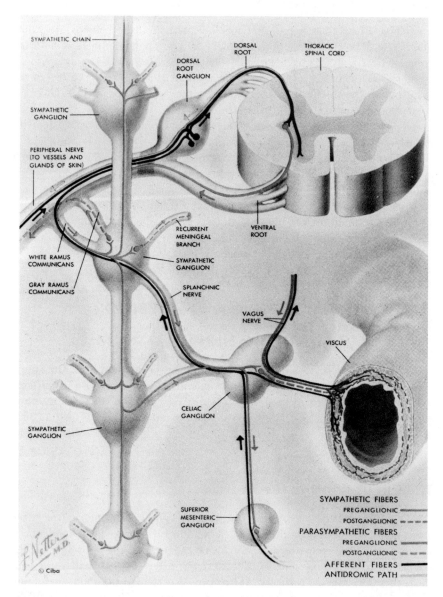

FIG. 22-2: The connections of the autonomic nervous system. (©1953, 1972 CIBA Pharmaceutical Co., Division of CIBA GEIGY Corp. Reproduced with permission from the CIBA Collection of Medical Illustrations by Frank H. Netter, M.D. All rights reserved.)

CHOLINERGIC AND ADRENERGIC FIBERS

Nerve fibers that secrete acetylcholine at their nerve endings are called cholinergic. The cholinergic fibers are (1) the preganglionic fibers of both the sympathetic and parasympathetic systems; (2) the parasympathetic postganglionic neurons; (3) all the skeletal nerve endings; and (4) a few of the postganglionic sympathetic fibers, such as to the sweat glands. Most, however, are adrenergic and secrete norepinephrine.

The acetylcholine released by the autonomic nervous system is metabolized by the enzyme cholinesterase just as it is in the skeletal muscles.

Norepinephrine, secreted by the adrenergic nerve endings, is methylated by the enzyme catechol O-methyl transferase, and the end product of its metabolism is 3-methoxy-4-hydroxymandelic acid (VMA). Part of the norepinephrine secreted is removed by reabsorption into the nerve endings. These are the main inactivating mechanisms responsible for terminating adrenergic effect. In addition, the enzyme monoaminooxidase is capable of deaminating amines, although the process is very slow (Chap. 27).

EFFECT OF STIMULATION AND INHIBITION OF THE SYMPATHETIC AND PARASYMPATHETIC NERVOUS SYSTEMS

The cerebral cortex, the hypothalamus, the brain stem, and the spinal cord all control the activity of the autonomic nervous system. Visceral reflexes play an important part in the function of this system. Both subdivisions of the autonomic nervous system can cause stimulation and inhibition of the functions of various organs.

The Circulation and the Heart

The sympathetic nervous system plays a major role in the control of the circulation. All vessels in the body, except the capillaries, have sympathetic innervation. The sympathetic nerve fibers can change the resistance of the vessels by changing the tone of the arterioles, arteries, and small veins and, thus, they alter tissue perfusion. They can also change the total circulating blood volume by changing the caliber of large vessels. The sympathetic fibers can cause both vasoconstriction and vasodilatation.

In some skeletal muscles, the stimulation of the sympathetic fibers releases acetylcholine and causes vasodilatation, whereas in other skeletal muscles, this stimulation releases norepinephrine and causes vasoconstriction. Stimulation of the sympathetics causes vasoconstriction in the kidneys, bowels, spleen, and skin.

The vasomotor center located in the lower portion of pons and upper portion of medulla controls the vasomotor activity. The center consists of excitatory and inhibitory portions and their stimulation increases or decreases the sympathetic vasoconstrictor tone. It also influences the heart activity through the vagus and the sympathetic nerves.

The vasomotor center is under control of the cerebral cortex and the hypothalamus. It can also be stimulated by accumulation of CO_2 or by ischemia.

The baroreceptors located in the large arteries respond rapidly to changes in arterial blood pressure. Stimulation of these baroreceptors causes inhibition of the vasomotor center and excitation of the vagus, resulting in a decrease of blood pressure.

THE LUNGS

Sympathetic stimulation causes bronchodilatation and mild pulmonary vasoconstriction.

The Gastrointestinal and Urinary Systems

The gastrointestinal system is mostly under the influence of the parasympathetic nervous system. Its stimulation increases the peristalsis and the secretion of many gastrointestinal glands.

The gallbladder, ureters, and bladder are inhibited by sympathetic and excited by parasympathetic stimulation.

Other Effects

The pupils of the eye dilate by sympathetic stimulation. Focusing of the lens is controlled entirely by parasympathetic activity.

The sympathetic nervous system stimulates glycolysis in the liver and thus increases the blood glucose concentration. It also has a stimulating effect on the basal metabolic rate.

The autonomic nervous system is also involved in regulating the sexual act.

In general, the sympathetic and parasympathetic systems are viewed as antagonists. The action of one system can be manifested by paralysis of the opponent system. However, in some organ functions, their actions can be indifferent, independent, or even synergistic.

SYMPATHETIC INNERVATION OF THE ADRENAL GLANDS

The cells of the adrenal medulla are derivatives of nerve tissue and actually are modified sympathetic ganglia. The sympathetic fibers entering the adrenal medulla are preganglionic, since they do not synapse in a paravertebral or collateral ganglion.

Stimulation of the sympathetic nervous system releases epinephrine and norepinephrine by the adrenal glands. The released epinephrine further potentiates the effect of stimulation of the sympathetic nerves. Thus, the organs actually are stimulated directly by the sympathetic nerves and indirectly by the adrenal hormones. This dual effect represents a safety mechanism, since one can substitute for the action of the other.

ADRENERGIC RECEPTORS AND SYMPATHOMIMETIC DRUGS

In 1948, Ahlquist[1] postulated that there are two types of adrenergic receptors, alpha and beta. The stimulation of alpha receptors causes vasoconstriction and intestinal relaxation. The stimulation of beta receptors causes vasodilatation in muscles, increased heart rate, and contraction as well as bronchial and myometrial relaxation.

Norepinephrine stimulates only the alpha receptors; epinephrine stimulates both. Low concentrations of epinephrine stimulate the beta receptors; high concentrations also stimulate the alpha receptors.[2]

The action of other sympathomimetic drugs can be predicted if the type of receptors on which they react is known. For example, isoproterenol (Isuprel) activates the beta receptors and has no effect on the alpha receptors. It increases the heart rate and the force of contraction, dilates the vasculature of the skeletal muscle, and relaxes the bronchial muscles. Phenylephrine activates mainly the alpha receptors, raises the blood pressure by causing peripheral vasoconstriction, but has little direct cardiac effect.

Lands et al described two types of beta receptors.[3] β_1-receptors, which are located in the heart and the small bowels; and β_2-receptors, which are found in the bronchi, the blood vessels, and the uterus. Some agents can selectively block one or the other.

Certain drugs can cause release of norepinephrine from its storage vesicles in the nerve endings and thus have indirect sympathomimetic action. To this group belong ephedrine, tyramine, and amphetamine. There is a group of drugs that block adrenergic activity. Reserpine prevents the synthesis and storage of norepinephrine at the nerve endings. Guanethidine prevents the release of norepinephrine. Phenoxybenzamine blocks the alpha receptors. Drugs like hexamethonium and trimethaphan block the transmission of impulses through the autonomic ganglia.

Parasympathomimetic Drugs

Directly acting parasympathomimetic drugs producing typical parasympathetic effect are also called muscarinic drugs. Pilocarpine is an example. Anticholinesterase agents like neostigmine and pyridostigmine inhibit cholinesterase activity and thus prevent rapid destruction of acetylcholine.

Anticholinergic Drugs

Atropine and scopolamine block the action of acetylcholine on cholinergic effector organs.

Nicotinic Drugs

Nicotine stimulates the postganglionic neurons of both systems; therefore, it has both sympathetic and parasympathetic effects. To this group belong acetylcholine itself, carbamylcholine, and metcholine. They produce sympathetic vasoconstriction in abdominal organs and extremities as well as a parasympathetic effect on the intestines. They also stimulate skeletal muscle.

"STRESS" REACTION

It is clear from the preceding discussion on the function of the sympathetic nervous system that it stimulates organic activity and functions in the body. Arterial blood pressure rises as does the blood glucose concentration and the basal metabolic rate. Mental activity is facilitated. It is responsible for what is known as the fight, flight, and fright reaction.

AUTONOMIC NERVOUS SYSTEM AND ANESTHESIA

The practice of anesthesia is closely related to the practice of clinical pharmacology. The large spectrum of agents used at present in anesthesia produces multiple changes and effects on the autonomic nervous system.

Surgical stimulation itself increases the activity of both components of the autonomic nervous system. The anesthesiologist has to balance the activity of the autonomic nervous system prior to and during administration of anesthesia. This starts with the preoperative visit, discussions, and preoperative medications. Sedatives, narcotics, antihistamines, and drying agents produce various effects on the autonomic nervous system either by direct action on the affected organs or by a central effect.

REFERENCES

1. Ahlquist RP: A study of the adrenotropic receptors. Am J Physiol 153:586, 1948
2. Goodman LS, Gilman A (eds): The Pharmacological Basis of Therapeutics, 5th ed. New York, Macmillan, 1975, p 484
3. Lands AM, Arnold A, McAuliff JP, et al: Differentiation of receptor systems activated by sympathomimetic amines. Nature 214:597, 1967
4. Best CH, Taylor NB: The Physiological Basis of Medical Practice. Baltimore, Williams & Wilkins, 1966

chapter 23

The Brain

The brain is conveniently divided into three parts: cerebrum, cerebellum, and brain stem.

CEREBRUM AND CEREBRAL FUNCTIONS

Sensory Functions of the Cortex

Neurons from various sense organs transmit impulses and terminate in the following sensory areas (Fig. 23-1):

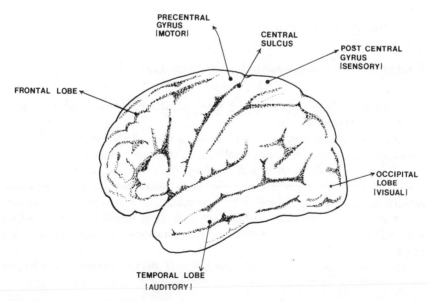

FIG. 23-1: Left cerebral hemisphere with representation of various localization areas.

1. The somesthetic association area is located in the postcentral gyrus of the parietal lobe. Proprioreceptive impulses, touch, and temperature sensations from the skin are conducted to this area.
2. The visual area is located in the occipital lobe.
3. The auditory area lies in the superior temporal lobe.
4. The receptor area for taste is located in the postcentral convolution. All pain impulses are also received in this area.

Motor Functions of the Cortex

PRECENTRAL MOTOR AREA

This is located next to the central sulcus and is the area in which all willed motions originate. Various parts of the body are represented contralaterally. The pyramidal tract has its origin here.

PREMOTOR AREA

This lies in front of the motor area and is the cortical extrapyramidal center.

FRONTAL ASSOCIATION AREA

This area is essential for mature judgment and abstract thinking. Fibers extend from this area to the dorsomedial nucleus of the thalamus. The operation called prefrontal leukotomy consists of disrupting this connection.

Thalamus, Hypothalamus, and Basal Ganglia

Thalamus, hypothalamus, and basal ganglia are defined areas of gray matter with specific functions.

The thalamus serves as a relay station for all afferent impulses. No conscious interpretation of sensory stimuli takes place in the thalamus.

The hypothalamus receives fibers from the thalamus and is also closely associated with the cerebral cortex. It exerts some control on the hormonal activity of the pituitary gland. The hypothalamus is considered to play an important part in the mechanism of emotion. It is also the center in which integration of all visceral functions of the autonomic nervous system takes place.

The functions of basal ganglia are not well defined; however, it is known that they inhibit the activities of the extrapyramidal system.

THE BRAIN STEM

The brain stem consists of the pons and the medulla. Since multiple neurons conducting sensory and motor impulses pass through, pathology in these areas manifests itself with multiple symptomatology. Centers regulating the heart activity, blood pressure, and respiratory functions are located in the brain stem.

The reticular formation consists of cells and nuclei scattered throughout the brain stem. The formation plays an important role in many visceral and somatic functions.[1] The motoneurons of the reticular formation are both excitatory and inhibitory. The cells, on the other hand, participate in the process of consciousness and attention. The reticular formation is also called the reticular activating system. The cerebral cortex and the higher centers exert their influence on the spinal cord activities through the reticular formation cells.

THE FEEDBACK THEORY
OF WAKEFULNESS AND SLEEP

The reticular activating system can be stimulated by peripheral sensory impulses or by the cerebral cortex. A large number of fibers from the motor regions of the cortex and from almost all parts of the cerebrum reach this system. These connections explain why motor activity is associated with wakefulness and also why other activities can also stimulate the reticular formation. In addition, increased activity of the reticular activating system raises the activity of the cerebral cortex. Hence, "feedback" mechanisms exist. The same relationship exists between the reticular activating system and the peripheral muscles.

Once the reticular system becomes activated, it will stay activated for a certain period of time due to the "feedback" mechanism. After awhile, many of the neurons of this system gradually develop fatigue and become less excitable. Thus, a vicious cycle is established and a depression of most components of the "feedback" system takes place, which results in the state of sleep.

SYNAPTIC TRANSMITTERS
OF THE CENTRAL NERVOUS SYSTEM
AND NEUROLOGIC MECHANISMS OF ANESTHESIA

Acetylcholine and norepinephrine are the main transmitters in the central nervous system.[2,3] They are widely and unevenly distributed.

Acetylcholine is the apparent transmitter for the reticular activating system. It depolarizes the postsynaptic membrane mainly by decreasing the permeability to potassium ions. Glutamic acid is the most likely transmitter for specific sensory pathways. It causes depolarization of the membrane mainly by increasing the permeability to sodium ion.

In addition, dopamine, serotonin, and 5-hydroxytryptamine probably serve as transmitters at certain sites in the central nervous system.

Several researchers have reported the existence and distribution of catecholamine (norepinephrine) and serotonin-containing nerve cell body in the central nervous system.[4-6] Norepinephrine-containing neurons plays a significant inhibiting role in sensory impulse transmission.

Gamma-aminobutyric acid (GABA) is considered the main inhibitory transmitter in the central nervous system.

General anesthetics may affect the synaptic transmission by:

1. Increasing membrane permeability to potassium ions, thus causing hyperpolarization and stabilization of the membrane potential together with decreased excitability
2. Blocking the action of acetylcholine and, therefore, causing loss of consciousness
3. Decreasing the uptake of GABA and, therefore, prolonging the synaptic inhibition

Effects of Anesthesia on the Reticular-Activating System and Cerebral Cortex

The reticular-activating system is extremely sensitive to the action of general anesthetics. Moruzzi and Magoun[7] and French et al[8] have established that anesthetics primarily affect the reticular formation and elicit the anesthetic state by abolishing its feedback mechanism. However, differences between the clinical and electroencephalographic patterns during general anesthesia established by different agents make doubtful that this effect is always related to inhibition of reticular formation activities.[9] On the one hand, the action of some agents like chlorpromazine is related to blockage of the relay of impulses to the reticular formation without influencing the activity of the formation per se.[10] However, they do not produce a state of general anesthesia. Ether, on the other hand, produces an early depression of the cortex. This is judged by depression of cortical potential and activity of the cortical neurons. There is no uniform mechanism of action of various general anesthetics on the central nervous system. Anesthetics like enflurane (Ethrane) enhance the activity of the reticular-activating system.

Although all anesthetic agents are classified as central nervous system depressants, their mode of action is different, and excitation and depression are simultaneously involved.[11]

Electroencephalography and the Effect of Anesthetics

The electroencephalogram (EEG) is recorded from multiple electrodes placed on the skull. Normally, there is no general pattern of EEG and different waves can be seen.

Alpha waves occur at a frequency of between 8 and 13 cycles per second. They are seen in the awake and resting states, and disappear during sleep.

Beta waves appear during activation of the central nervous system at a frequency of between 14 and 50 cycles per second.

Theta waves appear during emotional stress in some adults; otherwise, they are seen more commonly in children. They have frequencies of between 4 and 7 cycles per second.

Delta waves include all the waves with frequencies below 3½ cycles per second. They occur in deep sleep.

There is a very good correlation between the degree of brain activity and the frequency of the electroencephalographic rhythm. During epileptic seizure, the EEG is characterized by high voltage and spiking discharges over the entire cortex. There is no uniformity in the effect of various anesthetics on the EEG.[12]

Faulconer and Bickford found that changes in the EEG pattern are correlated with depth of anesthesia.[13] With the onset of anesthesia, the EEG pattern is dominated initially by fast-wave and high-voltage activities. However, deepening of anesthesia is manifested by slower EEG waves. Finally, a total electrical silence is produced.

Basically, there are two different types of slow waves recorded in an EEG that are induced by anesthetics.[14] The first type of slow wave is characteristic of barbiturates, halothane, and methoxyflurane. They elicit spindle-like bursts at a frequency of 10 to 12 Hz, then combine with slow waves of high amplitude and gradual flattening as the depth of anesthesia increases.

The second type is characterized by slow waves in light planes and high frequency and high amplitude EEGs in deeper planes. This type of EEG pattern is induced by ketamine, cyclopropane, and enflurane.

Effect of Hypoxia on EEG

The main effect of hypoxia is slowing of the wave frequency in the EEG. In acute anoxia, there might be an initial increase of frequency and amplitude. The cortical activities become slower and, by 18 to 20 seconds after anoxia, the EEG usually becomes a flat line.

Hockaday et al[15] classified the EEG in brain damage following cardiac arrest into five grades; from an almost normal EEG to a flat record and no EEG at all. The V6 grade with no EEG at all was later widely adopted as an EEG criterion for brain death. An isoelectric EEG due to hypoxia is reversible after up to 8 minutes of ischemia.

REFERENCES

1. Valdman AV: Pharmacology and Physiology of the Reticular Formation: Progress in Brain Research, Vol 20. New York, American Elsevier, 1967
2. Bradley PB: Pharmacology of the central nervous system. Br Med Bull 21:1, 1965
3. Hebb C: CNS at the cellular level: identity of transmitter agents. Annu Rev Physiol 32:165, 1970
4. Chu NS, Bloom FE: Norepinephrine-containing neurons: changes in spontaneous discharge patterns during sleeping and waking. Science 179:908, 1973
5. Anden NE, Dahlström A, Fuxe K, et al: Ascending monoamine neurons to the telencephalon and diencephalon. Acta Physiol Scand 67:313, 1966
6. Dahlström A, Fuxe K: Evidence for the existence of monoamine-containing neurons in the cell bodies of brain stem neurons. Acta Physiol Scand (Suppl) 232:1, 1964
7. Moruzzi G, Magoun HW: Brain stem reticular formation and activation of the EEG. Electroencephalogr Clin Neurophysiol 1:455, 1949
8. French JD, Verzcano M, Magoun IIW: Neural basis of anesthetic state. Arch Neurol Psychiat 69:519, 1953
9. Darbinjan TM, Golovchinsky VB, Plehotkina SI: The effects of anesthetics on reticular and cortical activity. Anesthesiology 34:219, 1971
10. Bradley PB: The central action of certain drugs in relation to the reticular formation of the brain. In Jasper HH, et al (eds): The Reticular Formation of the Brain. 1958, p 123
11. Mori K, Winters WD: Neural background of sleep and anesthesia. In Mori K (ed): Neurophysiological Basis of Anesthesia, International Anesthesiology Clinics. Boston, Little Brown, 13:67, 1975
12. Sadove MS, Becka D, Gibbs FA: Electroencephalography for Anesthesiologists and Surgeons. Philadelphia, Lippincott, 1967
13. Faulconer A Jr, Bickford RG: Electroencephalography in Anesthesiology. Springfield, Ill, Thomas, 1960
14. Mori K: Excitation and depression of CNS electrical activities by general anesthetics. In Proceedings of the 5th World Congress of Anesthesiology. Amsterdam, Excerpta, 1973, p 40
15. Hockaday JM, Potts P, Epstein E, et al: Electroencephalographic changes in acute cerebral anoxia from cardiac or respiratory arrest. Electroencephalogr Clin Neurophysiol 18:575, 1965

chapter 24

Physiology of the Cerebrospinal Fluid

FORMATION, CIRCULATION, AND ABSORPTION

The cerebrospinal fluid (CSF) is formed continuously by the choroid plexuses located in the lateral and third ventricles.[1] It is also partly formed from the extracellular fluid of the brain. The part produced in the lateral ventricle passes through the foramen of Monro into the third ventricle. From the third ventricle, the CSF circulates through the sylvian aqueduct into the fourth ventricle, from there into the cisterna magna, and passes into the spinal subarachnoid space via the foramina of Luschka and Magendie. CSF in the subarachnoid space is in communication with the part that flows around the brain stem and cerebral hemispheres (Fig. 24-1).

The cerebrospinal fluid is reabsorbed by the arachnoid villi into the venous circulation.[1] The reabsorption depends on the pressure gradient between CSF and venous blood. It is a mechanical process.

VOLUME AND COMPOSITION

The total volume of CSF is about 100 to 150 ml. The specific gravity varies between 1002 and 1009.

The composition of CSF differs from that of plasma. It has a lower concentration of protein, calcium, potassium, bicarbonate, urea, glucose, and phosphate than plasma. However, the concentrations of sodium and chloride are higher in CSF. Thus, CSF is not merely an ultrafiltrate of plasma but, as the evidence points out, it is also secreted.

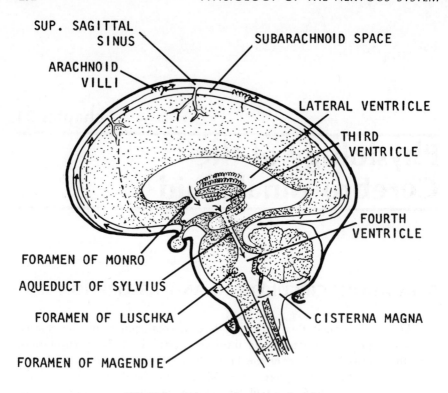

FIG. 24-1:   Pathways of cerebrospinal flow.

BLOOD–BRAIN BARRIER
AND PENETRATION OF DRUG

The interchange between blood and CSF is accomplished through the blood–CSF (blood–brain) barrier, which is composed of the endothelium of the capillary vessels in the brain. Besides this blood–CSF barrier, there is an additional one between the brain and CSF consisting of the ependymal layer of the ventricles.

The penetration of drugs through both barriers follows the same principles governing the penetration of drugs through other cell membranes. The un-ionized forms of drugs as well as the more lipid-soluble forms penetrate more readily. From the recognition of this fact the Mayer–Overton theory of anesthesia developed, basing the potency of various anesthetics on their lipid solubility. The speed of penetration is also related to the size of the molecules.

Barbiturates are highly lipid-soluble substances and penetrate the barriers quite well. Therefore, sodium pentothal, the most commonly used short-acting barbiturate, has a fast onset of action.

Most muscle relaxants possess low fat solubility and on physiologic pH are highly ionized.[2] Therefore, curare and succinylcholine cross the blood–brain barrier in very small amounts; however, gallamine crosses readily. Also, all analgesics, sedatives, and anesthetic agents readily pass through the blood–brain barrier.

CEREBROSPINAL FLUID PRESSURE

The normal pressure of CSF is between 150 and 200 mm water pressure measured through a lumbar puncture performed in a sitting position. The fluid is in a constant motion, and is affected by the pulsations of the brain vessels and by the respiratory cycle.

The CSF pressure is affected by several factors:

1. Rate of CSF formation and reabsorption. The rate of formation is around 0.3 ml per minute in normal conditions.
2. Cerebral blood flow. If cerebral bood flow increases, eg, during halothane administration, CSF pressure rises due to the concomitant increase in cerebral blood volume.
3. Arterial blood pressure. It does not affect CSF pressure within the normal range of autoregulation. However, it produces a systolic–diastolic fluctuation in CSF pressure.
4. Venous pressure. The pressure in the intracranial venous sinuses should be lower to allow continuous reabsorption at the arachnoid villi. In certain pathologic conditions, this pressure relationship can easily be disturbed, resulting in increased CSF pressure.

ACID–BASE OF CEREBROSPINAL FLUID

The pH of cerebrospinal fluid is approximately 7.3. It contains less bicarbonate and has higher CO_2 tension (bicarbonate 29 mEq/100 ml; P_{CO_2}, 48 mm Hg) than the arterial blood.

Experiments have shown that the reflection of changes in P_{CO_2} on CSF pressure occurs after a time lag. It takes even longer for changes in the arterial hydrogen ion and bicarbonate concentration to affect CSF pressure.[3]

The CSF pH is not altered significantly with changes in blood pH except when it is due to changes of blood P_{CO_2}. Carbon dioxide easily crosses the blood–brain barrier and produces rapid shifts in CSF pH. Thus, in conditions of acute metabolic acidosis when blood pH falls, the CSF pH rises because of the respiratory alkalosis accompanying the metabolic acidosis. However, in chronic conditions, compensatory mechanisms take place and CSF pH returns to normal values.

The CSF pH is an important factor in the control of respiration. The chemoreceptors located on the ventrolateral surface of the medulla are highly sensitive to changes in CSF pH.

CEREBRAL HEMODYNAMICS

The carotid and the vertebral arteries supply blood to the brain (Fig. 24-2). The anterior portion of the brain is supplied by the internal carotid arteries; the posterior portion is supplied by the vertebral arteries.

The main *branches of the internal carotid* artery are:

1. Anterior cerebral artery, which passes on the medial surface of the hemispheres and sends off branches to the frontal lobe. It anastomoses with the posterior cerebral artery.
2. Middle cerebral artery, which runs laterally in the sylvian fissure and which supplies blood to the internal capsule and part of the frontal and temporal lobes.
3. Posterior communicating artery, which anastomoses with the posterior cerebral artery (main branch of the basilar artery).
4. Choroidal artery.

The main *branches of the vertebral artery* (branch of the subclavian artery) are:

1. Posterior inferior cerebral artery, which is the most common site for thrombosis
2. Posterior spinal artery, which descends downward on the dorsal surface of the spinal cord
3. Anterior cerebral artery
4. Medullary arteries

The two vertebral arteries join and form the basilar artery. The main *branches of the basilar artery* are:

1. Anterior inferior cerebellar artery
2. Internal auditory artery
3. Superior cerebellar artery
4. Posterior cerebral artery

The *circle of Willis* is a ring formed by the anterior communicating artery connecting the two anterior cerebral arteries and by the posterior communicating arteries anastomosing the internal carotid and the posterior cerebral arteries.

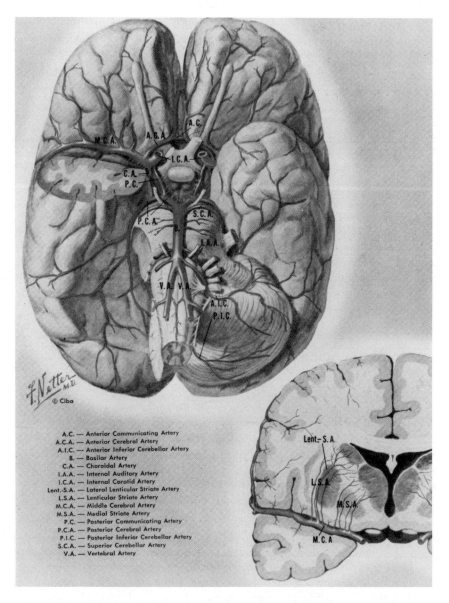

A.C. — Anterior Communicating Artery
A.C.A. — Anterior Cerebral Artery
A.I.C. — Anterior Inferior Cerebellar Artery
B. — Basilar Artery
C.A. — Choroidal Artery
I.A.A. — Internal Auditory Artery
I.C.A. — Internal Carotid Artery
Lent.-S.A. — Lateral Lenticular Striate Artery
L.S.A. — Lenticular Striate Artery
M.C.A. — Middle Cerebral Artery
M.S.A. — Medial Striate Artery
P.C. — Posterior Communicating Artery
P.C.A. — Posterior Cerebral Artery
P.I.C. — Posterior Inferior Cerebellar Artery
S.C.A. — Superior Cerebellar Artery
V.A. — Vertebral Artery

FIG. 24-2: Blood supply of the brain. (© 1953, 1972 CIBA Pharmaceutical Co., Division of CIBA GEIGY Corp. Reproduced with permission from the CIBA Collection of Medical Illustrations by Frank H. Netter, M.D. All rights reserved.)

The brain represents about 2 percent of the body's mass and normally receives about 15 percent of the cardiac output. The normal cerebral blood flow in the conscious adult is about 45 ml per 100 g brain tissue per minute. The gray matter has a higher flow of 80 ml per 100 g per minute and the white only 20 ml per 100 g per minute.

In 1945, Kety and Schmidt[4] described a technique for indirect measurement of cerebral blood flow in humans. Since then, it has been widely accepted and modified. Their technique and the modifications are based on the Fick principle, which states that the flow to a specific organ (Ft) is equal to the amount of substance taken up by the organ in a specific time (Qt) divided by the arteriovenous difference of that substance (Ca–Cv):

$$Ft = \frac{Qt}{Ca - Cv}$$

Nitrous oxide was the first substance used as an indicator. Lassen and Munck[5] used ^{85}Kr as an indicator. $^{133}Xenon$ has also been used for the same purpose. These radioactive indicators are injected into the carotid artery, then externally counted over the skull.

A thermodilution technique can also be used to determine cerebral blood flow as can electromagnetic flowmeters. The latter are of specific value during carotid artery surgery.

Factors Influencing Cerebral Circulation[6]

BLOOD PRESSURE

Cerebral autoregulation refers to the ability of the brain to keep blood flow constant in the face of alterations in cerebral perfusion pressure. Cerebral perfusion pressure is the mean arterial pressure minus the mean venous pressure. Normally, the autoregulation will maintain constant blood flow as long as the cerebral perfusion pressures range between 50 and 150 mm Hg[7]. This is accomplished by alterations in the caliber of the cerebral vessels. However, the cerebral autoregulation is abolished under the following circumstances:

1. During hypercapnia, when there is already an existing vasodilatation.[8]
2. During hypoxia when arterial oxygen saturation falls to 60 percent or less.
3. In patients who had an acute cerebral infarct.[9] The infarct is surrounded by an area that has lost its autoregulation.
4. In fairly severe hypotension, at values of one-third of normal levels, the cerebral blood flow falls and signs of cerebral ischemia are observed.[10]

Mechanism of autoregulation. The proposed theories concerning the mechanism of autoregulation can be classifed into three groups: (1) Metabolic theory. Certain metabolic changes in the brain are responsible for the maintenance of autoregulation. The autoregulation in response to a change in perfusion pressure is not immediate. It takes anywhere between 30 seconds and 2 minutes for the vessels to dilate and for the normal flow to be reestablished. During this period the CO_2 tension rises in the extracellular fluid (ECF) and the pH and the O_2 tension decrease. The proponents of this theory believe that the transient crop of pH causes vasodilatation. However, they have failed to show alkalosis of the extracellular fluid when perfusion pressure rises.

There is no direct evidence to suggest that CO_2 and O_2 tension are the factors causing this effect. In some situations, it has been found that the response of the cerebral circulation to CO_2 can be present in the face of lost autoregulation.

(2) Myogenic theory. Raising the pressure in a segment of an isolated artery leads to contraction of that vessel. This phenomenon has been observed on renal vessels.[11] (3) Neurogenic theory. Proponents of this theory[12] claim that sympathetic nerve denervation high up in the neck causes loss of autoregulation on that side.

In conclusion, the cause of autoregulation is yet to be determined.

BLOOD GASES

Carbon dioxide exerts profound effect on cerebral blood flow between 20 and 80 mm Hg arterial tension.[13] In this range, the increase of P_{CO_2} by 1 mm Hg is followed by a rise of cerebral blood flow of 2 ml per g brain tissue.[14] In the same range, P_{CO_2} has no measurable effect on the cerebral metabolic rate of oxygen. Minimal cerebral blood flow is reached at a P_{CO_2} of 10 to 20 mm Hg.[15] The hypoxia that develops at this level of P_{CO_2} limits further decrease of cerebral blood flow.[16] Several investigators[17-19] have suggested that the level of CO_2 in the blood alters the pH of the extracellular fluid, which in turn affects the smooth muscle tone of the cerebral arterioles. The pH of the extracellular fluid is determined by the concentrations of CO_2 and bicarbonate ions in CSF. The concentration of CO_2 around the artery mainly depends on the P_{CO_2} (respiration), whereas the concentration of the bicarbonate is related to the metabolic processes of the brain. However, as it has to be pointed out, in the presence of normal P_{CO_2}, alterations in arterial hydrogen or bicarbonate ion concentrations have little immediate effect on the cerebral blood flow.

Oxygen, per se, has a modest vasoconstrictive effect on cerebral vessels. If the partial pressure of oxygen in arterial blood is lowered, while the pressure of CO_2 is maintained constant, cerebral blood flow is unaffected until the P_{O_2} falls below 50 mm Hg.[20] At this point, cerebral vasodilatation occurs and cerebral blood flow increases. Thus, unlike continuous response to changes in Pco_2 the response of cerebral blood flow to decreased Po_2 is a threshold phenomenon. It also shows that the cerebral blood flow is not regulated to maintain constant Po_2.

The mechanism of action of oxygen on the cerebral circulation is not determined.[21] It has been shown that oxygen can act directly on isolated vessels and change their caliber. Hypoxia results in accumulation of acid metabolites in the extracellular fluid surrounding the cerebral arterioles, and they could be causing vasodilatation. However, alkalosis of the extracellular fluid does not cause vasoconstriction as hyperoxia does.

TEMPERATURE

Decreased temperature diminishes cerebral blood flow. When the body temperature is reduced to 28 C, there is a reduction of cerebral blood flow by 50 percent.[22]

AGE

The highest normal values of cerebral blood flow have been found in children between the ages of 3 and 10.[23] Lassen et al[24] reported that normal adults of a mean age of 72 years had unchanged cerebral blood flows. In persons who have suffered stroke or have senile dementia, the cerebral blood flow is decreased. In this situation, regional blood flow to the diseased areas assumes more importance than does the overall cerebral flow.

CEREBRAL FUNCTION

There is a slight increase in cerebral blood flow during sleep. This is attributed to a rise in Pco_2.

In normal subjects, there are no changes in the overall cerebral blood flow during any mental effort. However, there are changes in the regional distribution of blood. This regulation of regional cerebral blood flow is very likely to be mediated by local accumulation of metabolites, lactic acid, and also CO_2, which affect the pH of the extracellular fluid.[25] Changes in potassium concentration and hyperosmolarity in focal areas are also factors in redistribution of cerebral blood flow.

Cerebral blood flow increases during seizure activity. However, cerebral oxygenation remains adequate, provided ventilation and arterial blood pressure are maintained at normal levels.

Abnormalities of Response to Carbon Dioxide

The reactivity of vessels in areas surrounding cerebral infarcts and tumors is lost.[9] The vessels are in a state of maximal dilatation. Local accumulation of metabolic products is assumed to be the cause. This phenomenon is termed "luxury perfusion syndrome."[15] Since the cerebral vascular resistance in this area is at its lowest point, it cannot further decrease under the influence of CO_2 or hypotension.

If P_{CO_2} rises in patients who have brain areas with lost vessel reactivity, the blood will be shunted to the healthy areas. Hence, the hypercapnia will cause an increase of blood flow in normal areas of brain and a decrease in diseased areas. This phenomenon is called "intracerebral steal syndrome."[26]

The reverse, "Robin Hood" phenomenon,[27] happens in response to hypocapnia. The vessels in the ischemic areas will not constrict under the influence of low P_{CO_2}; however, the healthy areas will respond with an increase in vascular resistance. Therefore, blood will be shunted from the healthy to the diseased areas.

It is very important to note that the two phenomena described above do not occur in every patient with focal cerebral ischemia when P_{CO_2} is altered.

Alterations in Response to Blood Pressure Changes

It was pointed out in the paragraph above that the vessels in and around the ischemic areas of the brain are in a state of paralysis. The autoregulation in these areas is lost.

The autoregulation of cerebral blood flow in patients with hypertensive disease is present, but both the upper and lower limits are shifted upwards.[6] These patients might be very sensitive to small decreases in perfusion pressure. Also, the autoregulation is disrupted in hypoxia or hypercapnia.

Effects of Anesthetics on Cerebral Blood Flow

Cerebral blood flow and the effects of anesthetics on cerebral blood flow[28] as well as on intracranial pressure and various aspects of neuroanesthesia[29, 30] have been the subject of intensive review in the last few years.

All inhalation agents increase cerebral blood flow in anesthetic concentrations by causing some degree of cerebral vasodilatation. This effect varies with different agents and with their concentrations. Studies by Smith and Wollman[25] have shown excellent correlations between the concentration of the anesthetic agent, expressed as MAC multiples, and the ratio between cerebral blood flow and cerebral metabolic rate.

The response of cerebral blood flow to altered P_{CO_2} remains intact during general anesthesia.

Autoregulation of cerebral blood flow is maintained during the usual anesthetic concentrations of inhalational agents. However, when deliberate hypotension is induced, the autoregulation might be lost at the low levels of blood pressure.

Hyperventilation, before and during the administration of anesthetics, can markedly reduce the cerebral blood flow. In addition, the Bohr effect diminishes oxygen availability to the tissues.

Barbiturates, more than any other intravenous anesthetic agents, depress both cerebral blood flow and cerebral metabolic rate. Muscle relaxants like succinylcholine and curare can cause transient increases in cerebral blood flow. Pancuronium has a lesser effect.

Intracranial Hypertension and Relation to Anesthesia

The intracranial components are the brain, CSF, and the blood, and all of them are enclosed in a rigid box. The intracranial pressure is uniform as long as CSF can circulate freely.

Initially, a slow increase in the volume of one of the three components will cause reciprocal changes in the other two and, as a result, the intracranial pressure will not change. For example, in the presence of a space-occupying lesion in the brain, CSF is displaced from the intracranial compartment to the spinal subarachnoid space. The reabsorption of CSF is also augmented. After this compensatory mechanism is exhausted, the further increase in intracranial pressure compresses the venous channels in the brain. The arterial tree dilates in an effort to maintain cerebral blood flow during increased intracranial pressure. In this situation, the cerebral perfusion pressure is no longer represented by the difference between the mean arterial and the venous pressure, but becomes dependent on the intracranial pressure. Under these circumstances, the cerebral perfusion pressure becomes equal to mean blood pressure minus intracranial pressure.

These changes in arterial and venous resistance, and cerebral perfusion pressure eventually lead to edema formation. The edema further raises the intracranial pressure and, thus, a vicious cycle is established.

The anesthesiologist can alter the increased intracranial pressure through ventilation, blood pressure, and drugs.

VENTILATION

Moderate hyperventilation prior to and after induction of anesthesia is highly recommended for intracranial surgery. To avoid possibilities of hypoxia during hyperventilation, the Pco_2 should be kept above 20 mm Hg. This could be beneficial in avoiding the occurrence of the "intracerebral steal" syndrome.

BLOOD PRESSURE

Cerebral ischemia can occur above and below certain critical levels. If it is increased above the autoregulation level, breakthrough in the blood–brain barrier can occur with subsequent edema formation. The formation of edema is facilitated by dilation of the arterial vessels resulting from an inhalational anesthetic agent. Sudden hypotension can easily decrease the blood flow to areas in which autoregulation is lost. Thus, it is best to avoid fluctuations of blood pressure during induction and maintenance of anesthesia.

DRUGS

Inhalational anesthetic agents such as halothane, methoxyflurane, and ethrane cause an increase in cerebral flow, cerebral blood volume, and intracranial pressure. In healthy individuals, this is well tolerated. However, in patients with reduced intracranial compliance (increased intracranial pressure and cerebral ischemia) it can have detrimental effect.

Barbiturates produce proportionate reductions of function, metabolism, and flow. At present, they are the anesthetic agents of choice for neurologic procedures. The neuroleptic combination can produce a moderate decrease in intracranial pressure. Ketamine, on the other hand, increases the intracranial pressure with a resultant decrease in cerebral perfusion pressure.

REFERENCES

1. Cutler RWP, Page L, Galicich J et al: Formation and absorption of cerebrospinal fluid in man. Brain 91:707, 1968
2. Wylie WD, Churchill Davidson HC (eds): A Practice of Anesthesia. Chicago, Year Book, 1972, Chap 30
3. McDowall DG: Physiology of the cerebrospinal fluid. In McDowall DG (ed): Cerebral Circulation, International Anesthesiology Clinics, Vol 7, No 3. Boston, Little, Brown, 1969, p 507
4. Kety SS, Schmidt CF: Determination of cerebral blood flow in man by use of nitrous oxide in low concentrations. Am J Physiol 143:53, 1945

5. Lassen NA, Munck O: The cerebral blood flow in man determined by the use of radioactive krypton. Acta Physiol Scand 33:30, 1955

6. Lassen NA: Control of the cerebral circulation in health and disease. Circ Res 34:729, 1974

7. Harper AM: Regulation of cerebral circulation. In Scientific Basis of Medicine: Annual Review. London, Athlone, 1969

8. Harper AM, Glass HI: The effect of alterations in the arterial carbon dioxide tension on the blood flow through the cerebral cortex at normal and low arterial blood pressures. J Neurol Neurosurg Psychiat 28:449, 1965

9. Fieschi C: Regional cerebral blood flow in acute apoplexy, including pharmacodynamic studies. Scand J Clin Lab Invest 16:(Suppl 102):E, 1968

10. Finnerty FA, Witkin L, Fazekas JF: Cerebral hemodynamics during cerebral ischemia induced by acute hypotension. J Clin Invest 33:1227, 1954

11. Folkow B: Description of the myogenic hypothesis. Circ Res 15 (Suppl 1):279, 1964

12. James IM, Millar RA, Purves MJ: Extrinsic neural activity and the control of cerebral blood flow. Scand J Clin Lab Invest 6:(Suppl 102):E, 1968

13. Reivich M: Arterial pCO_2 and cerebral hemodynamics. Am J Physiol 206:25, 1964

14. Grubb RL, Raichle ME, Eichling JO, et al: The effects of changes in $PaCO_2$ on cerebral blood volume, blood flow, and vascular mean transit time. Stroke 5:630, 1974

15. Wollman H, Smith TC, Stephen GW, et al: Effects of extremes of respiratory and metabolic alkalosis on cerebral blood flow in man. J Appl Physiol 24:60, 1968

16. Alexander SC, Smith TC, Strobel G, et al: Cerebral carbohydrate metabolism of man during respiratory and metabolic alkalosis. J Appl Physiol 24:66, 1968

17. Betz E, Heuser D: Cerebral cortical blood flow during changes of acid–base equilibrium of the brain. J Appl Physiol 23:726, 1967

18. Lassen NA: The luxury-perfusion syndrome and its possible relation to acute metabolic acidosis localized within the brain. Lancet 2:1113, 1966

19. Severinghaus JW, Lassen NA: Step hypocapnia to separate arterial from tissue PCO_2 in the regulation of cerebral blood flow. Circ Res 20:272, 1967

20. Cohen PJ: The effects of decreased oxygen tension on cerebral circulation, metabolism and function. In Proceedings of the International Symposium on Cardiovascular and Respiratory Effects of Hypoxia. Basel, Karger, 1966 p 81

21. Kogure K, Scheinberg P, Reinmuth OM, et al: Mechanism of cerebral vasodilatation in hypoxia. J Appl Physiol 29:223, 1970

22. Albert SN, Fazekas JF: Cerebral hemodynamics and metabolism during induced hypothermia. Anesth Analg 35:381, 1956

23. Kennedy C, Sokoloff L: An adaptation of the nitrous oxide method to the study of the cerebral circulation in children; normal values for cerebral blood flow and cerebral metabolic rate in childhood. J Clin Invest 36:1130, 1957

24. Lassen NA, Feinberg I, Lane MH: Bilateral studies of cerebral oxygen uptake in young and aged subjects and in patients with organic dementia. J Clin Invest 39:491, 1960

25. Severinghaus JW: Outline of H^+ blood flow relationships in brain. Scand J Clin Lab Invest 8:(Suppl 102):K, 1968

26. Hoedt-Rasmussen K, Skinhoj E, Paulson O, et al: Regional cerebral blood flow in acute apoplexy. Arch Neurol 17:271, 1967

27. Lassen NA, Palvolgyi R: Cerebral steal during hypercapnia and the inverse reaction during hypocapnia observed by the [133]xenon technique in man. Scand J Clin Lab Invest 13:(Suppl 102):D, 1968

28. Smith AL, Wollman H: Cerebral blood flow and metabolism. Anesthesiology 36:378, 1972
29. Michenfelder JD, Gronert GA, Rehder K: Neuroanesthesia. Anesthesiology 30:65, 1968
30. Shapiro HM: Intracranial hypertension: therapeutic and anesthetic considerations. Anesthesiology 43:445, 1975

Section IV
The Endocrine System

INTRODUCTION

The endocrine system is composed of several glands, scattered throughout the body, with one common feature: their secretions are delivered internally into the bloodstream—hence, the name endocrine. This is in contrast to the other secretory glands whose products of secretion reach the skin or the hollow viscera by a series of ducts. Because in the endocrine glands the function of the ducts is performed by the blood, they are richly endowed with blood vessels. The product of the secretion of the endocrine glands is known as a hormone; by definition a hormone is a chemical substance that is released in small amounts directly into the bloodstream in response to a specific stimulus. On reaching its target cells, the hormone produces a typical physiologic response.

Although there is a large number of known hormones, the most important ones are those secreted by the pituitary, thyroid, parathyroid, pancreas, adrenals, placenta, and gastrointestinal mucosa. The first five are of special concern to the anesthesiologist because they can affect his daily practice.

The steroid hormones are synthesized from cholesterol inside the cytoplasm at the mitochondria, whereas the protein hormones are formed in the ribosomes and are attached to the endoplasmic reticulum. These hormones are stored as zymogen granules in the golgi apparatus. On stimulation, these granules are released into the interstitial spaces by fusing with the cell membrane.

Hormones do not act as substrates during metabolic reactions. They can only affect the rate of cellular reactions. Because they are not consumed (used up), in order to be effective, they must either be inactivated or excreted. Inactivation can be accomplished by reduction, oxidation, cleavage, or conjugation; excretion is mostly urinary, although in some cases it is biliary.

The biologic half-life of hormones in blood is variable, the average being 10 to 30 minutes. However, catecholamines have a very short half-life, on the order of seconds, while the half-life of thyroid hormone is a few days.

MECHANISM OF THE ACTION OF HORMONES

The way that hormones act at the cellular level seems to vary according to the size and characteristic of their molecules. For example, steroid hormones, which are small and lipid-soluble, can penetrate the cell membrane easily. Inside the cell, they bind to a receptor protein in the cytoplasm through which they reach nuclear receptor proteins on which they exert their action. However, most of the other hormones are protein in nature, have large molecules, and cannot penetrate the cell membrane. They perform their regulatory function by one of the following processes: (1) changing the permeability of the cell membrane or (2) producing a "second messenger" within the cell. Insulin is an example of the first process. It binds itself to the receptor of the cell, changing its permeability to glucose and amino acids. Most hormones affect cellular metabolism by an intracellular mediator (second messenger), which is cyclic 3'-5' adenosine monophosphate (cyclic AMP). The specific hormone binds at a receptor site on the cell surface that is part of the enzyme adenyl cyclase. This enzyme produces cyclic AMP using the substrate adenosine triphosphate (ATP). Cyclic AMP may alter cellular function by one of the following mechanisms: (1) changing the permeability of cell membranes to water, ions, and amino acids; (2) releasing intracellular hormones from their storage sites; or (3) forming new enzymes or changing the rate of their synthesis.

chapter 25

The Hypophysis and the Thyroid

The hypophysis, or pituitary gland, is located in the sella turcica at the base of the brain. It consists of two major parts: (1) the anterior pituitary, also called adenohypophysis, and (2) the posterior pituitary, or neurohypophysis. The pars intermedia is located between the two portions.

The function of the pituitary gland is under direct control of the hypothalamus. This is accomplished by two means: (1) nerve fibers extending between the hypothalamus and the neurohypophysis and (2) the hypothalamic-hypophyseal portal vessels.

The hypothalamus secretes substances called releasing factors, which stimulate the secretion of various adenohypophyseal hormones. (Fig. 25-1). These substances reach the hypophysis by way of the portal vessels.

The close relationship between the hypothalamus and the hypophysis is of prime importance, since the hypothalamus receives signals and collects information from various parts of the body.

Adenohypophysical Hormones and Abnormalities in their Secretion

The adenohypophysis secretes growth, adrenocorticotropic, thyroid-stimulating, follicle-stimulating, and luteinizing hormones.

GROWTH HORMONE

It stimulates the growth of the body cells as well as their mitosis. The effect of the hormone on the metabolism is very pronounced. It increases the protein synthesis as well as the use of fats for energy production and, conversely, it decreases the rate of carbohydrate metabolism. In order for the growth hormone to be effective, an adequate amount of carbohydrate should be available and an adequate insulin activity present.

An excess in growth hormone production results in gigantism or in acromegaly. Acromegaly is characterized by enlargement of hands, feet, and nose. Patients complain of excessive sweating, severe headaches, and have an abnormal glucose tolerance test. Prior to surgery, the glucose metabolism should be corrected with insulin if necessary. A deficiency of growth hormone in childhood results in short stature.

ADRENOCORTICOTROPIC HORMONE (CORTICOTROPIN, ACTH)

It controls the secretion of glucocorticoid and, partly, the mineralocorticoid hormones from the adrenal cortex (Fig. 25-1).

Excessive ACTH production results in bilateral adrenocortical hyperplasia and Cushing's syndrome. Bilateral adrenalectomy is indicated in most cases.

ACTH deficiency leads to a deficiency in cortisol secretion, which can precipitate a great anesthetic and surgical risk (Chap. 27). The adequacy of ACTH secretion is evaluated by the metyzapone test.[1] The treatment for ACTH deficiency should consist of full replacement doses of glucocorticoids.

Mineralocorticoid secretion is not under the primary control of ACTH and, therefore, hypoaldosteronism usually does not develop.

THYROID-STIMULATING HORMONE

It controls the secretion of thyroxine by the thyroid gland. Excess of thyroid-stimulating hormone is not known to cause the clinical syndrome of hyperthyroidism. However, deficiency causes hypothyroidism. If such a patient is to undergo surgery for removal of a pituitary tumor, he should be first rendered euthyroid.

FOLLICLE-STIMULATING AND LUTEINIZING HORMONES

They control the gonads. Abnormalities in their secretion do not represent any surgical or anesthetic problems. Replacement therapy is not necessary during and after surgery of the pituitary gland.

Most abnormalities of pituitary secretion are due to tumors. The symptomatology is caused by the expanding space-occupying lesion and by abnormal endocrine function. The expanding tumor exerts pressure on the optic nerve causing visual deficits and can exert pressure on the occulomotor, trochlear, and trigeminal nerves leading to disconjugate eye movements.

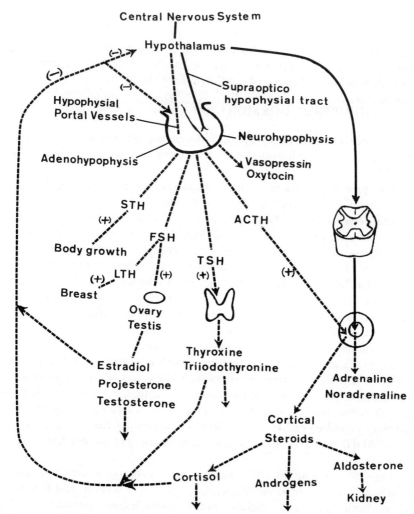

FIG. 25-1: Schematic representation of the neural control of the endocrine gland. Solid line indicates nerve pathway; dotted line, vascular pathway.

Neurohypophyseal Hormones and Abnormalities in their Secretion

The neurohypophysis secretes oxytocin and antidiuretic hormone.

OXYTOCIN

This hormone causes contractions of the pregnant uterus. Therefore, its normal secretion is an important factor for an effective delivery. It also stimulates milk secretion and ejection by the mammary glands.

ANTIDIURETIC HORMONE (ADH)

This hormone is secreted by the nerve ending of fibers originating in the supraoptic nuclei of the hypothalamus. It is stored and released by the pituitary gland.[2]

The primary functions of the antidiuretic hormone are regulation of osmotic pressure of extracellular fluid and regulation of blood volume.

The secretion of ADH is regulated by changes of osmotic pressure of blood.[3] When elevated, osmotic pressure stimulates the supraoptic nuclei of the hypothalamus and ADH is secreted. After absorption in the circulation, the hormone reaches the kidneys. The increased reabsorption of water dilutes the extracellular fluid and brings the osmotic pressure back to normal.[4]

Many factors and drugs influence the release of ADH. Pain and anxiety stimulate its secretion. The use of some narcotics and tranquilizers have the same effect as well as traction of abdominal viscera during surgery.

In studies in conscious patients during weaning from a ventilator, an increase in plasma ADH has been reported with intermittent positive pressure ventilation (IPPV).[5] Anxiety and stress with IPPV was offered as an explanation for this increase. Prolonged mechanical ventilation, at times, tends to cause water retention due to abnormal ADH release.[6] Addition of positive end-expiratory pressure (PEEP) has resulted in a significant rise in the amount of plasma ADH, which probably results from aortic and carotid baroreceptor stimulation.[7]

Excessive amounts of ADH secretion is a nonsurgical condition and is characterized by excessive water retention, low serum sodium, and low blood urea nitrogen. Lung and central nervous system lesions, porphyria, and a variety of other conditions can cause inappropriate ADH secretion.[8] If a patient with such a condition is to undergo surgical intervention, the water and sodium balance must first be corrected.

Deficit of ADH frequently occurs from tumor invasion of the posterior pituitary or the hypothalamus or during their surgical removal. In the absence of ADH the patient develops diabetes insipidus.[9] Large volumes of urine are secreted, leading to hypovalemia, azotemia, and hypernatremia. If the patient develops marked polyuria during the operation, adequate fluid replacement becomes very important to prevent circulatory collapse. This should be accomplished by intravenous doses of glucose and water to stabilize the sodium level. Diabetes insipidus, which develops during or immediately after pituitary surgery, is generally due to trauma of the neurohypophysis and is usually transient. However, if it persists and water replacement becomes a problem, treatment with aqueous vasopressin or Pitressin tannate should be instituted. Again, careful monitoring of patient input, output, and serum sodium should be carried on.

PANHYPOPITUITARISM

This is a condition that may develop after severe shock and arterial hypotension. It occurs mostly postpartum in cases of severe hemorrhage. Inadequate secretions by the adrenal cortex, thyroid, and ovaries result in apathy, weight loss, atrophy of breast, and genitalia.

If a patient is suspected of having inadequacy of the adrenohypophyseal system, substitution therapy with glucocorticoids should be provided before any anesthesia is administered and surgery is performed.

Anesthetic Problems Related to Surgery of the Pituitary Gland

The anesthetic problems are related to the basic pathology for which surgery is undertaken.[10] If surgery is performed because of intracerebral mass, the efforts of the anesthesiologist are directed toward preventing a further rise in intracranial pressure, adequate airway, ventilation, and fluid replacement, which are actually common problems for every craniotomy.

A resection of the pituitary gland may be undertaken in the course of treatment of metastatic carcinoma of the breast and complications of diabetes mellitus. Patients with advanced metastatic carcinoma are usually hypovolemic, anemic, and may have pulmonary metastasis.

The carbohydrate metabolism of a diabetic patient should be controlled with insulin prior to surgery.

Adequate replacement with steroid therapy should be provided before and after surgery for removal of the pituitary gland. Maintenance should also be carried throughout the lifetime of the patient.

THE THYROID GLAND

The thyroid gland normally synthesizes two hormones, thyroxine (T_4) and triiodothyronine (T_3). The synthesis can be divided into four phases; trapping, binding, coupling, and release:

TRAPPING

The iodide trapping is the transfer of iodides from the extracellular fluid into the follicles of the thyroid gland. The thyroid contains iodide in concentrations above the levels of plasma. The differential concentration of iodide between thyroid and serum is 20 or 30:1.

Pituitary thyrotropin stimulates the iodide pump mechanism. It can be depressed by thiocyanate.

BINDING

The first step in this process is the oxidative conversion of iodides to iodine, which in turn combines with the amino acid thyrosine to form T_4. In this process, first mono- and then diiodotyrosine are formed.

Inhibition of iodide oxidation or iodotyrosine formation can be achieved by propylthiouracil and methimazole, the most commonly used antithyroid drugs.

COUPLING

Two molecules of diiodothyrosine bind to form T_4. One molecule of each mono- and diiodothyrosine bind and form T_3.

STORAGE AND RELEASE

Thyroid hormones are stored in the form of thyroglobulin in the thyroid gland for a period of several weeks. Under thyrotropin stimulation, the thyroglobulin undergoes hydrolysis and subsequently the gland releases the thyroid hormones into the circulation. Iodide administration inhibits the release of hormones.

Transport of Thyroid Hormones to the Tissues

Thyroxine represents 95 percent of the active thyroid hormones entering the circulation; the rest is triiodothyronine.

Upon release into the circulation, thyroid hormones combine with the plasma proteins. The affinity of thyroxine to proteins is three times as much as the affinity of triiodothyronine. If both are injected intravenously in the same quantity, the amount of free triiodothyronine in the plasma is greater than that of the thyroxine. The protein-bound thyroid hormones can be precipitated from the plasma and the amount of iodine measured.

Interrelation Between Thyroid, Pituitary, and Adrenal Hormones

The control of normal thyroid gland activity rests with the thyrotropin of the anterior pituitary gland (Fig. 25-1). In turn, the concentration of thyroid hormones in blood control the secretion of thyrotropin, thus establishing a feed-back mechanism.[11]

The relationship of the adrenal cortex to the thyroid has been extensively investigated.[12] Cortisone administration for several weeks in euthyroid patients has caused depression of thyroid function.[13] Also, clinical euthyroid state has been established in some patients receiving steroid therapy for hyperthyroidism.[14]

Corticosteroids suppress the release of thyrotropin and, thus, diminish thyroid function.[15]

The relationship between the adrenal medulla and the thyroid is a complex one.[16] Reports about levels of circulatory catecholamines in hyperthyroid patients have been conflicting. However, there is a definite similarity between adrenergic hyperactivity and hyperthyroidism.

Thyroxine and Hyperthyroidism

Many questions concerning the etiology of hyperthyroidism remain to be answered. Increasing evidence suggests that immune factors participate in its pathogenesis. The presence of cell-mediated immunity has been clearly demonstrated in hyperthyroidism. The appearance of humoral immunoglobulins, such as long-acting thyroid stimulator (LATS), is probably secondary to the disturbance in cell-mediated immunity.

The principal effect of thyroxine is on metabolic rate of most tissues. It increases by as much as 60 to 100 percent above the normal level. The rate of protein synthesis and protein catabolism is increased. The growth of young persons, as well as their mental processes are accelerated.

Thyroid hormones increase the number and the activity of mitochondria as well as their size and total membrane surface.[17] The process of oxidative phosphorylation takes place in the mitochondria. The energy liberated by oxidation is transformed into the high energy bonds of adenosine-triphosphate (ATP). Thyroxine causes the uncoupling of oxidative phosphorylation. Hence, energy cannot be stored and heat production increases. Some of the clinical manifestations of hyperthyroidism (Graves' disease), such as sweating, tachycardia, and vasodilatation, are compensatory mechanisms for the elimination of excess heat.

The cardiac output is increased above the requirement of the metabolic state. The EKG changes are usually consistent with left ventricular hypertrophy. A patient with hyperthyroidism may show signs of arrhythmias or congestive heart failure. Tremor, dyspnea on exertion, increased appetite with weight loss, insomnia, and emotional disorders are some of the other manifestations of hyperthyroidism. Ocular pathology is also present in Graves' disease: upper lid retraction, infrequent blinking, lid lag are the more common. Thyroid myopathy is also a frequent symptom. Thyroxine, besides uncoupling the oxidative phosphorylation, also inhibits creatinine phosphokinase.

Hyperthyroidism, Anesthesia, and Surgery

Today, surgery for thyrotoxicosis should be an elective procedure, performed on a euthyroid patient. Propylthiouracil (Propacil) or methimazole (Tapazole) are the main antithyroid drugs used. They interfere with every step of thyroid hormone synthesis. The course of treatment is to render the patient euthyroid, and it lasts for 6 or 7 weeks.

Iodine is also administered for a week prior to contemplated surgery. It decreases the vascularity and the hyperplasia of the enlarged overactive thyroid gland. In addition, iodine inhibits the synthesis and secretion of the hormone through a direct effect on the gland.

Some patients are hypersensitive to the antithyroid drugs. They may develop skin disorders and agranulocytosis. If patients have to undergo emergency surgery for unrelated pathology, or if the enlarged thyroid is causing airway obstruction, simply put, there might not be enough time to achieve euthyroid state. Sympathetic blocking and sympatholitic drugs, in conjunction with steroids and iodine, are used to prepare the patient for emergency surgery. Although there is no evidence of any consistent rise in circulatory catecholamines in hyperthyroidism, there is increased reactivity of the adrenal medulla and peripheral noradrenaline stores. Definite clinical improvement is seen in patients receiving reserpine and guanethidine (Ismelin). Increased heart rate, blood pressure, and cardiac output are reduced toward normal. Improvement in the symptoms and signs occur very early in therapy.[18,19]

Alpha-methyldopa (Aldomet) exerts a centrally mediated antihypertensive effect, and interferes with the actions of biogenic catecholamine by forming a false transmitter. It slows the heart rate but has no effect on cardiac output and oxygen consumption in hyperthyroid patients.[20]

The cardiac output can be reduced in thyrotoxicosis and the heart rate decreased by propranolol (Inderal). Extreme caution should be used if propranolol (half-life, 4 to 6 hours) is discontinued 24 hours prior to surgery. In patients who depend on beta-adrenergic blockade to control cardiovascular symptomatology, the withdrawal of propranolol can precipitate thyroid crisis or cardiac decompensation; therefore, the discontinuation of the drug in this group of patients is not recommended.

Corticosteroid therapy is recommended for 1 week prior to surgery. Adequate steroid coverage during the operation should also be provided.

The combination of alpha and beta sympathetic block produces an improvement of thyrotoxic symptoms and a reduction of oxygen consumption by 12 percent.[21]

Investigations by Sutherland[22] shed some light on the interrelationship of thyroid function and catecholamine action. Hormones react with adenylcyclase on all membranes to catalyze the formation of cyclic AMP from ATP. In turn, cyclic AMP mediates many of the hormonal effects. Catecholamines react with adenylcyclase and form cyclic AMP. Thyroxine stimulates adenylcyclase production by increasing protein synthesis. Thus, in hyperthyroidism, the high levels of thyroid hormones facilitate the formation of cyclic AMP by catecholamines.

It is important to point out that all sympathetic blocking agents discussed above do not change the thyroid hormone secretion. The serum-bound iodine levels and the uptake of ^{131}I remain unchanged. These drugs have great value in the treatment of hyperthyroidism and, specifically, thyroid crisis, but they do not render the patient euthyroid.

Prior to surgery these patients should have adequate premedication.[23] Narcotics are theoretically contraindicated since they stimulate the sympathoadrenal axis.[24,25] Short-acting barbiturates and/or diazepam are preferable. Anticholinergic agents are omitted because they interfere with the sweating mechanism. However, atropine can be given if the patient is in a euthyroid state.

Cyclopropane and ether should not be used, since they also stimulate the sympathoadrenal axis. Halothane decreases circulatory catecholamine concentrations,[26] depresses sympathoadrenal activity,[27] and, therefore, can be used as the primary anesthetic agent with or without nitrous oxide.

Thyroid Storm

The condition known as thyroid storm rarely occurs today. It usually develops from 6 to 18 hours postoperatively and is manifested by tachycardia and severe hypotension. Physiologically, it is viewed as a decompensated thyrotoxic state[23] precipitated by sudden excessive release of thyroid hormones into the circulation. There is no therapeutic means of removing or inhibiting the action of circulatory thyroid hormones. Untreated, it results in a high mortality rate; however, improvement is usually seen a few hours after the initiation of treatment.

The only specific treatment is iodine, given as potassium iodine 500 mg i.v. Steroids and alpha-adrenergic blocking agents are also administered. Propylthiouracil 150 to 200 mg is given every 6 hours in order to prevent further synthesis of hormones. Administration of propranolol has proved useful in controlling the cardiac effect in crisis.

Symptomatic therapy consists of (1) lowering the elevated body temperature, (2) sedation, and (3) fluids.

Hypothyroidism

The characteristics of hypothyroidism are the opposite to those of hyperthyroidism. These include somnolence, muscular sluggishness, slowed heart rate, and decreased cardiac output and blood volume.

In hypothyroidism, there is an increase in blood lipids associated with increased arteriosclerosis. These patients are more prone to develop peripheral vascular disease, coronary sclerosis, and deafness.

The treatment of hypothyroidism is with thyroxine.

Less well appreciated is the effect of hypothyroidism on adrenal function. The hypothyroid patient has abnormal response to adrenergic stimuli, although the level of circulating catecholamines is normal. The myocardium is less sensitive to catecholamines. There is a decreased production of adrenal cortical hormone and evidence of atrophy of the adrenal cortex. Due to the inadequacy of adrenal function, complications such as shock and hypothermia can develop during induction and maintenance of anesthesia.

Probably the most important factor to the anesthesiologist is the delay of drug metabolism in hypothyroidism. Therefore, these patients are extremely sensitive to narcotics, barbiturates, and some inhalation agents. Their administration should be carefully titrated.

THE PARATHYROID

Anatomy

The parathyroid glands are located behind the thyroid glands, one behind each of the two upper and lower poles. In rare occasions they can be found in the mediastinum.

Physiology

The synthesis and the secretion of the parathyroid hormone is related to calcium concentration in the blood.

The parathyroid hormone stimulates the bone resorption by increasing the osteoclastic activity. Injection of the hormone causes elevation of serum calcium levels and depression of phosphate levels. The parathyroid hormone stimulates the reabsorption of calcium, magnesium, and hydrogen ions by the kidneys. The effect on the phosphate elimination is the opposite, it increases the excretion by decreasing the renal reabsorption.

The parathyroid hormone, in the presence of adequate amounts of vitamin D, stimulates the reabsorption of calcium from the intestines. Vitamin D and the hormone have a synergetic effect on bone metabolism.

Ionized Calcium and Regulation by Parathyroid Hormone

The physiologic importance of ionic calcium was first demonstrated by McLean and Hasting.[28,29]

Ionic calcium is identified with nerve conduction, bone formation and reabsorption, muscle contraction, cardiac, cerebral, and kidney functions, intestinal secretion and absorption, blood coagulation, enzyme function, hormonal release, and membrane and capillary permeability.

In serum, calcium is present in three forms: ionized calcium (Ca^{++}), which is the physiologically active form; nondiffusible protein-bound calcium; and diffusible nonionized calcium.

In a series of 60 normal subjects, a complete lack of correlation between serum Ca^{++} and serum total calcium concentrations was observed.[30] This important observation challenges the value of the customarily obtained total serum calcium, if the ionic form is physiologically more important. Serum protein, mainly albumin, determines the discrepancy between Ca^{++} and total calcium. A total serum calcium measurement is, therefore, an indirect measurement of the serum albumin level.[30] Direct measurement of serum Ca^{++} levels can be performed by the recently developed calcium-sensitive electrode.

Decrease in the Ca^{++} concentration in the extracellular fluid stimulates the synthesis and secretion of parathyroid hormone. This is easily seen to be the case in rickets. The opposite, an increase in Ca^{++} concentration, for instance, in cases of increased calcium intake from the diet, decreases the activity of the gland.

Calcitonin

Calcitonin is a hormone that has an opposite effect on blood calcium than does the parathyroid hormone. In the human, it is secreted by the thyroid gland and, therefore, it is also called thyrocalcitonin. Calcitonin inhibits the bone reabsorption.[31]

Calcitonin acts in a feedback system to control Ca^{++} concentration in a manner opposite to that of the parathyroid hormone. Since it operates very rapidly, it plays an important role in preventing the acute fluctuation of Ca^{++} concentration in the body fluids.

Hyperparathyroidism

The usual cause of hyperparathyroidism is a tumor (adenoma) of one of the parathyroid glands. Pregnancy and lactation, which cause low calcium levels for prolonged periods of time, stimulate the parathyroid hormone and may predispose to the development of a parathyroid tumor.

In hyperparathyroidism, the serum calcium level is elevated due to elevated osteoclastic activity in bone and accelerated calcium absorption from the gastrointestinal tract. The serum phosphate level is usually decreased due to increased renal excretion of phosphate. The increased calcium blood level causes hypercalcemia, stimulates formation of kidney stones, and ultimately leads to kidney damage.

Progressively developed hypercalcemia can be well tolerated by the patient. However, levels of 12 mg per 100 ml and above cause anorexia, nausea, vomiting, lethargy, confusion, and coma. The comatose patient is treated by hydration to correct the water and electrolyte inbalance, phosphate solutions, and corticosteroids.

Emergency surgical exploration of the parathyroid glands must be undertaken after regulating the electrolyte inbalance.

Hypoparathyroidism

In hypoparathyroidism, bone reabsorption is so depressed that the level of blood calcium decreases. Hypoparathyroidism is usually the result of surgical damage to the parathyroid glands during thyroid surgery. The calcium level in the blood falls from normal of 10 mg per 100 ml to 7 mg per 100 ml in 2 to 3 days. This results in tetany, muscle cramps, and may eventually lead to grand mal seizures.

Hyperparathyroidism and Anesthesia

The problems encountered during surgery are related to the degree of hypercalcemia. The main effect of hypercalcemia is on the heart function.

Bronsky et al[32] reports no change in cardiac rate or rhythm in a series of patients with hypercalcemia. The P-R interval is prolonged and the Q-T interval shortened on electrocardiogram in these patients. At levels higher than 16 mg per 100 ml, the same author reports disproportionally long Q-T intervals.

Calcium ions interfere with membrane transport and, therefore, may interfere with the action of muscle relaxants.[33] In the absence of calcium, muscle impulses arise spontaneously at the end plate. The responsiveness of the end plate to depolarization is lost. Calcium stimulates the release of acetylcholine at the neuromuscular junction.

Hypoparathyroidism may develop in the postoperative period. Transient tetany has been reported in about 30 percent of patients after removal of parathyroid tumors.[34] Neuromuscular irritability is related to the degree of hypocalcemia, and frank tonic contractions usually develop at blood calcium levels below 7 mg per 100 ml.

REFERENCES

1. Liddle GW, Estep HL, Kendall JW, et al: Clinical application of a new test of pituitary reserve. J Clin Endocrinol Metab 19:875, 1959
2. Kleeman CR, Fichman MP: The clinical physiology of water metabolism. N Engl J Med 277:1300, 1967
3. Moran WH, Zimmerman B: Mechanisms of antidiuretic hormone (ADH) control of importance to the surgical patient. Surgery 62:639, 1967
4. Kleeman CR: Water Metabolism. In Maxwell MH, Kleeman CR (eds): Clinical Disorders of Fluid and Electrolyte Metabolism. 2nd ed. New York, McGraw-Hill, 1972, p 215
5. Khambatta HJ, Baratz RA: IPPB, plasma ADH, and urine flow in conscious man. J Appl Physiol 33:362, 1972
6. Sladen A, Laver MB, Pontoppidan H: Pulmonary complications and water retention in prolonged mechanical ventilation. N Engl J Med 279:448, 1968
7. Kumar A, Pontoppidan H, Baratz RA, et al: Inappropriate response to increased plasma ADH during mechanical ventilation in acute respiratory failure. Anesthesiology 40:215, 1974
8. Bartter FC, Schwartz WB: The syndrome of inappropriate secretion of antidiuretic hormone. Am J Med 42:790, 1967
9. Coggins CH, Leaf A: Diabetes insipidus. Am J Med 42:807, 1967
10. Van Poznak A: Anesthesia for surgery of the pituitary gland. In Jenkins MT (ed): Anesthesia for Patients with Endocrine Disease. Philadelphia, Davis, 1963, p 118
11. Pearson OH: Endocrine consequences of hypophysectomy. Anesthesiology 24:563, 1963
12. Pittman JA: Adrenal cortex. In Werner SG, Ingbar SH (eds): The Thyroid, 3rd ed. New York, Harper & Row, 1971, p 644
13. Frederickson DA: Effect of massive cortisone therapy on thyroid function. J Clin Endocrinol Metab 11:760, 1951
14. Werner SC, Reatman SR: Remission of hyperthyroidism (Graves' disease) and altered pattern of serum-thyroxine binding induced by prednisone. Lancet 2:751, 1965

15. Ingbar SH: ACTH, cortisone and the metabolism of iodine. Metabolism 5:652, 1956
16. Crile GW: The interdependence of the thyroid, adrenals and nervous system. Am J Surg 6:616, 1929
17. Peachey LD, Greif RL: Alterations of mitochondrial structure induced by thyroid hormones in vivo and in vitro. Endocrinology 77:61, 1965
18. Gaffney TE, Braunwald E, Kahler RL: Effects of guanitidine on triiodothyronine induced hyperthyroidism in man. N Engl J Med 265:16, 1961
19. James ML: Endocrine disease and anaesthesia. Anaesthesia 25:232, 1970
20. Theilen EO, Wilson WR, Tutunji FJ: The acute hemodynamic effects of alpha-methyldopa in thyrotoxic patients and normal subjects. Metabolism 12:626, 1963
21. Stout BD, Wiener L, Cox JW: Combined alpha and beta sympathetic blockade in hyperthyroidism. Clinical and metabolic effects. Am Intern Med 70:963, 1969
22. Sutherland E: On the biological role of cyclic AMP. JAMA 214:1281, 1970
23. McArthur JW, Rawson RW, Means JH, et al: Thyrotoxic crisis, an analysis of thirty-six cases at The Massachusetts General Hospital during the past twenty-five years. JAMA 134:868, 1974
24. Stehling LC: Anesthetic management of patient with hyperthyroidism. Anesthesiology 41:585, 1974
25. Giesecke AH, Jenkins MT, Crout JR, et al: Urinary epinephrine and norepinephrine during innovar-nitrous oxide anesthesia in man. Anesthesiology 28:701, 1967
26. Roizen MR, Moss J, Henry DP, et al: Effects of halothane on plasma cate-cholamines. Anesthesiology 41:432, 1974
27. Skovsted P, Price ML, Price HL: The effects of halothane on arterial pressure, preganglionic sympathetic activity and barostatic reflexes. Anesthesiology 31:507, 1969
28. McLean FC, Hasting AB: Clinical estimation and significance of calcium ion concentration in the blood. Am J Med Sci 189:601, 1935
29. McLean FC, Hasting AB: The status of calcium in the fluids of the body. J Biol Chem 108:285, 1935
30. Moore EW, Studies with ion exchange calcium electrodes in biological fluids: Some applications in biomedical research and clinical medicine. In Durst RA (ed): Ion-Selective Electrodes. Washington D.C., U.S. Government Printing Office, National Bureau of Standards special publication 314, 1969, p 215
31. Munson PL: Thyrocalcitonin. In Astwood EB, Cassidy CE (eds): Clinical Endocrinology. New York, Grune, 1968, p 336
32. Bronsky D, Dubin A, Waldstein SS, et al: Calcium and the electrocardiogram. Electrocardiographic manifestations of hyperparathyroidism and of marked hypercalcemia from various other etiologies. Am J Cardiol 7:833, 1961
33. Foldes FF: Factors which alter the effects of muscle relaxants. Anesthesiology 20:464, 1959
34. Schafer M, Economov SG: Ode to an Indian rhinoceros, or the evaluation and preparation of patients for parathyroid surgery. Surg Clin North Am 50:227, 1970

chapter 26

The Endocrine Pancreas

The pancreas secretes two hormones, insulin and glucagon. They are secreted by the islets of Langerhans directly into the blood circulation. The alpha cells secrete glucagon and the beta cells secrete insulin.

INSULIN

It is a small protein composed of two amino acid chains. It plays a major role in the carbohydrate metabolism by enhancing the rate of glucose transport through cell membranes. As a result, insulin increases the rate of glucose metabolism and decreases blood glucose concentration and the stores of glycogen in various tissues.

Mechanism of Glucose Transport and the Effect of Insulin

Glucose cannot pass into the cell through the pores of the cell membrane, but enters by means of a transport mechanism. It probably combines with a carrier substance. The glucose transport through the cell membrane does not take place against a concentration gradient. The concentration outside of the cell should be higher than that of the inside of the cell. This means that the transport of glucose is one of facilitated diffusion.[1]

Insulin facilitates the glucose transport mechanism (Fig. 26-1). It is postulated that, in the absence of insulin, the transport of glucose is inhibited by an active process. Under normal conditions insulin counteracts the inhibitory effect of the active process.

The effect of insulin is not uniform on every organ in the body. It has no effect on the glucose transport in the brain, which depends on the diffusion through the blood–brain barrier. However, insulin is of great importance for glucose transport through the cell membrane in the skeletal muscles, the heart, and some smooth muscle organs.

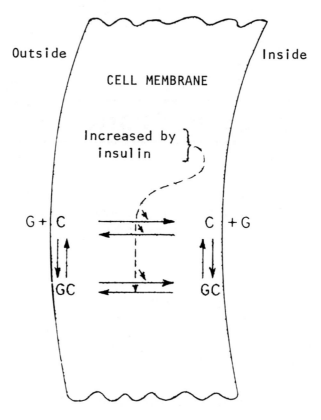

FIG. 26-1: Effect of insulin in increasing glucose transport in either direction through the cell membrane. (Reproduced with permission from Saunders.[1])

Effect of Insulin on Carbohydrate Metabolism in the Liver

Insulin increases the glycolysis in the liver and causes immediate release of glucose into the blood. The glycogen stores in the liver diminish.

The liver cells are highly permeable to glucose; therefore, insulin has minimal effect on the glucose transport through their membranes.

The effect of insulin on the carbohydrate metabolism and glucose transport is of extreme importance. When the muscles are in need of glycogen, it is rapidly transferred from the liver. If sufficient glucose is available in the diet, the glycogen is restored in the liver within a few hours.

Effect of Insulin on Protein and Fat Metabolism

Insulin increases the amount of protein stored in the tissues. Patients with diabetes mellitus suffer from decreased protein anabolism.

The effect of insulin on protein metabolism is mostly secondary to its effect on carbohydrate metabolism. Both proteins and fats are used to replace carbohydrate in energy production in the presence of insufficient insulin secretion.

However, insulin also exerts a direct effect on protein metabolism by increasing the transport of amino acids through the cell membrane.

In the absence of insulin, the free fatty acids, as well as all other lipids, increase in the plasma. In patients with severe diabetes, the increased cholesterol concentration in plasma is a major factor in the early development of arteriosclerosis.

The rapid utilization and mobilization of fats raise the quantities of acetoacetic acid and B-hydroxybutyric acid in blood, leading to ketosis.

Control of Insulin Secretion and Blood Glucose Concentration

Insulin secretion is regulated mainly by the glucose concentration in the plasma. There is an important feedback mechanism that exists between insulin secretion by the pancreas and blood glucose concentration.

In the case of decreased insulin production, less glucose is stored in tissue cells. As a result, the blood glucose concentration rises above the normal level of 90 to 100 mg per 100 ml in the fasting state. On the contrary, in the presence of insulin excess, the blood glucose concentration diminishes.

Liver is the main organ in which glycogen is stored. This glycogen undergoes breakdown (glycogenolysis) in the fasting state. As shown in Fig. 26-2 many other hormones stimulate glycogenolysis and also the synthesis of glucose from lactate (gluconeogenesis). In the fasting state, most of the energy needed is derived from lipolysis of neutral fat stored in adipose tissue. Insulin is the only hormone that stimulates the storage of these compounds.

In the discussion of regulation of glucose metabolism, it is important to put forward the glucose-buffering function of the liver. Liver cells can store glucose as glycogen very efficiently, as a response to increased blood glucose concentration. Conversely, when blood glucose concentration falls below normal, glycogen is quickly metabolized to glucose and released into the circulation.

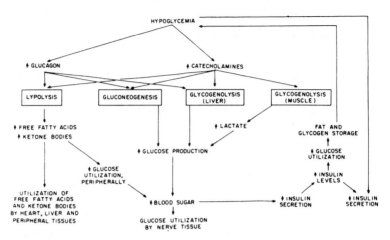

FIG. 26-2: The utilization of metabolic fuels in the fasting state. (Reproduced with permission from E. A. Brunner.[11])

In liver diseases, the regulation of blood glucose concentration is impaired. The liver cannot buffer well and, as a result, the blood glucose concentration fluctuates.

Sympathetic Nervous System
Control of Blood Glucose Concentration

Hypoglycemia stimulates the sympathetic nervous system and causes the release of epinephrine from the adrenal medulla. Epinephrine stimulates the glycogenolysis in the liver cell by activating the enzyme phosphorylase. Its effect is mediated by cyclic AMP.

The stimulation of the sympathetic nervous system also causes release of glucocorticoids from the adrenal glands. They enhance the conversion of amino acids into glucose (gluconeogenesis).

INTERACTION BETWEEN INSULIN AND OTHER HORMONES

ANTERIOR PITUITARY GLAND

The growth hormone elevates the blood glucose concentration because it reduces the rate of glucose utilization. Corticotropin stimulates the secretion of glucocorticoids and, therefore, increases the blood glucose concentration. The luteotropic hormone has the same effect as the growth hormone. The thyrotropic hormone increases blood glucose concentration by stimulating thyroxine production.

THYROID

Thyroxine stimulates the gluconeogenesis, however, to a lesser extent than the glucocorticoids.

ADRENAL CORTEX

Glucocorticoids increase the blood glucose concentration by stimulating gluconeogenesis and also by decreasing the glucose utilization of the cells.

DIABETES MELLITUS

Diabetes mellitus is a metabolic disease due to either insufficiency in insulin production or insensitivity to normally produced insulin. It is manifested by hyperglycemia and glycosuria. The disease causes degeneration of small blood vessels, mainly in the retina, the nervous system, and the kidneys.

Hereditary factors play an important role in the development of the disease. It is transmitted as a recessive genetic characteristic. There are two types of diabeties, juvenile (which is ketosis prone) and adult.

Lack of insulin results in several metabolic changes affecting carbohydrate, protein, and fat. The hyperglycemia is initially due to decreased peripheral uptake of glucose. The gluconeogenesis is stimulated. There is mainly an increased protein breakdown and amino acids are shunted into hepatic pathways of gluconeogenesis.[2] As the blood glucose level rises above the reabsorption capacity of the renal tubules, glucosuria results.

Plasma levels of free fatty acid are also increased. Metabolic acidosis may develop as a result of increased plasma levels of B-hydroxybutyrate and aceto-acetate. The high level of these in the blood is mainly due to hepatic over-production. However, the peripheral uptake of ketone bodies is insufficient in diabetes and contributes to the existing ketoacidosis.[3]

Diagnosis

The fasting blood glucose level in the morning, at least 8 hours after the last full meal, is normally 80 to 90 mg per 100 ml and the maximum upper limit is considered to be 120 mg per 100 ml.

If the fasting glucose is normal, the glucose tolerance test is the next step

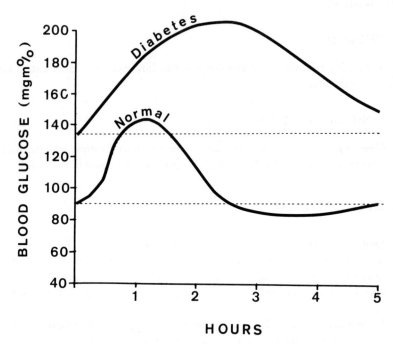

rIG. 26-3: Glucose tolerance curve. Note that in a normal person the blood glucose concentration returns to values below the fasting state. In a diabetic person, the blood glucose concentration level remains elevated for a prolonged period of time.

(Fig. 26-3). If a normal fasting person consumes 50 g of glucose, his blood glucose level rises to 140 mg per 100 ml and within 3 hours falls to normal. The diabetic response is characterized by a slow progressive rise in blood glucose levels for 2 to 3 hours and a return to the control value after 5 to 6 hours. However, it never falls below his/her control level.

Occasionally, diabetics have a normal fasting level of blood glucose concentration. However, in such instances, the glucose tolerance test is almost always abnormal.

An insulin tolerance test is performed to differentiate between diabetes mellitus resulting from insulin deficiency and hyperglycemia resulting from excess production of adrenocortical or anterior hypophyseal hormones. A small dose of insulin will cause a marked fall in blood glucose concentration in cases of diabetes mellitus of pancreatic origin. Also, hyperglycemia can be secondary to pancreatitis, pheochromocytoma, and hyperthyroidism. These possibilities should be considered in the differential diagnosis.

Treatment

DIET

The insulin requirement of the diabetic is established with the patient on a standard diet. In diabetics, the pancreas cannot adjust to an increase in carbohydrate intake, and, therefore, the insulin regimen should be adjusted accordingly.

Usually, the diabetic patient is placed on a single daily dose of one of the long-acting insulins. At meal times, when his glucose level tends to rise, additional quantities of regular insulin are administered.

It has not yet been clearly established whether strict control of blood sugar is sufficient to prevent or delay the serious small vessel changes in diabetics.

Surgery and Anesthesia in the Diabetic Patient

The main objectives during surgery on diabetic patients are to prevent the development of hypoglycemia, severe fluid loss, and ketoacidosis.

Preoperatively, on the day of surgery, one-half of the usual daily dose of insulin is given in the morning. If the operation is to be performed later in the day, one-third of the usual daily dose is given. Intravenous 5 percent dextrose in water is started. Additional doses of regular insulin (10 to 15 units) are administered, depending on the degree of glycosuria. The insulin can be mixed in the intravenous solution of 5 percent dextrose in water. No insulin should be given immediately prior to the operation.

The preoperative medication for the diabetic should generally be the same as that for the nondiabetic. Diabetic patients are more susceptible to the respiratory depressing action of narcotics.[4]

The effects of anesthetic agents on carbohydrate metabolism are far from clear.[5][6] The use of diethyl ether can cause hyperglycemia and a corresponding increase in lactic acid, pyruvic acid, citrate, ketone bodies, and serum inorganic phosphate. The hyperglycemia is a result of sympathetic stimulation that causes an increase in glycogenolysis in the liver.[7] Despite the effect of diethyl ether on carbohydrate metabolism, Greene[7] concludes that it is not absolutely contraindicated for the diabetic patient. Cyclopropane is similar in effect to diethyl ether. Under halothane anesthesia, mild hyperglycemia[5] as well as progressive hypoglycemia have been reported.[8] Thiopental in combination with nitrous oxide oxygen anesthesia has no effect on blood glucose concentration.[9]

Regional anesthesia also has no effect on carbohydrate metabolism. Frequently, surgery is performed on the lower extremities of diabetics because of vascular insufficiency. In these cases, subarachnoid or epidural block are satisfactory.[10]

In summary, selection of an anesthetic agent is not a major factor in the management of the diabetic patient. Mild hyperglycemia during surgery is not a dangerous phenomenon.

The most important objectives are to prevent acidosis, acetonemia, and hypoglycemia. This is accomplished by adequate administration of glucose and insulin. Respiratory and metabolic acidosis should be avoided.

Insulin-Secreting Tumors of the Pancreas

Hyperinsulinism does occur as a result of an adenoma of an islet of Langerhans. The best diagnostic test is the intravenous tolbutamide test: persistent hypoglycemia after 1 mg intravenous tolbutamide is good presumptive evidence. Surgical removal of this tumor is indicated, although they are usually benign. The blood sugar should be carefully monitored by the standard glucose oxidase method.

REFERENCES

1. Guyton AC: Textbook of Medical Physiology, 4th ed. Philadelphia, Saunders, 1971
2. Felig P, Owen OA, Cahill GF Jr: Role of plasma amino acids in the regulation of gluconeogenesis. J Clin Invest 47:32a, 1968
3. Basso LV, Havel RJ: Hepatic metabolism of free fatty acids in normal and diabetic dogs. J Clin invest 49:537, 1970
4. Galloway JA, Shuman CR: Profile, specific methods of management, and response of diabetic patients to anesthesia and surgery. In Statson JB (ed): International Anesthesiology Clinics, Vol. 5. Boston, Little, Brown, 1967, p 437
5. Greene NM: Inhalation Anesthetics and Carbohydrate Metabolism. Baltimore, Williams & Wilkins, 1963
6. Ngai SH, Papper EM: Metabolic Effects of Anesthesia. Springfield, Ill, Thomas, 1962
7. Greene NM: Carbohydrate metabolism and anesthesia. In Statson JB (ed): International Anesthesiology Clinics, Vol 5. Boston, Little, Brown, 1967, p 411
8. Galla SJ, Wilson EP: Hexose metabolism during halothane anesthesia in dogs. Anesthesiology 25:96, 1964
9. Henneman DH, Bunker JP: Effects of general anesthesia on peripheral blood levels of carbohydrate and fat metabolites and serum inorganic phosphorus. J Pharmacol Exp Ther 133:253, 1961
10. Katz J, Kadis LB: Anesthesia and Uncommon Diseases: Pathophysiologic and Clinical Correlations. Philadelphia, Saunders, 1963
11. Brunner EA: Anesthesia and the endocrine pancreas. Anesthesiology 41:1, 1974

chapter 27

The Adrenal Glands

Each adrenal gland is composed of two parts: the adrenal cortex and the adrenal medulla.

The division of *the adrenal cortex* into three zones is functional as well as structural:

1. The *zona glomerulosa* secretes mineralocorticoids, mainly aldosterone. Excessive production of this hormone results in aldosteronism.
2. The *zona fasciculata* secretes glucocorticoids, of which hydrocortisone is the main representative. Inadequate amounts of this hormone produce Addison's disease. Excessive production of glucocorticoids is responsible for the development of Cushing's syndrome. The function of zona fasciculata is under the influence of ACTH from the adenohypophysis.
3. The *zona reticularis* produces androgens and estrogens.

The *adrenal medulla* secretes epinephrine and norepinephrine in response to sympathetic stimulation. The effect of these two hormones on various body functions is similar to the effect of direct stimulation of the sympathetic nerves.

MINERALOCORTICOIDS

The most important effect of the mineralocorticoids is the decrease in the rate of tubular reabsorption of sodium. Without the mineralocorticoids, the sodium and chloride concentrations in the blood decrease. The volume of extracellular fluids also depends on the adequate mineralocorticoid secretion.

Aldosterone, corticosterone, and deoxycorticosterone are the three mineralocorticoids. Aldosterone is, by far, the main representative and exerts its effect on the distal tubule, collecting tubule, and part of the loop of Henle in the kidneys. Aldosterone has two basic effects: (1) it increases renal tubular reabsorption of sodium and (2) it increases renal excretion of potassium.

Inadequate production of aldosterone may be the result of either surgical removal or disease of the adrenal cortices. Primary hypoaldosteronism is a rare entity and hypoaldosteronism is on most occcasions accompanied by other corticosteroid deficiencies as well.

Regulation of Aldosterone Secretion

There are three (Fig. 27-1) theories concerning the mechanism of secretion of aldosterone: (1) renin–angiotensin mechanism, (2) direct stimulation of the adrenal cortex, and (3) neurosecretory regulation.

RENIN–ANGIOTENSIN REGULATION

Renin secretion is stimulated when circulation to the kidneys is inadequate. Renin acts and converts angiotensinogen to angiotensin I and

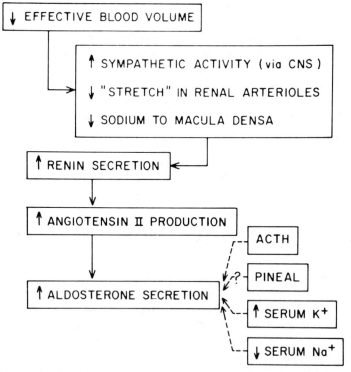

FIG. 27-1: Factors that stimulate secretion of aldosterone. (Reproduced with permission from Little, Brown.[19])

angiotensin II. Angiotensin II causes an increase in the aldosterone secretion rate. Aldosterone increases Na$^+$ reabsorption and restores effective renal blood volume.[1]

DIRECT STIMULATION OF ADRENAL CORTEX

The output of aldosterone increases when blood containing a low concentration of sodium and an excess of potassium is infused into the adrenal artery.

NEUROSECRETORY CONTROL OF ADRENOCORTICAL SECRETION

Corticotropin (ACTH) is the primary regulator of glucocorticoid secretion and, to a certain degree, that of aldosterone.

Hyperaldosteronism

Hyperaldosteronism may be the result of: (1) a single functioning tumor, (2) multiple ademomatous nodules, or (3) adrenocortical hyperplasia.

The classic features of hyperaldosteronism are hypertension, hypokalemia, and increased urinary secretion of aldosterone. Clinically, the full-blown disease manifests itself with muscular weakness, tetany, polydipsia, polyuria, paresthesia, and headaches.

ALDOSTERONE, SURGERY, AND ANESTHESIA

Surgery is performed to remove a single aldosterone-producing adenoma or, occasionally, to remove both adrenal glands with multiple adenomatous nodules.

Potassium loss creates the major problems with regard to anesthesia for patients with hyperaldosteronism. Metabolic alkalosis develops as a consequence of hypokalemia. There are difficulties in maintaining the water balance. The antihypertensive treatment with diuretics can contribute to the potassium depletion.

In preoperative preparation, the hypokalemia and the alkalosis should be corrected. This is done by administering large oral doses of potassium, despite the fact that this may further increase the secretion of aldosterone.

Postoperatively, careful monitoring of serum electrolytes, body weight, and salt and water balance should be done. If necessary, the patient should be placed on steroid replacement.

GLUCOCORTICOIDS

The main glucocorticoid secreted by the adrenal gland is cortisol, also known as hydrocortisone or compound F. Corticosterone and cortisone are also secreted in small amounts.

Regulation of Cortisol Secretion

Corticotropin (ACTH), secreted by the adenohypophysis, stimulates the adrenal cortex to secrete large quantities of glucocorticoids and small quantities of mineralocorticoids. The secretion of ACTH is mainly under the control of the hypothalamus and, if the hypothalamic–hypophyseal portal system is intact, the corticotropin secretion can be greatly enhanced by physiologic stress.

The adenohypophysis responds with decreased production of ACTH when the level of cortisol concentration in the blood is elevated. This is accomplished by the negative feedback mechanism that exists between the adenohypophysis and the adrenals.

Stress, whether physical or neurogenic, causes increased corticotropin secretion, followed by an increased secretion of cortisol. This reaction to stress is fast, and takes place within minutes.[2]

Effects of Cortisol on Carbohydrate, Protein, and Fat Metabolism

STIMULATION OF GLUCONEOGENESIS

The main metabolic effect of cortisol is to enhance the gluconeogenesis by the liver, often increasing it by as much as sixfold to tenfold, and to inhibit the utilization of glucose by the cells. The increased gluconeogenesis results in an increase in the glycogen found in the liver cells. The increased rate of gluconeogenesis and the resultant impaired glucose utilization lead to an increase in blood glucose concentration. Cortisol also stimulates the enzyme glucose 6-phosphatase in the liver, which catalyzes the dephosphorylation of glucose.

Excessive secretion of glucocorticoids leads to hyperglycemia and glycosuria, generally called "steroid diabetes." The administration of insulin for this condition lowers the blood glucose concentration somewhat.

Cortisol decreases the anabolism and increases the catabolism of proteins and, thereby, diminishes the protein stored in the cells.

Cortisol promotes fatty acid utilization instead of glucose for energy production.

Effect of Cortisol on Inflammation and Immunity

Large amounts of glucocorticoid administered to a person prevents the development of inflammatory reactions. Inflammatory processes are accompanied by a destruction of tissues because of the release of lysosomal enzymes. Cortisol and other glucocorticoids stabilize the membranes of cellular lysosomes and prevent the enzyme release.

Another factor of importance is the ability of cortisol to decrease the formation of bradykinin.

Cortisol decreases the permeability of the capillary membrane and, thus, prevents the leakage of protein into the inflamed tissues. Cortisol administration in large doses causes atrophy of all lymphoid tissue in the body and, hence, helps to diminish the production of antibodies.

ADRENAL SEX HORMONE

The adrenal cortex secretes mainly androgens and small quantities of progesterone and estrogens. Disturbance in the secretion of the adrenal sex hormone does not usually present a problem to the anesthesiologist.

Abnormalities of Adrenocortical Secretion

HYPOADRENOCORTICISM

Adrenocortical deficiency may develop as a result of (1) primary atrophy, tuberculous destruction, or cancer of adrenal corticies (Addison's disease); (2) ACTH deficiency, causing mainly insufficient secretion of glucocorticoids; or (3) prolonged administration of corticosteroids, which suppresses the patient's pituitary–adrenal axis.

The patient who is afflicted with Addison's disease has disturbances caused by mineralocorticoid and glucocorticoid deficiencies. Loss of aldosterone secretion leads to a decrease in extracellular fluid volume secondary to decreased sodium reabsorption. Chloride ions and water are lost into the urine. As a result, the plasma volume and cardiac output diminishes.

Loss of cortisol secretion causes a severe fall in blood glucose concentration between meals. Most metabolic functions of the body are depressed because of reduced mobilization of proteins and fats.

The patient with Addison's disease develops melanin pigmentation of the skin. The lack of glucocorticoid secretion makes the person very susceptible to infections. Any type of stress, even a mild one, can precipitate death.

The diagnosis is made by demonstrating low levels of steroids derived from the adrenals, either in the plasma or in a 24-hour urine specimen. However, to make a positive diagnosis, corticotropin (ACTH) is infused over an 8-hour period and the level of 17-hydroxysteroids in plasma or urine is measured. In Addison's disease, there will be no increase of 17-hydroxysteroids. If the failure of the adrenals is due to a failure of the adenohypophysis, the infusion of ACTH will cause normal secretion of 17-hydroxysteroids.

Deficiency of cortisol, regardless of the etiology, should be treated with large doses of corticosteroids before and during a surgical intervention. The equivalent doses of various glucocorticoids are as follows: cortisone, 5 mg; hydrocortisone, 4 mg; prednisone, 1 mg; prednisolone, 1 mg; methylprednisolone, 0.75 mg; betamethasone, 0.15 mg; and dexamethasone, 0.15 mg.

The normal physiologic output of the adrenal glands is equivalent to about 20 to 25 mg of cortisone a day; therefore, the daily maintenance dose of cortisone, in case of absence of any adrenal function, should not exceed this dose.

Preoperative and postoperative management. A patient with chronic hypoadrenocorticism is characterized by hyponatremia, hyperkalemia, low blood volume, hypotension, and hypoglycemia. Thus, such a patient is a very poor surgical and anesthetic risk, in whom acute circulatory collapse is imminent.

A patient who has been receiving steroids for any period of time may have depressed adrenal function and may develop acute circulatory collapse. Since the degree of adrenocortical suppression, following steroid treatment, cannot be accurately determined, administration of steroids prophylactically has been advocated.[3] The following regimen is suggested by Wylie and Churchill-Davidson:[4] On the day before surgery, administer 100 mg i.m. of cortisone acetate. On the day of surgery, administer the same amount of cortisone acetate and hydrocortisone sodium succinate 100 mg either i.m. 2 to 3 hours before surgery or i.v. during or immediately after surgery. On the day after surgery, administer 100 mg i.m. of cortisone acetate.

Postoperatively, the dose of cortisone acetate is decreased until a maintenance dose of 30 mg a day is achieved.

HYPERADRENOCORTICISM

Excessive levels of glucocorticoids may result from endogenous sources, such as from an excess of ACTH stimulation due to a basophilic adenoma of the pituitary or from hyperfunction of the adrenal cortex due to hyperplasia, adenoma, or carcinoma. The symptoms are the same, whether caused by endogenous secretion or by exogenous administration of corticosteroids. The clinical picture is that of Cushing's syndrome, with main features of a round, red face, arterial hypertension, impaired glucose tolerance, osteoporosis, muscle weakness, and impaired growth.

Intravenous cortisol should be given if bilateral adrenalectomy is performed. The function of the other adrenal gland is suppressed if adenoma or carcinoma of one adrenal gland is hypersecreting. In such cases, intravenous cortisol should be administered to enable the normal gland to resume function.

Operative and postoperative management. The majority of problems encountered in operative management of adrenal cortical hyperfunction are related to diabetes, hypokalemia, osteoporosis, and hypertension.[3]

If insulin is used prior to surgery, one-half to one-third of the dose of the long-acting insulin should be administered on the morning of the operation. Glucose solution with added crystalline insulin should be given intraoperatively.

The hypokalemia should be corrected with supplemental oral preoperative intake of potassium chloride. A low potassium condition, with muscle wasting, can interfere with adequate spontaneous ventilation; therefore, assisted or controlled ventilation is recommended.

Hypertension, polycythemia, and increased total blood volume can lead to congestive heart failure.

During the postoperative period, the same problems exist. The steroid therapy, if started prior to surgery, should be continued. A daily supplement of potassium chloride should be given intravenously, until fluids and electrolytes can be taken orally.

Premedication. Morphine[5] and short-acting barbiturates[6] have been thought to depress adrenocortical activity; however, in doses used for premedication, they do not inhibit the adrenocortical response to the stress of surgery.[7] Meperidine in combination with atropine used as premedication does not alter the cortisol level in the plasma.[8]

Anesthetic agents. Diethyl ether and cyclopropane stimulate the production of ACTH and cortisone. Induction with thiopental may decrease the rise in plasma levels of glucocorticoids following administration of an inhalation agent.[9]

Halothane and methoxyflurane administration tend to raise the plasma cortisol levels; halothane to a greater degree.[8]

Regional anesthesia prevents the adrenocortical hyperfunction that results from the operation.[10] However, this finding was not confirmed by Johnston,[11] who found plasma cortisol levels to be elevated in a patient during prolonged spinal anesthesia.

It has to be pointed out that changes caused by anesthetic agents and techniques are very insignificant when compared with the rise in the secretion of cortisol, which occurs during and after surgery.[12]

THE ADRENAL MEDULLA

The adrenal medulla synthesizes the catecholamines epinephrine and norepinephrine. Although nerve endings can also synthetize norepinephrine to a small extent, only the adrenal medulla is capable of methylating norepinephrine to epinephrine.

The half-life of both compounds in the circulation is less than 1 minute. The rapid metabolism is due to the action of monoaminooxidase and catechol-o-methyl transferase. The end products of the metabolism include 3-methoxy-4-hydroxymandelic acid (VMA), and metanephrine (Fig. 27-2).

Main Pharmacologic Actions of Epinephrine and Norepinephrine

Overall, the responses to epinephrine resemble the effects of stimulation of sympathetic nerves. The differences are due to norepinephrine, which has a predominant alpha effect, whereas epinephrine stimulates both the alpha and beta receptors.

BLOOD PRESSURE

Epinephrine has a very potent vasopressor effect. It constricts the vessels of the skin, mucosa, and kidney. It also causes direct myocardial stimulation that increases the contractibility and the rate of the heart. As a result, epinephrine raises the blood pressure. However, when epinephrine is administered in minute doses of 0.1 μg per kg it may cause a fall in blood pressure below the normal level.[13] This is due to the greater sensitivity of beta receptors in vascular beds dilated by the drug. Norepinephrine also raises the blood pressure.

VASCULAR EFFECTS

Epinephrine, as pointed out, constricts the blood vessels of the skin, mucosa, and kidney by acting on the alpha receptors, and dilates the vessels to the skeletal muscles, by acting on their beta receptors.

Norepinephrine predominantly acts on alpha receptors and has beta receptor action only on the heart. It increases the total peripheral resistance by constricting the vessels of most vascular beds.

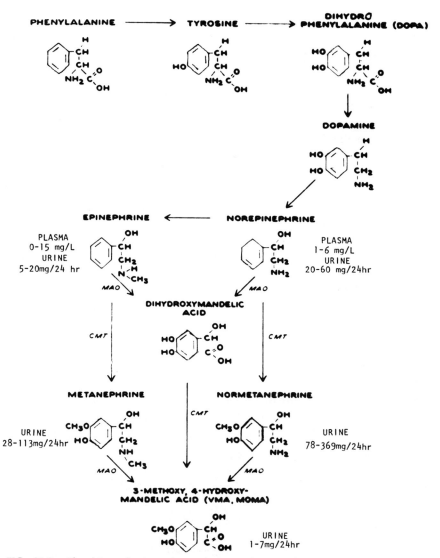

FIG. 27-2: The biosynthesis and metabolism of epinephrine and norepinephrine. (Reproduced with permission from A. Goldfien.[20])

CARDIAC EFFECTS

Epinephrine stimulates the heart by acting directly on beta receptors of the myocardium, pacemaker, and conducting tissue. The heart rate increases and the systole is shorter and more powerful; as a result, the cardiac output is enhanced.

Norepinephrine does not change the cardiac output. The coronary blood flow is increased due to coronary dilatation and elevated blood pressure.

RESPIRATORY EFFECTS

Epinephrine stimulates the respiration to a certain degree and has powerful bronchodilatatory action. Norepinephrine causes slight increase in respiratory volume.

METABOLIC EFFECTS

Epinephrine has a potent hyperglycemic effect. This action is attributed to stimulation of glycogenolysis in the liver. It also raises the concentration of free fatty acids in the blood (Fig. 27-3).

The epinephrine secreted by the adrenal medulla increases the metabolic rate often twice that of the normal.

Norepinephrine has similar metabolic effects. The adrenal medulla secretes about 75 percent epinephrine and about 25 percent norepinephrine.

Importance of Adrenal Medulla

The value of the adrenal medullae is that they are capable of supporting and even substituting for the action of the sympathetic nerves. The secreted catecholamines are also capable of stimulating structures that have no direct sympathetic innervation.

INNERVATION OF ADRENAL MEDULLA

Only preganglionic fibers from the sympathetic nervous system reach the adrenal medulla, and they secrete acetyl choline at the synapses.

PHEOCHROMOCYTOMA

This is a tumor of chromaffin tissue which usually originates in the adrenal medulla, but may also be found in aberrant tissue along the sym-

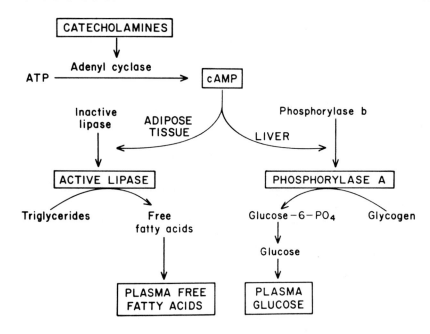

FIG. 27-3: Some metabolic effects of catecholamines: the mechanism of stimulation of lipolysis and glycogenolysis. (Reproduced with permission from Little, Brown.[19])

pathetic nerve chain. Most of the pheochromocytomas are physiologically active and secrete epinephrine and norepinephrine in varying proportions.

Clinical symptoms and signs. The classic picture is the pale calming agitation of the hypertensive crisis.[14] The patient complains of sweating, palpitations, and headache. The diagnosis may be suspected during an operation for an unrelated disease when blood pressure becomes very unstable.

If untreated, pheochromocytoma eventually leads to permanently elevated systolic and diastolic pressures. The basal metabolic rate frequently is increased and a misdiagnosis of hyperthyroidism may be made.

Diagnosis. The history is frequently very suggestive. The normal value of total catecholamine concentration in plasma is 0.3 to 0.6 μg per liter. Epinephrine is usually less than 0.1 μg per liter and norepinephrine is 0.3 to 0.5 μg per liter.

However, in the majority of cases, a 24-hour urine specimen for determination of VMA or catecholamines is enough to make the diagnosis. Normal values for VMA are between 2 and 6 mg per 24-hour urine; catecholamines, 300 mg per 24-hour urine. The test of choice is the quantity of metanephrine excreted per 24-hour urine, which normally is 0.5 to 1.3 mg. Occasionally, the histamine and phentolamine (Regitine) tests are also used.

Preoperative preparation and anesthesia.   The preoperative preparation of the patient with pheochromocytoma is aimed at minimizing the risk from
hypertension, hypotension, and ventricular arrhythmia.

Hypertension is preoperatively best controlled by treatment with the
alpha-blocking agents phentolamine (Regitine) and phenoxybenzamine (Diben-
zyline). The patient may have marked reduction of blood volume due to
continuous vasoconstriction.[15] The pretreatment with alpha-blocking agents
helps to restore normal blood volume.

The ventricular arrhythmias commonly encountered can be controlled
with lidocaine or propranolol.

In the premedication order, atropine should be avoided.[16,17] The choice of
anesthetic agents is less important than is the understanding with which they
should be used. Smooth induction and intubation should be performed without
hypoxia and hypercapnia. Excellent muscle relaxation should be provided to
enable the surgeon to expose the retroperitoneal tumor with minimal manipu-
lation and retraction.

Hypertensive episodes during the operative procedure are best controlled
by phentolamine. It is usually administered in increments of 2.5 mg i.v. at
intervals of 45 to 60 seconds until blood pressure is lowered to the desired level.
An infusion of phentolamine can also be used.

Hypotension usually occurs after the ligation of the venous drainage of the
tumor, because the concentration of norepinephrine and epinephrine in the
blood falls rapidly. This condition should be treated with rapid administration
of blood, plasma, and electrolyte solution. The central venous pressure should
be carefully monitored. Norepinephrine or metaraminol (Aramine) have been
recommended under certain hypotensive conditions.[18]

REFERENCES

1. Dobson EL: The Regulation of volume in body fluid homeostasis. Presented at the
   16th Postgraduate Assembly on Anesthesiology, New York, New York State Society
   of Anesthesiology, 1962
2. Liddle GW, Island DP, Meador CK: Normal and abnormal regulation of
   corticotropin secretion in man. Rec Prog Horm Res 18:125, 1962
3. Cahill CF, Jr, Thorn GW: Preoperative and postoperative management of adrenal
   cortical hyperfunction. Anesthesiology 24:472, 1963
4. Wylie WD, Churchill-Davidson HC (eds): A Practice of Anesthesia. Chicago, Year
   Book, 1972, p 1363
5. Briggs FN, Munson PL: Studies on the mechanism of stimulation of ACTH secretion with the aid of morphine as a blocking agent. Endocrinology 57:205, 1955
6. Vandam LD, Moore FD: Adrenocortical mechanisms related to anesthesia.
   Anesthesiology 21:531, 1960
7. Van Brunt EE, Ganong WF: The effects of preanesthetic medication, anesthesia
   and hypothermia on the endocrine response to injury. Anesthesiology 24:500, 1963

8. Nishioka K, Levy AA, Dobkin AB: Effect of halothane and methoxyflurane anaesthesia on plasma cortisol concentration in relation to major surgery. Can Anaesth Soc J 15:441, 1968
9. Oyama T, Shibata S, Matusmoto F, et al: Effects of halothane anaesthesia and surgery on adrenocortical function in man. Can Anaesth Soc J 15:258, 1968
10. Hume DM, Bell CC, Barter F: Direct measurement of adrenal secretion during operative trauma and convalescence. Surgery 52:174, 1962
11. Johnston IDA: Endocrine aspects of the metabolic response to surgical operation. Ann R Coll Surg Engl 35:270, 1964
12. Brown PS, Clark CG, Crooks J, et al: Thyroid and adrenocortical responses to surgical operation. Clin Sci (Lond) 27:447, 1964
13. Goodman LS, Gilman A (eds): The Pharmacological Basis of Therapeutics, 5th ed. New York, MacMillan, 1975, p 484
14. Ross EJ: Pheochromocytoma: medical aspects. Proc R Soc Med 55:427, 1962
15. Brunjes S, Johns VJ, Crane MG: Pheochromocytoma: postoperative shock and blood volume. N Engl J Med 262:393, 1960
16. Rosenberg JC, Varco RL: Physiologic and pharmacologic considerations in the management of pheochromocytoma. Surg Clin North Am 47:1453, 1967
17. Cooperman LH, Engelman K, Mann PEG: Anesthetic management of pheochromocytoma employing halothane and beta adrenergic blockade. Anesthesiology 28:575, 1967
18. Mathews WA, Crandell DL: Pheochromocytoma. In Jenkins MT (ed): Anesthesia for Patients with Endocrine Disease. Philadelphia, Davis, 1963, p 92
19. Sawin CT: The Hormones, Endocrine Physiology. Boston, Little, Brown, 1969
20. Goldfien A: Pheochromocytoma: diagnosis and anesthetic and surgical management. Anesthesiology 24:463, 1963

Section V

The Kidney and Body Fluids

chapter 28

Body Fluids and Electrolytes

Water is the most abundant single constituent of the body, representing more than half of the body weight. The percentage of body water relative to body weight diminishes with the increase in age of the individual, the highest being at the newborn stage, when it represents 70 percent of his mass. In the adult male, it constitutes 60 percent of his weight whereas in the female it is 50 percent.[1] The main reason for this sex difference is that females tend to have a greater percentage of adipose tissue, and fat, being an essentially anhydrous tissue (water content 10 to 20 percent), contributes more to the weight than the water content of the body.[2]

Water is very important for the viability of the body organism; it is the medium in which all the metabolic reactions occur, and all the nutrients and the solutes of the body are dissolved or suspended in it. Body water content is remarkably constant in healthy individuals despite its rapid turnover rate.

BODY FLUID COMPARTMENTS

Traditionally, the body fluid has been divided into two major compartments according to their location relative to the cell membrane.

Intracellular Fluid

This fluid represents all the water with its solutes present inside the cells. It is in this medium that all the essential chemical reactions of the body occur. The water present inside the red cell is a part of this compartment.

345

Extracellular Fluid

This fluid represents all the fluids surrounding the cells. The extracellular fluid space is further divided into two major compartments by the capillary membrane: plasma volume and interstitial fluid. The interstitial fluid also include the lymph and the extracellular portion of the dense connective tissues such as bone and cartilage. Another small compartment (1 to 2 percent of body weight) incorporated in a few of the techniques that measure the extracellular fluids is the "trancellular compartment," which consists of the fluids present in the body cavities, such as the secretions of the gastrointestinal tract, the urine in the bladder, and the cerebrospinal and the intraocular fluids.

Measurement of Body Fluid Compartments

The measurements of body fluid compartments are based on the *indicator dilution principle,* in which a measured amount of the indicator is given, and after an equilibrium is reached, the plasma is analyzed for the concentration of the indicator. By knowing the distribution characteristics of the indicator within the compartments of the body water, the volume distribution of the substance can be determined by the following formula:

$$\text{Volume of compartment} = \frac{\text{Amount administered}}{\text{Concentration}}$$

For this technique to be accurate, the indicator should meet certain basic conditions:

1. It should be distributed evenly in the measured compartment and should not enter other compartments.
2. Its plasma concentration should be similar to the compartment that is being measured.
3. If this drug is excreted during the equilibration period, it should be amenable to measurement, in order to apply the appropriate correction.
4. It should be nontoxic and by no means interfere with the normal distribution of the body water.

The total body water is the easiest and most accurate measurement that can be performed in the human being by this technique. The main reason is that trace forms of isotopic water such as heavy water, deuterium oxide (D_2O), and tritiated water behave essentially as water does, ie, they distribute, as water does, equally in all compartments (Fig. 28-1).

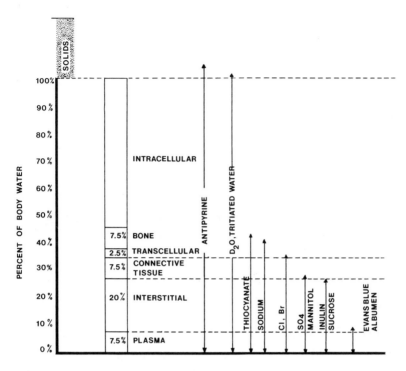

FIG. 28-1: The body water compartments and the surmised distribution of the indicators used in determination of these spaces.

In contrast to total body water, the extracellular volume is more difficult to measure. Because there is no one indicator that gives exactly the same volume as the other. The basic assumption here is that the indicator will diffuse through the capillary membranes and equilibrate throughout the interstitial fluid spaces and be halted by the cell membranes of every tissue of the body. However, not all capillary and cell membranes are alike. The substances used are either large molecular crystalloids, such as mannitol, inulin, and sucrose, or radioactive ions such as bromide, chloride, sulphate, or sodium. The first group gives a smaller volume because of their large molecules. The second group of the smaller ions penetrate the connective tissue spaces more rapidly than the larger molecules. It appears that the chloride (or bromide) space is the closest to true extracellular space, which also includes the connective tissue water that is in equilibrium with the extracellular space. Being divalent, sulphates are less likely than chloride to enter cells, and the former is the indicator used by Shires et al in their original studies[3] on fluid distribution in extracellular fluid associated with surgery.

The extracellular water represents about 18 percent of total body water. This is an estimated value that falls between the values measured with nonelectrolyte indicators and monovalent anions. The extracellular space is in dynamic equilibrium with the capacitance side of the vascular compartment. It is an available reservoir from which the water and electrolytes can be mobilized into the circulation. Conversely, it can accept large amounts of water and electrolytes if they are in excess.

For determination of plasma volume, the radioiodinated human serum albumin (RISA) or Evan Blue dye are commonly used. These two techniques give slightly inaccurate results because a small amount of these indicators is lost in the extravascular compartment. A more accurate measurement of blood volume can be performed by using tagged red cells. A radioactive molecule of chromium, iron, or phosphorus is incorporated in the erythrocyte and is injected intravenously. By measuring the radioactivity after it is thoroughly mixed in blood, the red cell volume is determined and the total blood volume is derived from the hematocrit.

There is no absolute way to determine the intracellular fluid volume. The only way is to subtract the extracellular fluid volume from the total body water.

Electrolyte Distribution

The distribution of electrolytes differs markedly from one compartment of the body to another. The major cations of plasma are sodium with small amounts of calcium, potassium, and magnesium; in contrast, the major cations of the cell are potassium with significantly larger amounts of magnesium and smaller amounts of sodium (Fig. 28-2).

Divalent ions such as calcium and magnesium (Ca^{++} and Mg^{++}) carry two charges in their molecules, in contrast to monovalent ions which carry only one charge. Thus 1 mmol of calcium carries double the electrical activity of 1 mmol of sodium and potassium.* Thus, 1 mmol of divalent cation equals 2 mEq. Whereas 1 mmol of monovalent ions such as Na^+ and K^+ is equivalent to 1 mEq.

In any of the body fluids for the maintenance of electrical neutrality, the number of positive charges should equal the number of negative charges. This does not imply that the number of particles with a positive charge (cations) should equal the number of particles with a negative charge (anions), eg, plasma proteins have several negative charges. Therefore, several cations are present opposite each molecule of protein.

The distribution of cations in the intracellular fluid spaces differs markedly from the extracellular spaces, potassium being the major cation inside the cell, whereas sodium is the major cation outside the cell. Thus, there is a large potassium gradient across the cell membrane from inside to outside, and a large sodium gradient in the opposite direction. The cell membrane is permeable to

* *mmol per liter is one-thousandth of the molecular weight of the substance in grams dissolved in 1 liter of water. mEq per liter = mmol per liter/valency.*

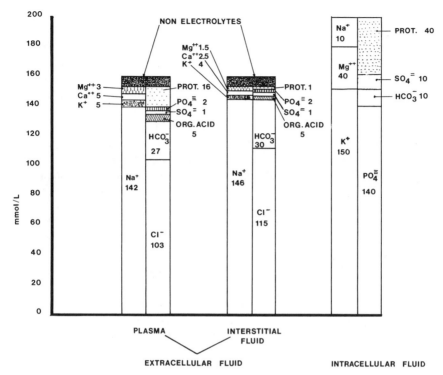

FIG. 28-2: Comparison of ionic compositions of extracellular and intracellular fluids (approximate).

these cations, but the difference in the concentration between these two is maintained by an active metabolic process through a set of pumps that can discriminate between these two ions. This unequal distribution of ions results in the setting up of a potential across the cell membrane with the interior of the cell being negative to the exterior.

The Osmotic Characteristics of Body Fluids

Osmosis is the movement of solvent (liquid) molecules across a semipermeable membrane from an area of lower concentration of the solute (solid) to an area of higher concentration, the semipermeable membrane being permeable to the solvent phase but not to the solute. The pressure necessary to prevent the migration of the solvent is known as the effective osmotic pressure of the solution. The osmotic properties of the solution depend on the number of particles (solvent) in a solution, regardless of the size or the charge of the particle.

The unit most commonly used for expression of osmotic property is the milliosmole (mOsm), which is a measure of particle concentration: mOsm = mmol × n, where n is the number of electrolyte particles produced by dissociation of 1 mmol of a given substance. For example, as sodium chloride dissociates in solution into two ions, Na^+ and Cl^-; therefore, n for sodium chloride is 2. Thus, 1 mmol of sodium chloride yields an osmotic pressure of 2 mOsm whereas glucose, which does not dissociate its mmol, produces an osmotic pressure of 1 mOsm. Calcium chloride, which dissociates into three particles (one calcium, two chlorides) yields 3 mOsm.

In the plasma, sodium is the most important cation, because it contributes the most to plasma osmolality. The contribution of potassium is minimal, whereas the contribution of calcium and magnesium are negligible because of their low concentration. Also half of the calcium is osmotically ineffective because it is bound to plasma proteins. On the anionic side, chloride and bicarbonate are the biggest contributors, each providing 1 mOsm for each 1 mEq, whereas the contribution of plasma proteins is minimal (less than 1 mOsm) because of their large molecular size, despite their high concentration. Of the nonelectrolyte solutes, glucose and urea are the biggest contributors, each providing about 5 mOsm.

Thus, more than 90 percent of the 290 mOsm per liter of plasma is made up of sodium and its accompanying cations, chloride and bicarbonate. Thus, an approximate osmolality of plasma can be obtained by multiplying the plasma sodium concentration by 2. A better formula that takes into consideration both blood glucose and urea nitrogen is:

$$\underset{\text{(mOsm per liter)}}{\text{Osmolality}} \quad = \quad \underset{\text{(mEq per liter)}}{2 \, [Na]^+} \quad + \quad \underset{\text{(mEq per liter)}}{2 \, [K]^+}$$

$$+ \quad \underset{\substack{2.8 \\ \text{(mg/100 ml)}}}{[BUN]} \quad + \quad \underset{\substack{18 \\ \text{(mg/100 ml)}}}{[Glucose]}$$

This method of calculating plasma osmolality is inaccurate in advanced hyperlipemic conditions. In this condition, a large amount of the plasma will be replaced by solids, and the plasma will contain less water (eg, 5 ml of each 100 of plasma will be solids). Although the sodium concentration of the available plasma will be normal, because sodium concentration is expressed as liters of whole plasma, the sodium concentration will be artificially low (120 mEq per liter). However, hyperlipemia of such an advanced degree can be readily recognized from the milky white color of plasma.

The sum of all the components of plasma contributing to its osmolality is about 300 mOsm per liter. However, plasma is not an ideal solution. Not all electrolytes are dissociated completely in it, and the ionic interaction diminishes the number of free particles that exert an osmotic effect. Thus, the effective osmotic pressure of plasma is 290 mOsm per liter.

Solutions that are administered to patients are classified according to tonicity, ie, their effective osmotic pressure relative to plasma. Thus, an isotonic solution exerts the same osmotic pressure as plasma. Those with a higher pressure are known as hypertonic and those with low pressures are known as hypotonic. Thus, a solution of 0.9 NaCl or 5 percent glucose is isotonic with plasma. However, as glucose becomes metabolized, the end result will be a hypotonic solution. Conversely, a solution of 5 percent dextrose in lactated Ringer's solution is initially a hypertonic solution (about 560 mOsm), but as glucose is taken up and metabolized, the hypertonicity diminishes.

THE EXTRACELLULAR SPACE

The functional extracellular space (interstitial lymph water)[1] is part of extracellular cells outside the vascular bed that is in dynamic equilibrium with the capacitance side of the vascular compartment. It contains about 20 percent of total body water and is a reservoir that can accept or donate large amounts of water and electrolytes. It consists of a gelatinous ground substance traversed by collagen fibers.[4] The pressure in this space is negative, varying between −4 to −8 mm Hg. As long as the pressure in this space is negative, it can retain a large amount of fluid in its gelatinous matrix in an immobile form. However, as fluid continues to accumulate in this space, the pressure in it increases. When it reaches near zero, its compliance increases rapidly and edema forms. This is one of the reasons that when large volumes of crystalloids are given to a normal man, the central venous pressure does not rise at the initial stages. However, once this space starts to be saturated, the venous pressure rises at a fast rate.

Besides this functional extracellular fluid space, there are two other pools of extracellular water, ie, the dense connective tissue and the bone water, each representing about 7 percent of total body water (equivalent to plasma volume). They appear to be in slow equilibrium with intracellular water and the functional extracellular volume. However, the connective tissue space is in more dynamic equilibrium with the interstitial spaces and sometimes is included as part of extracellular fluid space.

As a general rule, almost all chronic diseases are characterized by a fall in intracellular fluid volume and concomitant expansion of the extracellular space.

WATER BALANCE

Water is so important for the body that its intake as well as its output are closely regulated. Some of the water losses of the body, such as in evaporation or in feces are obligatory and cannot be altered. Whereas the urinary output and the voluntary intake of water are variable within a wide range.

The average water intake of an individual is between 2 and 3 liters per day or about 1 ml per kcal of food intake. About 15 percent of the daily water requirement of the body is derived from the nutrient metabolism through the oxidation of the hydrogen molecule, whereas the remainder is from the water present in the solid foods and, from drinking water and beverages, each contributing 40 to 50 percent of the fluid intake.

Under basal conditions, 40 percent of the water lost by the body is through the feces, skin, and expired air, while the remaining 60 percent is through the urine. A considerable amount of solute-free water is lost from the body by evaporation through the skin and the respiratory passages. Inspired air contains small amounts of water, whereas the expired air is fully saturated with water vapor. The amount of water lost by this route depends on the temperature and the humidity of the inspired air. In any condition in which the pulmonary ventilation is increased (eg, exercise, fever), the water lost by this route is increased.

Insensible perspiration is water lost from the body through evaporation from the moist tissues beneath the skin. It amounts to about 500 ml per day in the adult. Evaporation is a very efficient way of losing heat from the body. Evaporation of 1 ml of water requires 575 cal. It is estimated that in febrile states the caloric requirement is increased by 12 percent for every celsius degree rise in body temperature. Thus, in these people the fluid intake should be increased 12 percent for every Celsius degree rise in core temperature. Evaporation is a function of body surface area. Therefore, the insensible water loss is more important in infants in whom this ratio of body surface to volume is much higher than in adults.

Sweat is the secretion of the sweat glands of the skin. In contrast to insensible perspiration, which is pure water, sweat contains a significant amount of electrolytes and urea. Sweat is hypotonic (sodium, 48 mmol per liter; chloride, 40 mmol per liter; urea 28 mg/100 ml). Thus, excessive sweating will lead to hypertonicity of the body fluids if they are not adequately replaced. The amount of water lost through sweating is minimal in a person resting in a cool environment. However, it might be secreted at a rate of 2 liters per hour if heavy work is performed in an extremely hot environment.

Gastrointestinal Loss

Although a tremendous amount of water (about 8 liters) is secreted in the gastrointestinal tract, very little is excreted through the feces (only 50 to 200 ml per day). The remainder is reabsorbed in normal situations. Of these 8 liters, 1500 ml is saliva, 2500 ml is gastric secretion, 500 ml is bile, 700 ml is pancreatic secretions, and the largest component is the secretions of the small intestine, which amounts to 3000 ml. With the exception of saliva, which is hypotonic, all the secretions of the gastrointestinal tract are isotonic with the extracellular fluid space. A marked difference exists between the electrolyte composition of these fluids, eg, the main anion of the stomach is H^+, whereas the main anion in the secretion of bile and the small intestine is sodium. All of them contain an appreciable amount of potassium (5 to 10 mmol per liter). Almost all of the cations in the stomach are chlorides, whereas in the lower gastrointestinal secretions about one-third of the cations are in the form of bicarbonate, and the remainder are mostly chlorides (Fig. 28-3).

Adjustments of Water Balance

The two major variables regulating body water are thirst and renal tubular reabsorption of water.

THIRST

Thirst is a subjective sensory impression referred to the pharynx that leads to the desire for ingesting water. When a person is deprived of water, his salivary secretions are diminished, which results in the dryness of the mucous membrane of his mouth and throat. Atropine, which depresses salivary secretion, gives the same type of feeling. The hypothalamic thirst center can be stimulated from changes of the tonicity of the extracellular fluid relative to its

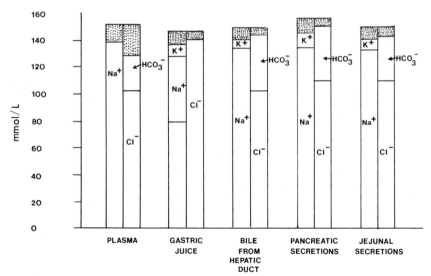

FIG. 28-3: Approximate composition of gastrointestinal secretions. (Adapted from Gamble.[25])

own osmotic pressure. For example, urea, which diffuses easily inside the cell, does not lead to increased water ingestion because it does not lead to changes in the ratio of extracellular to intracellular tonicity. This is in contrast to concentrated salt solutions that increase the tonicity of extracellular space and lead to the sensation of thirst. Thirst is also stimulated by several other mechanisms, such as loss of extracellular volume as in hemorrhage. The sensation of thirst in the human being is more complicated because several other factors contribute to its sensation beside water requirement. Emotional stress leads to thirst, and there are several cultural and social factors leading to drinking. If a person is allowed free access to water he will drink more than he needs to stay in balance, thus not exposing his kidneys to their maximum concentrating capacity.

RENAL WATER EXCRETION

Of the 120 ml of glomerular filtrate filtered every minute, only 20 ml reaches the collecting tubules. The volume of urine excreted can vary between 0.5 and 20 ml per minute depending on the presence of antidiuretic hormone (ADH). ADH is produced in the hypothalamus, stored in the posterior lobe of the thalamus, and released in circulation by the same mechanism that leads to the sensation of thirst. With extracellular hypertonicity, ADH is released, leading to water retention. Conversely, if the person is overhydrated, ADH secretion is suppressed and the water excretion increases. Also, in hypovolemia ADH secretion is increased, probably initiated from receptors in the left atrium. Conversely, alcohol inhibits ADH secretion, leading to polyurea.

Under normal conditions, urinary volume as well as its solute content can be varied independently. However, there is a maximum limit for the concentrating ability of the kidney. The minimum urinary volume will depend on the amount of solute (urea and electrolytes) presented to the kidney. The normal kidney can concentrate urine up to 1400 mOsm per liter (specific gravity, 1.035). Therefore, to be able to excrete the average daily solute load presented to the kidney, the minimal urinary volume should be 100 to 500 ml per day.

INTRACELLULAR FLUID

The intracellular fluids represent about two-thirds of the total body water. The composition of intracellular fluid is extremely difficult to measure directly and usually is derived indirectly also, its composition varying from one site to another.

Potassium is the most important intracellular cation. In the skeletal muscle its concentration is about 150 mmol per liter. This is in contrast to 4 mmol per liter of extracellular or plasma potassium. Thus, the plasma potassium levels reflect very poorly the total-body potassium. The body potassium content diminishes with the increase in age of the individual, indicating a progressive loss of lean body mass. Intracellular potassium can be determined by measuring the 24-hour exchangeable radioactive potassium (^{142}K). The potassium present in the leukocytes seems to be the most readily accessible for serial measurement and correlates better with total exchangeable potassium.[5]

In contrast to potassium, the calcium content of intracellular fluid is low (less than 0.1 mmol per liter) and most of this calcium is concentrated around the mitochondria and endoplasmic reticulum. Magnesium seems to be distributed in a similar manner.

The intracellular pH is more acidic than extracellular fluid, ranging from 6.8 to 7.2.[6]

The important anions of intracellular spaces are the proteins and the phosphate. The anionic content differs markedly from cell to cell, eg, skeletal muscles contain virtually no chloride, while red cells contain an appreciable amount. The intracellular anions are mostly polyvalent and too large to pass through the cell membrane. To prevent disruption of the cell membrane, intracellular fluids should be isotonic with the extracellular fluids, and the anionic charges should be equal to cationic charges intracellularly as well as extracellularly.

The only cation present inside the cell available for neutralizing these large anionic molecules is potassium. Although sodium is present in large amounts in the extracellular space, it is excluded from inside the cell because of the relatively low permeability of the cell membrane to sodium and by the sodium pump. Chloride also can move inside the cell, but is prevented by the high concentration of large molecular anions of the cells, which cannot move out. Thus, the only way to achieve electrical and osmotic equilibrium is by having a high level of intracellular potassium and a low chloride level. This discrepancy between the potassium and chloride is largely responsible for the recorded transmembrane potential, which is −60 to −80 mV.

The Sodium Pump

The cell membrane is less permeable to sodium than potassium. However, because of the high concentration of sodium in the extracellular space it continuously oozes into the cell. This is counterbalanced by the *sodium pump,* which is an energy-utilizing mechanism derived from adenosine triphosphate (ATP)[7] that pushes Na^+ outward and K^+ inward. The ratio of K^+ to Na^+ moved is about 2:3. This active transport (ATPase) mechanism is activated by Na^+ and K^+ and is inhibited by cardiac glycoside.

MAINTENANCE OF EXTRACELLULAR VOLUME

The body adjusts the volume of extracellular space by sensing its osmolality and its volume. The main sensor for osmolality is located in the hypothalamus. If an individual ingests a moderate amount of salt, it will be absorbed and the plasma and extracellular osmolality will rise. This rise in the osmolality of extracellular space, according to osmotic principles, will result in a shift of clear water from the intracellular to extracellular space. Thus, the intracellular space will shrink, which in turn will stimulate the thirst mechanism and the individual will drink more water. The shrinkage of the cells in the osmoreceptors of the hypothalamus leads to the release of ADH from the posterior pituitary, which in turn will lead to an increase in water reabsorption at the distal convoluted tubule. Thus, the urine osmolality (and concentration) will rise and its volume will fall. The net result of this mechanism (or loop) is an increase in the extracellular volume in an effort to keep its osmolality constant. The body then has to compensate for the rise in extracellular fluid compartments. This is accomplished through another mechanism (volume loop). The sensor of this loop is probably located in the left[8] or the right atrium.[9] Stretching the atria will stimulate the receptors in their walls, which will lead to diminution of aldosterone secretion, resulting in an increase in the sodium loss.

The atrial receptors do not seem to be the only afferents for aldosterone secretion, eg, diminution in the renal perfusion can be detected by the juxtaglomerular cells of the kidney that lead to the release of renin,[10] which in turn stimulates angiotensin II production, which is a powerful stimulant of aldosterone secretion.

The time constants of these salt and volume adjustments are different. The osmolality loop has a rapid time constant, the typical example being the prompt diuresis after excessive water drinking. The volume loop has a much slower course, eg, patients after isotonic saline infusion excrete it at a much slower rate within a few hours. However, changes in sodium excretion from changes in posture occur in a few minutes, while changes in sodium excretion after parenteral aldosterone occur after a lapse of at least 1 hour. Also, if aldosterone is given continuously, the body adjusts to the new situation. The extracellular volume increases up to a certain point; thereafter, additional administration of aldosterone does not lead to any further sodium retention.

ABNORMALITIES OF FLUID
AND ELECTROLYTE CONTENTS OF THE BODY

Dehydration

The condition of pure water deficiency is relatively rare in human beings. Most of the conditions leading to fluid loss in man are associated with electrolyte loss. Pure water deficiency occurs in pituitary diabetes insipidus, which results from distortion of the antidiuretic hormone mechanism. It can also occur when an individual is unable to drink either from loss of consciousness, paralysis or when water is simply unavailable. Because water is freely diffusible in all body compartments, the dehydration occurs in the extracellular as well as the intracellular compartments of the body. The plasma osmolality increases and the rise of intracellular osmolality stimulates the thirst mechanism. Occasionally, this condition is termed hypertonic or hyperosmotic dehydration, and the serum sodium concentration rises. When the total fluid loss is more than 10 percent of body weight, drowsiness followed by coma ensues. Individuals with diabetes insipidus can compensate by drinking a hugh quantity of water. However, if for any reason they are unable to ingest water, decompensation occurs rapidly.

Water Excess

Water excess can occur in renal failure (acute tubular necrosis) when the kidneys are unable to excrete the water taken in. It is also seen with some disorders of the anterior pituitary. In the condition known as inappropriate antidiuretic hormone (inappropriate ADH) secretion, which may occur after surgery, head trauma, or in certain tumors, the abnormal ADH is not under the control of the posterior pituitary. Thus, the level of the ADH is high despite the low plasma Na^+ and osmolality, and conversely the urine osmolality is high despite the low plasma osmolality. This syndrome is usually self-limiting and can be treated by restriction of fluid intake.

In all conditions of water excess, the plasma sodium level is decreased as well as its osmolality. There is cellular swelling and the consequences of this swelling become more manifest in the intracranial cells, where the volume is limited by the cavity of the skull. A rise of intracranial pressure occurs, which manifests as nausea, vomiting, headache, and coma.

Water overload can sometimes be seen in personality disorders in which the person compulsively drinks excessive amounts of water. This can be differentiated from true diabetes insipidus by the fact that plasma osmolality is lower than normal in this condition (higher than normal in diabetes insipidus), and water deprivation leads to a more concentrated urine than antidiuretic hormone administration.

Sodium Deficiency

Sodium deficiency is the most common situation that the anesthesiologist is confronted with. It occurs frequently when fluid is lost through the gastrointestinal tract, such as in protracted vomiting, intestinal obstruction, biliary and pancreatic fistula, or severe diarrhea. The fluids lost in these conditions are isotonic with plasma, but since the patient is drinking clear water or the fluids administered are hypotonic, part of the water loss is replaced while the sodium loss is not. The patient becomes more sodium depleted than water depleted. A solution of 5 percent dextrose is isotonic with plasma when transfused; therefore, hemolysis does not occur. As the glucose is taken up by the cells, the patient is left with an excessive hypotonic fluid load, and cellular overhydration occurs. A similar situation can be seen during excessive sweating. Sweat is hypotonic; however, if the sweat is replaced by drinking large quantities of water, then hyponatremia occurs, which is usually manifested as muscular cramps or fainting.

In conditions in which the cause of sodium loss is extrarenal in origin, the increase in aldosterone secretion leads to reabsorption of all the sodium present in the collecting tubules. Urine is virtually free from sodium. This is in contrast to sodium deficiency from intrinsic renal sources in which aldosterone is not very effective in reducing the sodium losses.

A large amount of sodium is lost in diabetic ketoacidosis, from vomiting and urinary excretion. A large part of the excreted ketoacids are accompanied by sodium and potassium in an effort by the kidney to neutralize these acids. Certain patients with chronic renal failure have an obligatory salt loss. Therefore, if their intake is diminished, they will end up with decreased sodium reserves.

Because sodium is the major cation of the extracellular space, the main effect of sodium depletion is a diminution of the extracellular volume. This condition usually manifests as postural hypotension, in which a fall of blood pressure of more than 5 mm Hg can be observed on standing. This is probably due to the inability of the capacitance vessels (venous) to respond by vasoconstriction. In the presence of diminished blood volume, thirst and oliguria are frequently seen. In the later stages, hypotension, tachycardia, and sweating occur, with a rise in blood urea levels. A characteristic feature of this condition is marked desaturation of venous blood from the sluggish circulation, which manifests as peripheral cyanosis.

Sodium Excess

Chronically ill patients with normal kidneys have a tendency to have raised body sodium stores, the exception being Addison's disease. Sodium retention is almost always accompanied by water retention. It occurs in any condition in which the drainage of fluid is impeded, ie, whenever there is increased pressure on the venous side of circulation, as in congestive heart failure or in lymphatic obstruction. It is also seen in hypoalbuminemia of the nephrotic syndrome. In the latter, the low plasma oncotic pressure will have a tendency to lower circulating blood volume, and through the stimulation of the renin–angiotensin–aldosterone mechanism, sodium and water retention occurs. Sodium retention also occurs in liver cirrhosis by two different mechanisms: first, the metabolism of aldosterone is impaired, and second, the increased pressure in the portal veins leads to a transudation of fluid in the peritoneal cavity, resulting in ascites. If the obstruction in the liver is postsinusoidal, the ascitic fluid is higher in protein content because of the high permeability of the sinusoids of the liver to proteins.[11]

Fluid Shifts during Surgery

The initial work of Shires et al,[3] in which they measured the functional extracellular fluid volume by radioactive sulfate during surgery, showed that there was marked diminution in the extracellular space on the order of 3 to 4 liters, which varied with the degree of trauma. This was assumed to be due to a shift of this part of the extracellular volume to another site, probably the operative site. However, there can be another explanation that has been neglected, namely that surgery might interfere with the distribution of the isotope. This study led to the overenthusiastic use of lactated Ringer's solution during surgery. Later studies failed to demonstrate such large changes of extracellular volume during surgery.[12]

However, moderate amounts of salt solutions have the advantage that they counteract the severe oliguria that occurs during surgery. Most authorities have agreed to providing moderate amounts of Ringer's lactate during surgery of about 2½ liters per day.[13] This is in addition to the replacement given for the blood loss during surgery. However, if one decides to replace moderate amounts of blood loss with electrolytes during surgery, the volume of the electrolyte solution should be about three times the amount of blood loss. Because of the administered salt solution, only one-third remains in circulation, while the remainder is distributed in the extracellular space.

Hypernatremia

Hypernatremia is defined as an increase in plasma sodium concentration and is frequently seen by the anesthetist in two conditions: (1) In overzealous administration of sodium bicarbonate during cardiopulmonary resuscitation, this hypernatremia with the associated hyperosmolarity is more hazardous in the newborn infant, in whom it can lead to intracranial hemorrhage.[14] (2) Relative hypernatremia from water depletion in which the water lost is in excess of the sodium lost. Thus, despite the rise in the serum sodium levels, the body sodium is diminished. This is frequently seen in comatose patients in whom concentrated protein feedings are given by an intragastric tube, and this is aggravated by the repeated administration of the diuretic mannitol. The associated hyperventilation and fever aggravate it further from increased fluid loss through evaporation.

The main danger in these patients is giving them a rapid infusion of 5 percent dextrose, which might lead to water intoxication.

Potassium Depletion

Trauma and acute as well as chronic diseases are associated with progressive potassium loss. A patient undergoing surgery loses about 100 mmol potassium in the first 2 days after surgery and later on loses about 25 mmol per day. This potassium loss is through the kidney.[15]

Potassium is lost whenever there is loss of gastrointestinal fluids either through excessive vomiting, fistulae, or severe diarrhea. In paralytic ileus, a large amount of potassium is held in the dilated nonperistaltic bowels. The most frequent cause of potassium depletion in clinical practice is iatrogenic, resulting from diuretic therapy. Most of the diuretics cause potassium depletion. This also occurs during primary aldosteronism. Potassium depletion is usually associated with Cl^- depletion, which can either be from the primary factor or from excessive Cl^- loss through the kidney.

To differentiate hypokalemia (potassium less than 3 mmol per liter) of renal origin from secondary hypokalemia as in gastrointestinal loss, the measurement of urinary potassium levels are very useful. If the 24-hour urine collection contains more than 20 to 30 mmol per liter of potassium, the hypokalemia is renal in origin, in contrast to patients with gastrointestinal potassium loss, who excrete far lesser amounts of potassium.[16]

The effect of hypokalemia is most dramatically manifested in the cardiac function. Depression of the S-T segment is seen and prolonged Q-T interval and U-waves are noted (Fig. 2-15). The incidence of cardiac arrhythmias, especially in the presence of digitalis, is increased; this includes multiple extrasystoles, tachycardia, and eventually ventricular fibrillation. Hypokalemia depresses the contractility of smooth muscles, perpetuating a paralytic ileus. It also might lead to tetany. Potassium losses of up to 10 percent of total body potassium are well tolerated. In severe depleting conditions, almost half of the total body potassium may be lost.

Hyperkalemia

In contrast to sodium, there is no known disease in which the total body potassium content is increased. An excess of potassium load is very effectively handled by the kidney. The only possible situation in which total body potassium can be raised is iatrogenic when potassium administration is continued on in the presence of impaired renal function. Hyperkalemia is seen with excessive muscle injury in which large amounts of potassium are liberated into the circulation. Succinylcholine in a severely burned patient or severely traumatized patients leads to a marked rise in plasma potassium levels. Hyperkalemia can also occur after the administration of intravenous solutions with high potassium content, during renal failure, or in the absence of aldosterone.

There is a very close distribution of the hydrogen ions and potassium ions at the cell membrane. Acidosis, particularly metabolic in origin, is associated with hyperkalemia and, conversely, alkalosis is associated with hypokalemia. The mechanism by which these changes occur is not well defined; it is partly renal and partly from the distribution of potassium between inside and outside the cell in an effort to keep the ratio of hydrogen and potassium ions constant intracellularly as well as extracellularly.[17]

The effect of hyperkalemia can be counteracted by increasing the serum calcium and sodium concentration and by administering insulin and glucose, which help in the movement of potassium from the extracellular to the intracellular space.

Fluid Redistribution after Hemorrhage

The immediate response of the body to a sudden reduction in blood volume is to maintain the blood supply to the vital organs, such as the heart and the brain. This is achieved by constricting the vascular bed, redistributing the blood from the nonvital areas, such as the splanchnic and skin vessels, to the vital areas, and by more efficient use of the remaining blood, ie, by circulating it at a faster rate (increasing the cardiac output).

As the blood volume is diminished, the plasma volume is refilled at the expense of the interstitial fluid volume. This is a much slower process and lasts for about 24 hours. The rate of refilling is higher at the beginning and slows down as it reaches the original blood volume.[18, 19] At this time the plasma protein and the hematocrit are diluted. The classic explanation of the refilling of the plasma volume is based on the original Starling concept (Chap. 5).

When the blood loss is moderate, there is no significant reduction in blood pressure, but there is slight diminution (1 to 2 cm H_2O) in the central venous pressure. This diminution of the venous pressure will reflect at the venous end of the capillary, leading to a diminution of its hydrostatic pressure. Therefore, transcapillary absorption will increase. Also the increased production of aldosterone and antidiuretic hormone helps the hemodilution and at the same time diminishes the urinary excretion of water and sodium.

The plasma proteins are diluted after hemorrhage. However, their dilution is less than that of the red cells, indicating that there is a net gain of intravascular albumin. This results from increased synthesis, decreased catabolism, and an increase in the albumin flow from the interstitial spaces into the blood through the thoracic ducts.[20]

THE RESPONSE OF THE BODY
TO SURGICAL TRAUMA

The metabolic response of the body to uncomplicated surgery is usually divided into three phases:[21] catabolic, early anabolic, and late anabolic. Obviously, the extent and duration of these responses depend on the magnitude of surgery and the associated trauma, blood loss, and complications.

Catabolic Phase

This stage lasts for about 5 to 7 days. The immediate response of the body to anesthesia, and surgery, with the associated pain and hemorrhage, is a transient increase in the secretion of adrenergic hormones and antidiuretic hormone. This is followed by a more prolonged increase in the secretion of adrenocortical hormones. Thus, in the first day or two after surgery, the urinary output is diminished, while its osmolality increases because of the antidiuretic hormone release and the changes in renal hemodynamics. This is associated with a Na^+ retention from the increased secretions of the adrenocortical hormones.

The metabolic rate is increased in the postoperative period, and this is often accompanied by a mild rise in body temperature. There is a negative nitrogen balance, which is more pronounced than what is seen during starvation. Body protein is catabolized at a rate of 75 to 150 g per day representing losses of 300 to 600 g of lean body mass (primarily muscle).[22] This negative nitrogen balance is directly related to the extent of surgery and is much more marked in extensive surgical procedures. This catabolic state and the increase of adrenocortical hormones lead to an increase in the urinary potassium loss. A surgical patient loses about 100 mmol of K^+ in the first 36 to 48 hours after a major surgical procedure, and later on this stabilizes to a constant of about 25 mmol per day.[23] The urinary ratio of K^+ to nitrogen exceeds the usual value of 3.0.

It has been long assumed that during the perioperative period the principal source of energy is glucose derived from liver glycogen, gluconeogenesis, and intravenous glucoses. However, recently it has been demonstrated that fatty acids and ketone bodies are the primary metabolic fuel in several organs (ie, myocardium, liver, and muscle)[24] and that fatty acid metabolism does not seem to be affected to the same extent as carbohydrate metabolism during anesthesia. An average person loses 2 to 4 kg in the postoperative period, and of the energy utilized in this interval, 25 percent is derived from fat, whereas the remainder is from intravenous solutions and from the lean tissues (average nitrogen loss, 16 to 18 g per day).

Early Anabolic Phase

This stage lasts for a few weeks. Because of the positive nitrogen balance, the nitrogen excretion diminishes. The K^+ balance becomes positive as new tissues start to form. The glucosteroid secretion becomes normal. In the early stages of this phase, the weight loss will continue for a short time because of the return of mineralocorticoid secretion towards the normal with less fluid and salt retention.

The beginning of this stage is considered to be the turning point in recovery from surgery, indicating that there is no more catabolism and no complications such as infection. It is interesting to note that wound healing takes priority. Even if the patient is in a catabolic state, the wound healing will continue at the expense of other tissues.

The metabolic rate is near normal at this stage. However, the rate of protein buildup is low (2 to 3 g per day). Thus, if the patient is given extra calories at this stage, it is deposited as fat. Several weeks are required to replenish all the tissues of lean body mass.

Late Anabolic Phase

This is a much slower phase in which the body weight returns to normal and all the lost fat depots are replenished.

REFERENCES

1. Edelman IS, Leibman J: Anatomy of body water and electrolytes. Am J Med 27:256, 1959
2. Bradbury MW: Physiology of body fluids and electrolytes. Br J Anaesth 45:937, 1973
3. Shires GT, Williams J, Brown FT: Acute changes in extracellular fluid associated with major surgical procedures. Ann Surg 154:803, 1961
4. Guyton AC, Scheel K, Murphree D: Interstitial fluid pressure: its effect on resistance to tissue fluid mobility. Circ Res 19:412, 1966
5. Patrick J, Bradford B: A comparison in leucocyte potassium content with other measurements in potassium depleted rabbits. Clin Sci 42:415, 1972
6. Waddell WN, Bates RG: Intracellular pH. Physiol Rev 49:285, 1969
7. Whittam R, Wheeler KP: Transport across cell membranes. Ann Rev Physiol 32:21, 1970
8. Ledsome JR, Linden RJ: The role of left atrial receptors in the diuretic response to left atrial distention. J Physiol (Lond) 198:487, 1968
9. Kappagoda CT, Linden RJ, Snow HM: The effect of stretching the superior vena caval-right atrial junction on right atrial receptors in the dog. J Physiol (Lond) 227:875, 1972

10. Vander AJ: Control of renin release. Physiol Rev 47:359, 1967
11. Orloff MJ: Pathogenesis and surgical treatment of intractible ascites associated with alcoholic cirrhosis. Ann NY Acad Sci 170:213, 1970
12. Gauer OH, Henry JP, Behn C: The regulation of extracellular fluid volume. Ann Rev Physiol 32:547, 1970
13. Moore FD, Shires GT: Editorial. Moderation. Surgery 166:300, 1967.
14. Simmons MA, Adcock EW, Bard H, et al: Hypernatremia and intracranial hemorrhage in neonates. N Engl J Med 291:6, 1974
15. Moore FD, Ball MR: The Metabolic Response to Surgery, American Lecture Series: 132 Springfield, Ill, Thomas, 1952
16. Harrington JT, Cohen JJ: Measurement of urinary electrolytes. Indications and limitations. N Engl J Med 293:1241, 1975
17. Brown EB, Goott B: Intracellular hydrogen ion changes and potassium movement. Am J Physiol 204:765, 1963
18. Lister J, McNeil IF, Marshall VC, et al: Transcapillary refilling after hemorrhage in normal man: basal rates and volumes. Effect of norepinephrine. Ann Surg 158:698, 1963
19. Moore FD: The effects of hemorrhage on body composition. N Engl J Med 273:567, 1965
20. Zollinger RM, Skillman JJ, Moore FD: Alterations in water, colloid and electrolyte distribution after hemorrhage. In Fox CL, Nahas GG (eds): Body Fluids Replacement in the Surgical Patient. New York, Grune, 1970
21. Kinney JM, Moore FD: Surgical metabolism in metabolism of body fluids. In Bland JB (ed): Clinical Metabolism of Body Water and Electrolytes. Philadelphia, Saunders, 1963
22. Felig P: Intravenous nutrition: fact and fancy. N Engl J Med 294:1455, 1976
23. Moore FD, Brennan MF: Current concepts in intravenous feeding. N Engl J Med 287:862, 1972
24. Biebuyck JB: Anesthesia and hepatic metabolism. Anesthesiology 39:188, 1973
25. Gamble DR, Wilbur DL: Chemistry of Digestive Diseases. Springfield, Ill, Thomas, 1961

chapter 29

The Kidney

The kidneys are among the most important organs of the body because their main function is to maintain a constant composition and volume of body fluids. The importance of their function is exemplified by the fact that despite their small weight of 300 g, which represents about 0.5 percent of total body weight, they receive about 20 percent of the resting cardiac output.

The kidneys are the flexible controllers of body water and electrolyte content. They maintain its osmolality and acidity constant. Through their intricate mechanisms, essential body nutrients, such as glucose and amino acids, are retained, whereas unwanted products, such as urea, uric acid, and creatinine, are excreted. They detoxify drugs besides excreting them and also produce hormones such as erythropoetin and renin.

FUNCTIONAL ANATOMY

The functional unit of kidney is the nephron. Each human kidney contains about 1,200,000 nephrons, and the number of nephrons does not increase after birth. In situations of compensatory hypertrophy, such as after nephrectomy, the increase in kidney size is due to increase in size of the nephrons, not the number. The main components of the nephron are the glomerulus, proximal convoluted tubules, the loop of Henle, and the distal convoluted tubule (Fig. 29-1).

The *glomerulus* is formed by invagination of a tuft of capillaries into the dilated blind end of the nephron (Bowman's capsule). The glomeruli are only found in the cortex of the kidney. The tuft of glomerular capillaries arises from an afferent arteriole and is drained by an efferent arteriole. Thus, the glomerular capillaries have a unique anatomic arrangement in which they are interposed between two sets of arterioles. Consequently, the hydrostatic pressure inside these capillaries can be varied by changing the tone of each of these arteriolar systems.

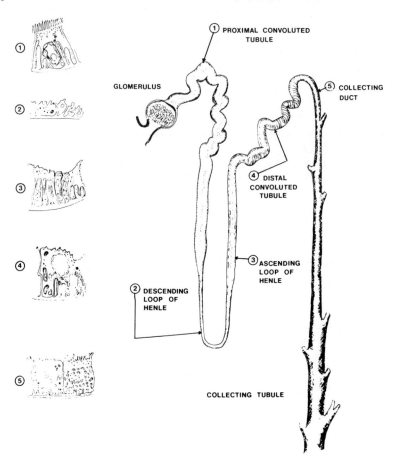

FIG. 29-1: A juxtamedullary nephron showing the basic structure of each segment.

The lumen of Bowman's space is in direct continuity with that of the proximal tubule. The ultrafiltrate present in Bowman's capsule is separated from the blood in the capillaries by three layers, ie, the capillary endothelium, the epithelium formed by the cells of Bowman's space, and the basement membrane interposed between these two layers (Fig. 29-2).

The cardiac action produces a hydrostatic pressure of about 50 mm Hg in the glomerular capillaries. This hydrostatic pressure pushes water, crystalloids, and low molecular weight substances into Bowman's space, whereas cells and substances with large molecular weights, such as plasma proteins, are held back. The cytoplasm of the capillary endothelial cells is attenuated and is riddled with pores. These pores have a diameter of about 1000 Å. The epithelial cells that form the visceral layer of Bowman's capsule are provided with foot-like processes known as podocytes. From these podocytes a multitude of small

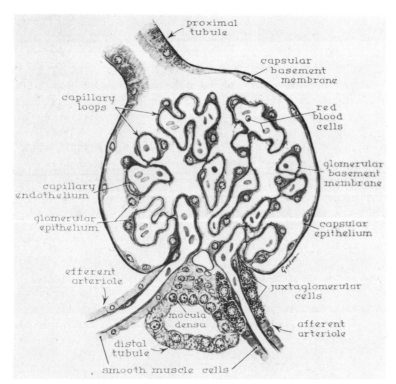

FIG. 29-2: Semidiagrammatic drawing of a renal corpuscle showing the juxta-glomerular apparatus. (Reproduced with permission from Lippincott.[1])

processes arise and plant themselves on the basement membrane of the capillary following its curvature. Protein particles with molecular weights less than 40,000 can easily pass through the three layers of the glomerulus, whereas protein particles with large molecular weights after passing through the endothelium and basement membrane are impeded in their further passage by the slits between the feet of the podocytes that rest on the basement membrane.[1]

The *proximal convoluted tubule* forms the major portion of the renal parenchyma, is in continuation with Bowman's capsule, is about 15 mm long (12 to 24 mm), and is highly convoluted. Most of it is located next to its own glomerulus, except the last part, which extends toward the medulla and is relatively straight (pars recta). The proximal convoluted tubular cells are composed of a single layer of interdigitating epithelial cells. The sides of these cells facing the lumen of the tubule have a prominent brush border made up of a very large number of microvilli. These microvilli increase tremendously the surface area of the membrane in contact with the tubular fluid.

Most of the sodium and chloride filtered in Bowman's capsule is reabsorbed in the proximal tubule (60 to 80 percent) into the blood through the peritubular capillaries via the tissue fluid at the base of these cells. The transfer of sodium is an active transport mechanism. This transfer of sodium and water in these tubules is isotonic, ie, the fluid reabsorbed has the same tonicity of plasma, indicating that concentration of solutes has not occurred yet.

Glucose is also actively reabsorbed in the first part of the proximal tubule. However, there is a maximum rate of transfer of glucose across the tubule (threshold). Above this threshold level, the system is saturated and glucose appears in the urine. Other substances are also actively transported across the tubular lumen. These include potassium, phosphate, amino acids, creatine, uric acid, and ketone bodies, and each of them has a different threshold level.

The proximal tubules are actively involved in the formation of hydrogen ions and ammonia. They also secrete into the urine the metabolic products of endogenous hormones and exogenous drugs.

The *loop of Henle* is the continuation of the straight segment of the proximal tubule. The descending limb is formed by thin epithelial cells that are relatively impermeable to sodium and chloride. The length of the thin segment of the loop varies between 2 and 14 mm. The last segment of the loop is composed of cuboidal cells. The thick ascending limb of the loop of Henle ends near its own glomerulus. At this point the cells are narrower and their nuclei are closely packed. This is known as the *macula densa*. The depth that the loop dips into the medulla varies according to the location of the glomerulus from which it is derived. About 85 percent of the loops are derived from cortical nephrons whose glomeruli are located in the outer two-thirds of the cortex, have short loops, and dip only for a short distance into the medulla before turning back to the cortex. The remaining 15 percent of the loops are derived from *juxtamedullary glomeruli* whose loops are long and penetrate deeply to near the tip of the papilla before turning back.

The ultrafiltrate formed at the glomerulus is isotonic with plasma. However, as the fluid passes along the descending loop of Henle, it becomes hypertonic, reaching its maximum osmolality at the top of the loop. The reason for this increase in osmolality is the outward diffusion of water and inward diffusion of solutes, mainly sodium, chloride, and urea. The osmolality of the fluid inside the loop of Henle is higher in the presence of antidiuretic hormone.

Animals living in a dry atmosphere, such as desert rodents, have the longest and the most developed loop of Henle, with a thick ascending portion. Thus, they can concentrate urine much more effectively.

The *distal convoluted tubule* begins at the macula densa. It is formed by convolutions similar to that of the proximal convoluted tubule. However, its length is about one-third of the proximal tubules and its epithelium is lower in height and lacks the brush border. The distal end of several of the convoluted tubules join together to form the *collecting ducts*. The distal tubule can reabsorb sodium and water at different rates, can exchange sodium for potassium and hydrogen ions, and can reabsorb calcium, chloride, and water. However, it is impermeable to urea. The osmolality and the volume of the luminal fluid in the distal tubule and the collecting duct are under the control of the antidiuretic hormone. It increases the permeability of the epithelium of the distal tubules and the collecting ducts to water. Thus, a small volume of concentrated urine is excreted. In its absence, a large amount of fluid remains in the collecting ducts. The urinary output increases while its osmolality drops to about 30 mOsm per liter.

The *juxtaglomerular apparatus* (Fig. 29-2) is the name given to the complex aggregation of the cells next to the glomerulus. It consists of the afferent and efferent arterioles, the macula densa, and some interstitial cells (juxtaglomerular mesangium). The cells in the media of the afferent arterioles contain granules. These granules contain the enzyme renin, which is synthesized within them and released in the circulation during hypotension or renal ischemia in an effort by the kidney to restore its own blood flow. The release of renin is influenced by several other factors, including anesthesia, sodium content of tubular fluid, and the pressure inside the afferent arterioles.[2] The beta receptors seem to be the sympathetic component involved in the release of renin and are stimulated by isoproterenol and blocked by beta blockers such as propranolol.[3]

THE RENAL CIRCULATION

The total renal blood flow is about 1.2 to 1.3 liters per minute, ie, one-quarter to one-fifth of the cardiac output. Each renal artery divides into two main branches. From each of these branches arise the interlobar arteries, which run between the pyramids of the medulla to the junction of the cortex with the medulla. At this level, they turn and run a more horizontal course, forming arterial arches known as arcuate arteries. From these arcuate arteries arise the interlobular arteries, which run outward through the cortex (Fig. 29-3). The interlobular arteries are known to be end arteries, ie, there is no anastomosis between them. However, blockade in one of them leads to the development of collaterals, mainly from capsular vessels.

The afferent arterioles arise from the interlobular arteries. They are short and muscular. They enter a glomeruli and break up into a tuft of glomerular capillaries, and these join together to form the efferent arterioles. The course of the blood beyond the efferent arteriole depends on the location of the glomeruli. In the outer and midcortex, the efferent arterioles subdivide into a capillary network surrounding the tubules of the same nephron before joining the confluent veins. In the inner cortex, the blood leaving the juxtamedullary glomeruli may take one of two pathways (Fig. 29-4):

1. A course similar to outer cortical peritubular vessels, ie, peritubular capillaries around the loop of Henle and the collecting ducts in the inner cortex and outer medulla, and then back to the interlobular veins

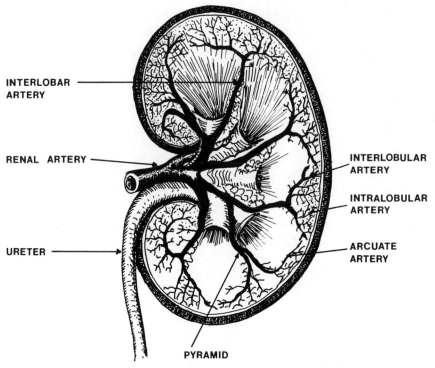

FIG. 29-3:   The distribution of the arteries in the kidney.

2.   Descend directly to inner medulla through the long descending vasa recta and return as the ascending vasa recta in the medullary bundles to the arcuate veins [4]

These long vessels are essentially the sole blood supply to the papilla. Also in these juxtamedullary nephrons, the efferent arteriole does not distribute itself around the convoluted tubule of the same nephron. They may be completely dissociated.

In the human kidney, the cortex receives about three-fourths of the total renal blood flow, which amounts to 4 ml per g of kidney tissue per minute, whereas juxtamedullary cortex and the outer medulla receive only one-fifth of the blood supply, amounting to 1 to 2 ml per g per minute in the outer medulla and less than 0.3 ml per g per minute in the inner medulla.

In the microcirculation of the renal cortex, fluid exchange occurs at very high rates in two anatomically and functionally distinct capillary systems. The first is at the glomeruli, in which net ultrafiltration occurs at the glomerulus at a rate of 125 ml per minute; 99 percent of this ultrafiltrate is reabsorbed during

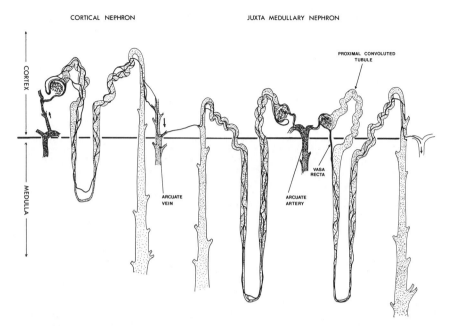

CORTICAL NEPHRON   JUXTA MEDULLARY NEPHRON

PROXIMAL CONVOLUTED TUBULE

VASA RECTA

ARCUATE VEIN

ARCUATE ARTERY

CORTEX

MEDULLA

FIG. 29-4: Diagrammatic representation of the blood distribution of a cortical (**A**) and juxtamedullary nephron (**B**). Note the two possibilities that the efferent artery from the juxtamedullary nephron can pursue: a similar course of an artery supplying a cortical nephron or dipping directly into the medulla as vasa recta.

its passage along the renal tubules and is returned to the circulation by a second set of capillaries, ie, the peritubular capillaries. This is in contrast to the peripheral circulation, in which the exchange occurs across the arterial and venous ends of the capillaries, whereas in the kidney it occurs across two distinct sets of capillaries connected in series by the efferent arteriole.

A subject that has perplexed nephrologists is the fact that renal blood flow may be reduced to one-third of normal in chronic renal failure with an adequate renal function to sustain life, whereas a similar reduction in acute situations such as hypotension or intravascular hemolysis leads to oliguria and renal insufficiency. One of the explanations is that during chronic renal failure, in which the number of functioning units is diminished, the remaining nephrons receive an adequate blood supply for filtration of a sufficient quantity of fluid, whereas an inadequate blood flow throughout the cortex invariably leads to oliguria. Also, the large vessels that branch in the subcapsular region supply the superficial part of the renal cortex. These vessels are very sensitive to sympathetic vasoconstrictor influence and may be the major vessels involved in superficial cortical ischemia.[4]

The *renal plasma flow* is measured by using Fick's principle. A substance with a high extraction ratio is used. The most commonly used agents are paraaminohippuric acid (PAH) or Diodrast. Ninety percent of a small dose of PAH is cleared through one circulation of the kidney. Thus, for practical purposes, the arterial and urinary PAH are determined by urinary volume measured, and from these effective renal plasma flow is calculated according to the formula:

Effective renal plasma flow

$$= \frac{\text{Urinary PAH level (mg per ml)} \times \text{urine volume (ml per minute)}}{\text{Plasma PAH (mg per ml)}}$$

Knowing the extraction ratio (90 percent for PAH), the renal plasma flow can be computed, and by knowing the hematocrit, the total renal blood flow can be estimated. By this technique, the total renal blood flow is 1 to 1.2 liters of blood per minute.

The sympathetics are vasoconstrictors to the renal blood vessels. Severe hypoxia leads to renal vasoconstriction, and this is mediated through the chemoreceptors. Small doses of catecholamines have more vasoconstrictor effects on the efferent arterioles than on the afferent ones. Thus, the glomerular filtration rate is maintained. However, in large doses they decrease the renal blood flow precipitously as well as the glomerular filtration rate.

Medullary Blood Flow

The main source of the renal medullary blood supply is the vasa recta derived from the efferent arteries of the juxtamedullary glomeruli. The blood flow in the renal medulla is rather poor compared to the cortex, representing about 6 to 7 percent of the total renal blood flow. The reason for this low flow is probably due to high resistance provided by these extraordinary long vessels. This circulation plays an important role in the countercurrent mechanism by controlling the rate of solute removal from the interstitium. Through these long loops of vessels, the osmolality of the renal medulla is kept high, at about 1200 mOsm at the tip of the renal papilla. This is achieved by shifting medullary solute from the hypertonic ascending limb to the interstitium and from there into the less concentrated descending limb.[5]

Autoregulation is the ability of the kidney to keep its blood flow constant within a wide range of mean arterial pressures of from 70 to 180 mm Hg. This is an intrinsic mechanism of the kidney, because it occurs in denervated as well as in innervated kidneys. It is prevented by drugs that paralyze smooth muscle, such as cyanide, or relax them, such as procaine or papaverine. In addition to the renal blood flow, the glomerular filtration is also regulated, by changes in the tone of preglomerular vascular segment.[6] This autoregulation seems to be absent during general anesthesia.[7]

GLOMERULAR FILTRATION

The cardiac action produces a hydrostatic pressure of about 50 mm Hg in the glomerular capillaries. This hydrostatic pressure is the driving force for filtration inside the glomeruli. The autoregulation of renal blood flow keeps the glomerular filtration constant by maintaining the hydrostatic pressure. The filtration in the glomeruli is opposed by the plasma oncotic pressure, the hydrostatic pressure inside Bowman's capsule, and the resistance of the glomerular wall.

The hydrostatic pressure inside the glomerular capillaries is higher than that of other capillary beds because the afferent arterioles are relatively short and direct branches of the large interlobular arteries. A further diminution in pressure occurs in the efferent arterioles, and the pressure in the peritubular capillaries drops to about 10 mm Hg.

The permeability of the glomerular capillaries is 100 times more than the peripheral (muscle) capillaries.[8] Proteins with small molecular weights like plasma proteins and hemoglobin (molecular weight, 68,000) are held by the podocytes. However, if the concentration of hemoglobin rises above a certain level, they are excreted in urine (hemoglobinuria).

Measurement of Glomerular Filtration Rate

The rate at which a substance is filtered through the glomeruli can be calculated by multiplying its concentration in plasma by the rate of formation of glomerular filtrate. Similarly, the rate of the excretion of this substance is the product of urine output and its concentration in urine. Glomerular filtration in man is measured by the above principle, and the marker which is used is inulin. Inulin is a polysaccharide, a polymer of fructose with a molecular weight of 5400, which is freely filtered through the glomerulus. Usually, inulin is given at a loading dose followed by a maintenance dose to keep the arterial level constant. After equilibration, the urinary as well as the plasma level of inulin are determined and the urine output is measured. Because all inulin present in the renal blood is excreted in one passage through the glomeruli and is neither reabsorbed nor secreted in the tubules, its filtration rate equals its excretion rate. Thus, the inulin clearance or, in other words, the glomerular filtration rate becomes:

Inulin clearance (ml/minute)

$$= \frac{\text{Urinary inulin conc. (mg/ml)} \times \text{urinary output (ml/minute)}}{\text{Plasma inulin conc (mg/ml)}}$$

In the normal man, the glomerular filtration rate determined by this technique is about 125 ml per minute. In females it is about 10 percent less. Thus, out of 660 ml per minute of plasma (1200 ml per minute blood) reaching the kidney, about 16 to 20 percent is filtered as glomerular filtrate. Sometimes this ratio is known as the filtration fraction.

If a substance is filtered through the glomeruli and its clearance is less than inulin, that indicates it is reabsorbed in the tubule. If it is higher than inulin, then it is also secreted in the tubule.

Clinically, creatinine clearance is used more frequently because it is a normally occurring substance with similar properties to inulin, ie, filtered freely through the glomeruli. But a small amount of creatinine is secreted by the tubules. However, the effect of this secreted part of creatinine is cancelled out during the calculation of its clearance because small amounts of other substances are included in the chromagenic determination of plasma creatinine.

TUBULAR FUNCTION

The function of the renal tubules can be classified into two main categories: reabsorption and secretion.

Tubular Reabsorption

About 80 percent of the sodium, chloride, and water filtered through the glomeruli is reabsorbed at the proximal tubule from inside of the tubules to the peritubular capillaries. The transfer of sodium from inside the cell, through the cell membrane, into the tissue fluid at the base of the cell, where the capillaries are located, is against a gradient. The only way to move this solute against this gradient is through a pump mechanism (sodium pump), and this requires energy. This reabsorption of sodium represents the greatest energy expenditure of the kidney. The transfer of chloride and water is passive. They follow the sodium ions in an effort to preserve the electroneutrality and isotonicity of the ultrafiltrate; therefore, the intraluminal fluid leaving the proximal tubule is still isotonic with plasma.

Glucose is another important metabolic product completely reabsorbed at the proximal tubule. It is also actively transported because glucose is an uncharged molecule, and its reabsorption is against a chemical gradient. The mechanism of glucose transport across the tubular cells is still obscure; supposedly a "carrier" exists, which combines with glucose at the luminal side of the cell and discharges it into the peritubular space. This glucose transport mechanism has a maximum capacity beyond which it becomes saturated. This maximum capacity point is known as T_m. The T_m for glucose in man is about 350 mg per minute, which is equivalent to arterial plasma glucose levels of 200 mg per 100 ml (venous 180 mg per 100 ml). Beyond this threshold point glucose appears in urine. This glucose transfer mechanism is inhibited by the glycoside phlorhizin, which leads to the appearance of glucose in the urine at a much lower plasma concentration (renal glycosurea).

A small amount of protein usually leaks through the glomeruli. The protein is reabsorbed at the tubules by a process of pinocytosis. Little membranous vesicles containing protein are found at the cell membrane. These are pinched off between the microvilli and pass into the cytoplasm of the cells, where lysosomes digest them to amino acids, which in turn are absorbed into the capillaries.[1]

Phosphate is also actively reabsorbed at the proximal tubule, and this is under the control of parathormone, which decreases its reabsorption, ie, increases its excretion. Uric acid is also reabsorbed at the proximal tubule, but this is complicated by the fact that it is also secreted by the tubules. Its reabsorption is inhibited by probenecid and phenylbutazone. Other substances actively reabsorbed at the tubule include potassium, sulfate, ascorbic acid, acetoacetic acid, and betahydroxybutyric acid.

Tubular Secretion

The process by which materials present in the peritubular fluid are transferred to the tubular lumen is known as tubular secretion.

The first substance in which tubular secretion was demonstrated was phenol red. Other substances such as hippuric acid, penicillin, sulfonphthaleins, and several compounds used in intravenous pyelography, such as Diodrast, are secreted by tubules. It is interesting that all these compounds are not normal constituents of the body. Paraaminohippuric acid, which is used for renal blood flow measurement, is also secreted by the tubules. Metabolic products of steroids and glucoronides are also secreted by the tubules.

Nonionic Diffusion

Some ionic compounds may appear in the urine in concentrations that suggest that they are actively secreted, but this is not true because many of these are weak acids or bases in the un-ionized form, which make them readily diffusible across the cell membrane. However, in the tubular fluid at the appropriate pH, they become ionized (thus not diffusible), ie, become trapped in the tubular lumen.

A typical example is phenobarbital, which is a weak acid and diffuses across the biologic membrane in un-ionized form. Thus, in barbiturate intoxication, if the urine is made alkaline, the barbiturate will ionize in the tubular lumen and be trapped in there, and its excretion enhanced.

THE COUNTERCURRENT MECHANISM

A countercurrent mechanism is a system in which the inflow to that particular area is in parallel, in close proximity, and in the opposite direction to outflow from that area. A typical example of the countercurrent heat exchange is the blood supply to the legs of a bird living in a cold environment, in which the arterial blood loses heat to the venous blood as it goes down to the leg, while the venous blood gains heat from the arterial blood on its way up. Thus, the legs of the animals are kept at a temperature lower than body temperature, while excessively cold blood from the periphery is warmed up before joining the central circulation. A similar but more complicated exchange occurs at the loop of Henle in the kidney. The main theoretical advantage of the countercurrent theory is that all the water movements in the kidney can be explained as being secondary to the movement of solutes, and there is no need to postulate an active transport mechanism for water in the process of the formation of concentrated urine.

The ultrafiltrate at the glomerulus is isotonic with plasma. Similarly, the intraluminal fluid in the proximal tubule is isotonic despite the fact that more than two-thirds of sodium is absorbed at this level. Since the proximal glomeruli are highly permeable to water, water is reabsorbed pari passu with solute reabsorption. The amount of salt and water reabsorbed at this stage is independent of the presence of antidiuretic hormone.

In the thin descending loop of Henle, the tubular fluid becomes hypertonic because there the tubules are highly permeable to water but impermeable to solute, and because the osmolality of the interstitium is higher than the tubular fluid, the fluid by an osmotic gradient moves outward from the descending limb to the interstitium. The osmolality of the interstitium varies. It is less near the cortex than near the papillae. Thus, the nephrons with the longest loops reaching the papilla can achieve the highest concentration of urine. The highest concentration of the intraluminal fluid is achieved at the bend of the loop. Beyond this point, the fluid becomes more dilute because the ascending limb actively transports chloride out of the tubular fluid (sodium following passively) while it is impermeable to water. Thus, as the fluid passes up in the ascending tubule, its osmolality diminishes from the loss of solute, and it becomes hypoosmotic. By this mechanism the hypertonicity of the interstitium of the renal medulla is maintained (Fig. 29-5).

The permeability of the distal tubule and the first portion of the collecting tubules to water depends on the presence of the antidiuretic hormone, but they

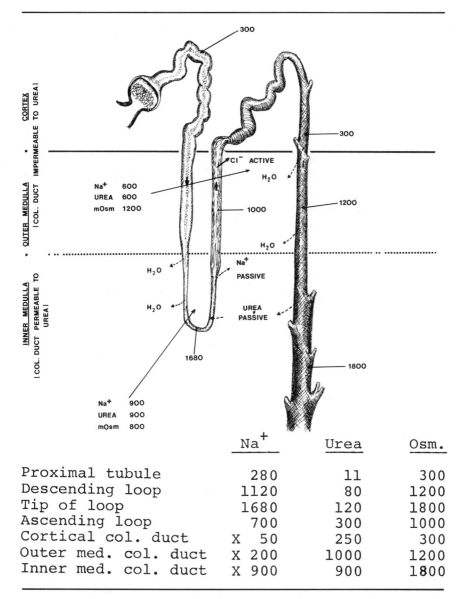

	Na$^+$	Urea	Osm.
Proximal tubule	280	11	300
Descending loop	1120	80	1200
Tip of loop	1680	120	1800
Ascending loop	700	300	1000
Cortical col. duct	X 50	250	300
Outer med. col. duct	X 200	1000	1200
Inner med. col. duct	X 900	900	1800

FIG. 29-5: A schematic representation of the countercurrent mechanism in a juxta-medullary tubule. (Modified after and reproduced with permission from Kokko and Rector.[18]) All the values are expressed as mOsm per liter. The numbers on the drawing represent the osmolality in that particular area. X is nonreabsorbable solutes.

are basically impermeable to urea. In the presence of the antidiuretic hormone, the permeability of these tubules is increased. Thus, water diffuses out of the lumen, and the urea concentration increases markedly.

As the collecting ducts pass to the inner medulla, they become permeable to urea. Therefore, some of the urea passes into the interstitium, maintaining its high osmolality. Also, additional water is removed, the amount depending on the presence of the antidiuretic hormone. Thus, the urine emerging from the collecting ducts can have an osmotic concentration similar to the surrounding interstitium. Therefore, by this complex countercurrent mechanism a hyperosmolar urine is formed without any requirement for active transport of water.

This osmotic gradient in the medulla of the kidney would not have existed if the blood supply to this area of the kidney was similar to other areas of the body. This high concentration of sodium and urea would have been washed out by circulation. Its gradient is maintained because of the peculiar arrangement of the vasa recta. While flowing into the descending vasa recta, the blood becomes more hypertonic because of diffusion of solutes to the inside of the capillary, while the water diffuses out. This water and solute movement are passive due to the osmotic gradient. The opposite occurs on the ascending limb, ie, water diffuses in while solute diffuses out. Therefore, the loss of solute by this mechanism is minimal. The sluggishness in the flow in the vasa recta will tend to keep this osmotic gradient constant. An increase in the flow of the vasa recta will tend to wash out this osmolality gradient and diminish urine concentration.

This countercurrent hypothesis can explain several observations made in the past, eg, animals with long loops of Henle are the only ones that can excrete a concentrated urine, and animals living in deserts have a very long loop and have a very high concentrating ability. The highest urinary concentration achieved depends on the length of the longest loop present in the kidney and not the percentage of nephrons with long loops.

SODIUM EXCRETION

As mentioned previously, about 80 percent of the sodium present in the glomerular filtrate is actively transported across the proximal tubular wall. This sodium transfer is accompanied by chloride and water. The reabsorption of salt in the proximal tubule is obligatory, ie, not related to the body requirement for salt and water.

It seems that sodium ions enter the tubular cell passively down an electrochemical gradient but are actively expelled against this electrochemical gradient to the peritubular space. Recently, it has been postulated that sodium is transported through the extensions of the interstitial spaces (lateral intercellular spaces). In the loop of Henle, sodium is transported as part of the countercurrent system. In the thin descending limb, there is passive movement of sodium ion toward the lumen, whereas in the ascending limb chloride is actively transported (followed by sodium).[9] The reabsorption in the distal convoluted tubule and collecting ducts is more variable depending on several factors, including the state of hydration, the hydrostatic pressure of the peritubular capillaries, circulating level of aldosterone, and adrenocortical hormones.

It seems that two separate types of sodium pumps exist in the renal tubules[10] (Fig. 29-6):

1. Electrogenic sodium pump, which pumps out the sodium, keeping the interior of the cell electronegative. The chloride ion follows the sodium ion passively. This mechanism is inhibited by ethacrynic acid.
2. Coupled exchange pump through which a potassium moves in for every Na^+ expelled out of the cell. Thus, there is no net change in the charge. This pump is inhibited by ouabain or low extracellular potassium.

POTASSIUM EXCRETION

Potassium is unique among the normal constituents of the blood in that it is both reabsorbed and secreted by the renal tubules. Most of the filtered

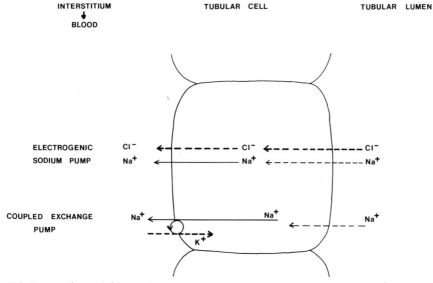

FIG. 29-6: The possible mechanism of sodium, chloride, and potassium transfer in the distal tubules. Solid line represents active transport, and dashed line possible active or passive transport.

potassium is reabsorbed in the proximal tubule, and the filtrate reaching the distal tubules has a very small amount of potassium in it. Most of the potassium excreted is derived through secretion in the distal convoluted tubule and continues into the collecting system.

Potassium ion is secreted in exchange for sodium ion. This exchange does not have to be in a one-to-one ratio because sodium can be exchanged for hydrogen ions also. For example, during systemic acidosis, when hydrogen ions are more available, they are excreted in preference to potassium ions. Therefore, acidosis depresses potassium secretion, whereas alkalosis increases it. Because excretion of potassium and hydrogen ions depends on the availability of sodium, in case of dehydration or hyponatremia the secretion of potassium is diminished.

The amount of potassium secreted depends on the intracellular potassium content, particularly of the renal tubular cell. The effect of extracellular potassium concentration has little effect on potassium excretion because it is basically an intracellular ion.

In Addison's disease, in the absence of mineralocorticoids, the sodium reabsorbing capacity is diminished with the increase in sodium loss, potassium is retained, and hyperkalemia results. The ability of the kidney to conserve potassium is strong, but it is less efficient than sodium conservation. In situations of excessive potassium ingestion, the urine potassium excretion is increased.[11]

RENAL REGULATION OF ACID-BASE BALANCE

The average diet is richer in acidic metabolites than alkalotic ones. The most abundant of the acids is carbonic acid, which is excreted by the lung. However, the diet provides a continuous source of nonvolatile acids that cannot be handled by the lung, such as phosphoric, sulfuric, and other organic acids. Few diets are alkali producing. Fruits and vegetables are sources of alkali because they contain salts of organic acids. These organic acids are oxidized to CO_2 and water, whereas the basic radicals, such as sodium and potassium, remain in circulation in association with the bicarbonate. As a result, the kidney is provided most of the time with an excess load of acid. The kidney excretes this excess load by two main mechanisms:

1. Exchanging a hydrogen ion for a sodium ion, thus acidifying the urine. The capacity of this system is limited because the lowest pH that the kidney can achieve is a urine pH of 4.5. This by itself is a remarkable achievement considering that this constitutes a 1000-fold increase in hydrogen ion concentration.
2. Synthesis and excretion of ammonia and substitution of NH_4^+ for each sodium ion.

Hydrogen Ion Secretion

The renal tubular cell, similar to the gastric cell, is capable of secreting hydrogen ions, which are actively transported into the lumen. For each hydrogen ion secreted, a sodium ion enters passively into the cell from the peritubular fluid. The exact source of this hydrogen ion secreted is not definitely known, but is probably derived from carbonic acid, which dissociates to bicarbonate and hydrogen ion by the following formula:

$$H_2O + CO_2 \overset{\text{carbonic anhydrase}}{\rightleftharpoons} H_2CO_3 \rightleftharpoons H^+ + HCO_3^-$$

The regeneration of carbonic acid from CO_2 and water is rather fast in the kidney because of the presence of the enzyme carbonic anhydrase in the renal cell. Thus, if carbonic anhydrase is inhibited, the ability of the kidney to acidify urine diminishes. Therefore, for each hydrogen ion secreted, one bicarbonate ion becomes available and a sodium ion enters the cell from the intraluminal fluid, both of which are eventually discharged into the circulation (Fig. 29-7). The hydrogen ion present in the urine may react with the filtered bicarbonate, thus forming CO_2 and water, or may react with dibasic phosphate HPO_4^{--} to form monobasic phosphate $H_2PO_4^-$. The latter occurs mostly in the distal tubules. It also reacts with the other buffer anions.

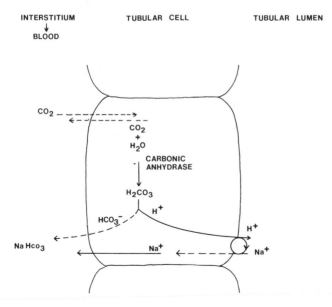

FIG. 29-7: A possible mechanism of hydrogen ion transport in the proximal tubule.

Excretion of Ammonia

The distal tubules are capable of forming ammonia. Most of the ammonia is derived from the amino acid glutamine, and this reaction is catalyzed by the enzyme glutaminase and glutamine dehydrogenase. Ammonia also can be synthesized from other amino acids, such as alanine and glycine and also can be derived directly from blood. Ammonia is lipid-soluble and diffuses freely across the cell membranes into the surrounding fluids. It reacts with hydrogen ions to form ammonium ions, which are water-soluble and do not cross cell membranes easily.

$$NH_3 + H^+ \rightarrow NH_4^+$$

The amount of ammonia excreted depends on the pH of urine. In an alkaline urine it is virtually absent, whereas it is high in maximally acid urine (pH 4.5). In chronic acidosis, the maximum amount of ammonia production is reached within 3 to 5 days, brought about by an increase in glutaminase activity.

Bicarbonate Excretion

Normally the kidneys keeps the plasma bicarbonate concentration at 28 mEq per liter (mmol per liter). It seems that the maximum reabsorption capacity (T_m) is at this plasma level. At higher concentrations, it is excreted in urine and the urine becomes alkaline. However, this arterial bicarbonate level is not absolute; during CO_2 retention the plasma bicarbonate may rise over this 28 mmol per liter, and during potassium or chloride deficiency, more bicarbonate is reabsorbed.

Factors Affecting Hydrogen Ion Secretion

CARBON DIOXIDE

In the presence of CO_2 retention, in an effort to minimize the acidity of plasma, the kidney reabsorbs a higher amount of bicarbonate and the plasma bicarbonate rises. The rise in hydrogen ion excretion will lead to an increase in ammonia production and excretion. With the increased bicarbonate reabsorption, chloride reabsorption diminishes, and Cl^- excretion increases. The reverse of these reactions happens with respiratory alkalosis.

POTASSIUM

It appears that cells can exchange hydrogen ions to a certain degree for potassium ions. This occurs during potassium deficiency, in which the cellular uptake for hydrogen increases. In the renal tubular cells this cellular acidosis will stimulate a rise in the bicarbonate reabsorption. Thus, alkalosis will result with an acid urine. Therefore, hypokalemia is usually associated with alkalosis and paradoxical aciduria. Conversely, hyperkalemia is associated with systemic acidosis and alkaline urine.

CARBONIC ANHYDRASE

If inhibited, acid secretion in urine is decreased because the formation of carbonic acid is not accelerated.

ALDOSTERONE AND OTHER ADRENOCORTICAL STEROIDS

By enhancing the reabsorption of sodium they will lead to an increase in the secretion of H^+ and K^+.

METABOLIC ACIDOSIS

Chronic metabolic acidosis is frequently found in diabetes mellitus. These nonvolatile acids are buffered through the bicarbonate system and plasma bicarbonate is reduced. The drop in pH stimulates respiration and a diminution in P_{CO_2}. As a result, the amount of bicarbonate filtered through the kidney is diminished, which raises the urinary titratable acidity. Also the ammonia secretion is increased.

METABOLIC ALKALOSIS

This may be due to ingestion of a large amount of alkali or from intractable vomiting of acidic material. Because of the increase in bicarbonate content of plasma, respiration is depressed and CO_2 retention occurs. If the intake of sodium and potassium is adequate, the acidity of urine will decrease and may even be alkaline, containing a large amount of sodium and potassium. However, in vomiting or in continuous loss of gastric secretion through a nasogastric tube, there is an associated loss of potassium and sodium. As the body exchanges H^+ for K^+ and the stimulus for conserving K^+ is stronger, part of the sodium will be exchanged for H^+ (instead of K^+) at the renal tubule and urine will become acidic. This progressive acid loss will make the alkalosis worse. This situation is an exception to other types of metabolic acid–base disturbances in which the urine pH shifts in the same direction as the pH of plasma. In metabolic alkalosis with potassium deficiency an acid urine occurs despite the alkaline plasma.

UREA EXCRETION

Urea is the main end-product of nitrogen metabolism. Because of its high lipid solubility, it is freely diffusible through all the membranes of the body except the blood–brain barrier. It easily crosses the glomerular membrane and is also reabsorbed in the tubules. Its rate of reabsorption depends on the concentration of the tubular urine. Thus, the urinary excretion of urea depends mostly on urinary flow. During oliguria only 10 to 20 percent of the filtered urea is excreted, whereas with high urinary flows 50 to 70 percent will appear in urine. The countercurrent mechanism will produce a high concentration of urea in the interstitium of the medullary portion of the kidney. Although some urea leaks in the interstitium of the medullary portion of the kidney from the collecting tubules, this is not as easily washed out as in the cortex because of the countercurrent mechanism. Because of its high solubility, ease of diffusion, and high concentration, urea is very important in the concentrating mechanism of the kidney.

The amount of urea excreted depends on the dietary intake of protein. This indirectly affects the capability of the kidney to produce concentrated urine, because the diffused urea increases the osmolality of the medullary portion of the kidney, which in turn raises its concentrating ability. As the urea secretion depends on urinary flow, in hypovolemia and oliguria the blood urea level rises.

ANESTHETICS AND RENAL FUNCTION

As a general rule, all anesthetics, as well as the stress of surgery, inhibit renal function. This is usually manifested as a decrease in urinary output with a diminution in renal blood flow and glomerular filtration rate. The electrolyte excretion is also decreased. The magnitude of these changes vary with the extent and duration of surgery and to a lesser extent with the anesthetic agent.[12] The effects of general anesthetics on urinary function are apparently transitory, since urinary function returns to normal levels on terminating anesthesia, whereas the effects of the surgical insult linger on for a longer duration, depending on the extent of surgery. Several factors contribute to this depression of renal function during anesthesia.

Cardiovascular Effects

Almost all anesthetic agents are myocardial depressants. Whether hypotension occurs or not depends on the compensatory vasoconstriction. Ether and especially cyclopropane[13] cause peripheral vasoconstriction and a marked increase in the renal vascular resistance, which leads to a diminution in renal blood flow and glomerular filtration rate with a consequent drop in urinary volume and a rise of its osmolality. Similar but less marked effects have been observed with thiopental, nitrous oxide, and morphine anesthesia with neuromuscular blocking agents.[14] Halothane[15] and methoxyflurane are anesthetic agents known for their lack of increased sympathetic activity, but they produce renal vasoconstriction, probably by activation of the renin–angiotensin system. However, the possibility of other vasoactive substances or ADH effect on renal vasculature cannot be ruled out. If anesthesia is supplemented with drugs known to have alpha-blocking properties, such as droperidol or chlorpromazine, the renal flow does not change appreciably because the renal vascular bed is dilated from the alpha blockade, despite the presence of systemic hypotension.

Sympathetic Nervous System

The kidney is supplied with sympathetic vasoconstrictor fibers from the T_4 to the L_4 spinal segments. No functional parasympathetic fibers are seen in the kidney. The sympathetics as well as catecholamines cause a marked renal vasoconstriction, which is more pronounced in the efferent than in the afferent vessels. During anesthesia and surgery, if a stress situation exists, such as with hemorrhage or hypoxia, the renal blood diminishes at the initial stage and the glomerular filtration is kept constant by an increase in the tone of efferent glomerular vessels. With severe stress, the glomerular filtration and overall urinary function diminishes and oliguria results. In an adult, oliguria implies that 24-hour urinary output is below 400 ml.

Spinal anesthesia with sensory levels of T_2, which produces complete renal sympathectomy, causes a mild reduction in renal plasma flow that parallels the drop in arterial blood pressure (about 10 percent) without any change in renal vascular resistance and glomerular filtration rate.[12]

Antidiuretic Hormone (ADH)

Because of the marked depression in Na^+ and Cl^- excretion relative to K^+ excretion, it has been suggested that morphine as well as general anesthetics lead to an increase in the antidiuretic hormone production. However, this is a matter of dispute, but it seems that both antidiuretic hormone secretion and changes in renal vascular dynamics are responsible for the antidiuresis seen during anesthesia.

INAPPROPRIATE ADH SECRETION

This is usually seen in elderly patients who have undergone major surgery and is manifested by a variety of neurologic symptoms. These patients show hyponatremia associated with low serum osmolality, while the urine is hypertonic. These patients respond to sodium chloride administration.

Aldosterone

Anesthetics are known to induce aldosterone release by various mechanisms:

1. Sensitization of the baroreceptors.
2. Affects on the renin–angiotension mechanism.
3. Release of ACTH by ADH.

These in turn stimulate aldosterone release. Despite the aldosterone release, the serum sodium falls during general anesthesia. This is said to be due to the predominance of the ADH effect.

Methoxyflurane and Renal Failure

After prolonged methoxyflurane anesthesia, several incidences of renal failure were reported that were manifested by marked polyurea, diminished urinary concentrating ability even after the administration of the antidiuretic hormone, hypernatremia, plasma hyperosmolality, and an increase in plasma BUN and creatinine. This nephrotoxicity is dose-related and depends on the amount of inorganic fluoride produced from the biodegradation of this anesthetic agent.[16]

Because other anesthetic agents are fluorinated hydrocarbons, it has been suggested that these might also cause fluoride nephropathy, eg, enflurane is partially defluorinated in the body to a greater extent than isoflurane but less than methoxyflurane. Because the rate of defluorination is low, in man renal dysfunction will not occur except in patients with renal disease.[17] However, halothane is not defluorinated in the body. Thus, its nephrotoxic potential is remote.

DIURETICS

Diuretics are a group of drugs that increase the urinary output of water and electrolytes. Their main indications include:

1. Excessive water and electrolyte retention from any of several conditions, eg, congestive heart failure, renal or hepatic disease, or endocrine disorders
2. As a measure to prevent renal ischemic changes, such as during aortic cross clamping or in myoglobinuria, the reason behind this being the preservation of renal blood flow and a continuous glomerular filtration to prevent "plugging" of the tubules

OSMOTIC DIURETICS

When a large amount of unreabsorbed solutes is presented to the renal tubules, by their osmotic effect they will retain a larger amount of sodium and water inside the lumen of the tubule and diuresis will ensue. A similar situation occurs during diabetes mellitus in which the increased level of glucose in the renal tubule (beyond its maximum reabsorbing capacity T_m) will lead to decreased water and electrolyte reabsorption. Osmotic diuresis also is seen after the administration of dyes for arteriography and intravenous pyelography, because of their very high osmotic pressures.

The most commonly used drug in this group is mannitol. This drug, besides decreasing the reabsorption of water and sodium, has been demonstrated to increase renal plasma flow and glomerular filtration. This effect is especially notable when the renal perfusion is decreased and is the reason why 20 percent mannitol has been advocated in patients undergoing abdominal aortic surgery as a preventive measure to decrease the incidence of postoperative renal complications.

Urea has occasionally been used as an osmotic diuretic but it is less effective than mannitol because it is reabsorbed by the renal tubules.

CARBONIC ANHYDRASE INHIBITORS

Carbonic anhydrase inhibitors such as acetozolamide act by inhibiting the enzyme carbonic anhydrase present at the brush border of the proximal tubule cell. Therefore, the H^+ secretion is diminished.

Instead of H^+, sodium and potassium ions are excreted. However, after a short while, because of the increased reabsorption of chloride, hyperchloremic metabolic acidosis develops, which counteracts the effect of the diuretic.

THIAZIDES

Thiazides inhibit sodium reabsorption in the distal tubules as well as in the ascending loop of Henle. They also decrease glomerular filtration. Thus, they should be avoided whenever glomerular filtration is reduced or if there is a potential that it will be reduced. Potassium depletion also occurs.

MERCURIALS

Mercurials inhibit the reabsorption of sodium at the ascending loop of Henle. They also lead to increased aldosterone secretion, which leads to alkalosis, decreasing the effectiveness of this drug. Administration of acidifying salts such as ammonium chloride counteract the alkalosis and help to maintain diuresis. Hypokalemia is not marked with mercurials.

FUROSEMIDE AND ETHACRYNIC ACID

These drugs inhibit the reabsorption of sodium at the loop of Henle and also inhibit the sodium–potassium exchange. Thus, there is marked loss of potassium with these drugs. A special feature of these two drugs is that they are effective in the presence of hypovolemia. Also, furosemide, like mannitol, can counteract the diminution of renal perfusion after a stressful situation. In animals, they have demonstrated that they can deplete myocardial potassium, making them vulnerable for arrhythmias.

SPIRONOLACTONE, TRIAMTERINE, AND AMILORIDE

These agents interfere with the sodium–potassium exchange in the distal convoluted tubule and collecting ducts. The first is a competitive inhibitor of aldosterone, ie, aldosterone antagonist. These drugs have the advantage of causing an increase in the acidity of the plasma and have a tendency to retain potassium. Thus, they are good drugs to alternate with the thiazides and furosemide to counteract their alkalotic and hypokalemic effects.

REFERENCES

1. Ham AW: Histology, 7th ed. Philadelphia, Lippincott, 1974, pp 759–763
2. Vander AJ: Control of renin release. Physiol Rev 47:359, 1967
3. Peart WS: Renin–angiotensin system. N Engl J Med 292:302, 1975
4. Barger AC, Herd JA: The renal circulation. N Engl J Med 284:482, 1971
5. Deen WM, Robertson CR, Brenner BM: Transcapillary fluid exchange in the renal cortex. Circ Res 33:1, 1973

6. Waugh WH, Shanks RG: Cause of genuine autoregulation of the renal circulation. Circ Res 8:871, 1960
7. Larson CP, Jr, Mazze RI, Cooperman LH, et al: Effects of anesthetics on cerebral renal and splanchnic circulations. Anesthesiology 41:169, 1974
8. Pappenheimer JR: Passage of molecules through capillary walls. Physiol Rev 33:387, 1953
9. Rocha AS, Kokko JP: Sodium chloride and water transport in the medullary thick ascending limb of Henle. J Clin Invest 52:612, 1973
10. Giebish G: Coupled ion and fluid transport in the kidney. N Engl J Med 287:913, 1972
11. Kallen RJ, Rieger CH, Cohen HS, et al: Near-fatal hyperkalemia due to ingestion of salt substitute by an infant. JAMA 235:2125, 1976
12. Deutsch S: Effects of anesthetics on the kidney. Surg Clin North Am 55:775, 1975
13. Deutsch S, Pierce EC, Vandam LD: Cyclopropane effects on renal function in normal man. Anesthesiology 28:547, 1967
14. Deutsch S, Bastron RD, Pierce EC, Jr, et al: The effects of anaesthesia with thiopentone, nitrous oxide, narcotics and neuromuscular blocking drugs on renal function in normal man. Br J Anaesth 41:807, 1969
15. Deutsch S, Goldberg M, Stephen GW, et al: Effects of halothane anesthesia on renal function in normal man. Anesthesiology 27:793, 1966
16. Cousins MJ, Mazze RI: Methoxyflurane nephrotoxicity: a study of dose response in man. JAMA 225:1611, 1973
17. Cousins MJ, Greenstein LR, Hitt BA: Metabolism and renal effects of enflurane in man. Anesthesiology 44:44, 1976
18. Kokko JP, Rector FC: Countercurrent multiplication system without active transport in inner medulla. Kidney Int 2:214, 1972

Index